D1551593

Electrophysiology of Vision

of Vision

Clinical Testing and Applications

Electrophysiology of Vision

Clinical Testing and Applications

Byron L. Lam
Bascom Palmer Eye Institute
University of Miami School of Medicine, Florida, U.S.A.

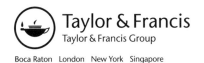

Taylor & Francis
Taylor & Francis Group

Boca Raton   London   New York   Singapore

Published in 2005 by
Taylor & Francis Group
6000 Broken Sound Parkway NW, Suite 300
Boca Raton, FL 33487-2742

© 2005 by Taylor & Francis Group, LLC

No claim to original U.S. Government works
Printed in the United States of America on acid-free paper
10 9 8 7 6 5 4 3 2 1

International Standard Book Number-10: 0-8247-4068-8 (Hardcover)
International Standard Book Number-13: 978-0-8247-4068-9 (Hardcover)

Library of Congress Cataloging-in-Publication Data

Catalog record is available from the Library of Congress

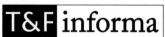

Taylor & Francis Group
is the Academic Division of T&F Informa plc.

Visit the Taylor & Francis Web site at
http://www.taylorandfrancis.com

Preface

This book was written to provide the clinician with practical information of visual electrophysiologic tests in an accessible and understandable format. Personnel involved in electrophysiologic testing and ophthalmic trainees may also find this book beneficial. The book is organized into two sections keeping in mind that the majority of clinical users of visual electrophysiologic tests do not perform the tests themselves. The first section consists of six chapters that discuss clinical recording techniques and physiologic origins of electroretinogram (ERG), electro-oculogram (EOG), and visual evoked potential (VEP); the section ends with a chapter that focuses on the effects of maturation and aging on these tests as well as electrophysiologic testing in infants. The second section consists of 11 chapters dealing with the clinical applications of ERG, EOG, and VEP testing. The first chapter of this section is an overview from a clinical perspective. The electrophysiologic findings of specific clinical conditions are discussed in subsequent chapters with an emphasis on when and why a specific test should be considered. The clinician will find the second section particularly useful in everyday patient care.

ACKNOWLEDGMENTS

The completion of the book wouldn't have been possible without the support of my family and colleagues. Dr. Mu Liu assisted immensely in many of the figures and tables. Rick Stratton helped substantially in the preparation of figures. Ailin Rodriguez provided excellent secretarial support. Dr. Sheridan Lam reviewed drafts and gave valuable advice.

I wish to thank my family for their support and encouragement during the writing of this book. In particular, I deeply appreciate Diane, my lifetime soul mate and best friend, for her loving sustenance. The book is dedicated to my family.

Byron L. Lam

Contents

Electrophysiology of Vision

of Vision

Clinical Testing and Applications

1

Full-Field Electroretinogram

The full-field electroretinogram (ERG) records the summed transient electrical responses from the entire retina elicited by a flash stimulus delivered in a full-field dome Fig. 1.1. The ERG was discovered in excised animal eyes in the middle 1800s, and ERG recording in humans was first reported in 1920s. The clinical use of full-field ERG began in the 1940s, and in 1989, standard for clinical full-field ERG was established by the International Society for Clinical Electrophysiology of Vision ISCEV (1). The ERG standard is reviewed every three years, and the most updated version is available on the ISCEV Internet site. No major revision of the standard has occurred over the years, and the standard is summarized in Table 1.1. This chapter discusses ERG assuming an understanding of basic retinal anatomy and physiology detailed at the end of the chapter.

CLINICAL USE OF FULL-FIELD ERG

The full-field ERG measures the overall rod- and cone-generated retinal responses and is the only electrophysiologic

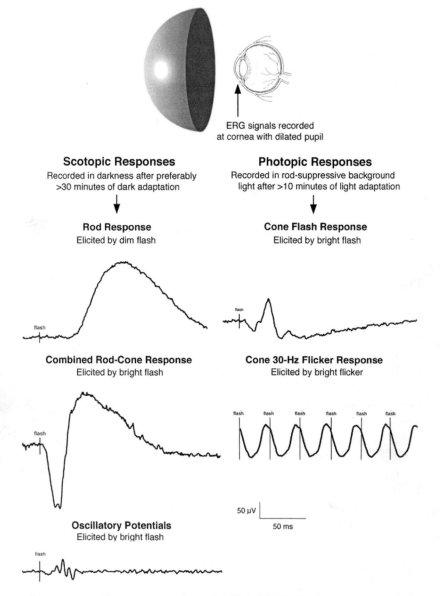

Figure 1.1 Basic principles of full-field ERG. A summary of the international standard for clinical full-field ERG is provided in Table 1.1.

Table 1.1 Summary of International Standard for Clinical Full-Field Electroretinography (ERG)

Clinical protocol	
Preparation of patient	
Pupillary dilation	Maximally dilated with eye drops
Pre-adaptation to light or darkness	$\geq$20 min dark adaptation before recording rod responses
	$\geq$10 min light adaptation before recording cone responses
Pre-exposure to light	Avoid fluorescein angiography or fundus photography before ERG; $\geq$1 hr of dark adaptation needed before ERG after these procedures
Fixation	Fixation point incorporated into stimulus dome
ERG measurement and recording	
Measurement of the ERG	Amplitudes and implicit times
Averaging repetitive responses	Not ordinarily required, helpful to identify very weak responses; artifact rejection must be a part of averaging system
Normal values	Each laboratory establishes limits of normal values for specific ERG responses and provides median and 95% confidence limits from direct tabulation of normal responses
Reporting of ERG	Display waveforms with amplitude and timing with normal values and variances; strength of stimulus and level of light adaptation given in absolute values
Pediatric ERG recording	
Sedation or anesthesia	With or without anesthesia; full anesthesia may modify responses, less effect on ERG with sedation or brief, very light anesthesia
Electrodes	Pediatric size electrodes
Normal values and measurement	ERG responses mature during infancy, interpret with caution; pediatric ERG responses compared to normal subjects of the same age

(Continued)

Table 1.1 Summary of International Standard for Clinical Full-Field Electroretinography (ERG) (*Continued*)

Specific responses (Fig. 1.2)	1. Rod single-flash response after dark adaptation with flash 2.5 log unit dimmer than standard flash (≥ 2 sec between flashes)
	2. Maximal combined rod and cone single-flash response after dark adaptation (≥ 10 sec between flashes) with standard flash
	3. Oscillatory potentials with standard flash (15 sec between scotopic flashes or 1.5 sec between photopic flashes, bandpass of amplifier changed to 75–300 Hz)
	4. Cone single-flash response after light adaptation with standard flash (≥ 0.5 sec between flashes)
	5. Cone 30-Hz flicker response after light adaptation with standard flash
Basic technology	
Light diffusion	Full-field ("ganzfeld") stimulation with full-field dome
Electrode	
Recording	Contact-lens type electrodes or electrodes on cornea or nearby bulbar conjunctiva, topical anesthesia needed for contact-lens type electrodes
Reference	Incorporated into contact-lens electrode or a separate reference skin electrode placed temporally near orbital rim or on forehead
Ground	Skin electrode connected to ground, typically placed on forehead or ear
Skin electrode characteristics	Skin electrodes for reference or ground, ≤ 5 KΩ impedance measured between 10 and 100 Hz
Stability	Stable baseline voltage in the absence of light stimulation
Cleaning	Cleaned and sterilized after each use
Light sources	
Duration	Flash with duration of ≤ 5 msec
Wavelength	Color temperature near 7000° K used with dome or diffuser that are visibly white

Table 1.1 (*Continued*)

Strength	$1.5–4.5\,cd\,s\,m^{-2}$ at surface of ganzfeld bowl, a flash of this strength is called a standard flash (SF)
Background	For photopic recording, white background with even and steady luminance of $17–34\,cd\,m^{-2}$
Light adjustment and calibration	
Adjustment of stimulus and background intensity	System capable of attenuating flash strength from the SF over a range of at least $3\log$ unit in steps of $\leq 0.3\log$ unit without changing wavelength composition
Stimulus and background calibration	Flash strength measured by an integrated photometer at location of eye; separate calibrations for single flash and repeated flashes. Background luminance of Ganzfeld bowl measured with photometer in nonintegrating mode
Recalibration	Frequency of recalibration depending on system used
Electronic recording equipment	
Amplification	Bandpass of amplifiers and preamplifiers include range of $0.3–300\,Hz$ and adjustable for recording oscillatory potentials: impedance of preamplifiers $\geq 10\,M\Omega$
Display of data and averaging	Waveform displayed promptly; system able to represent full amplifier bandpass without attenuation
Patient isolation	Electrically isolated

test that assesses rod-generated activity. The full-field ERG is essential in the diagnosis of numerous disorders including cone dystrophy, retinoschisis, congenital stationary night blindness, Leber congenital amaurosis, rod monochromatism, and paraneoplastic retinopathies. The ERG should be used in conjunction with a thorough ocular examination and when necessary other tests such as visual field and fluorescein angiography. The full-field ERG provides no topographical information about localized defects, and an isolated macular lesion is unlikely to decrease the full-field ERG response substantially. In such cases, testing with focal or multifocal ERG is helpful.

RETINAL ELECTRICAL RESPONSES

The ERG response is produced by light-induced movements of ions in the retina. This activity is measured indirectly at the cornea with a recording electrode. The extracellular movement of predominantly positive potassium (K^+) and sodium (Na^+) ions occurs as a result of opening (depolarization) and closure (hyperpolarization) of channels of the cellular membranes. The small size and short axons of the retinal cells are such that a change in ionic activity of one part of the cell is adequate to affect its synaptic activity. Both neuronal and non-neuronal retinal cells contribute to this light-evoked electrical current. The full-field ERG receives virtually no contributions from retinal ganglion cells that form the optic nerve. The ganglion cells utilize conventional all-or-none spike action potentials and are more response to the stimulus of the pattern ERG.

CLINICAL RECORDING OF FULL-FIELD ERG

Scotopic and Photopic Recordings

Dark-adapted or *scotopic* ERG responses are recorded after a period of at least 20 min of dark adaptation but a period of 30–40 min is preferable to allow more complete dark adaptation of the rods. Scotopic recordings are rod-driven although cones also contribute if bright stimuli are used. Light-adapted or *photopic* ERG responses are recorded with a lit white background after at least 10 min of light adaptation (2). Light adaptation is achieved with exposure to ambient room light or alternatively can be better standardized by exposing the patient to 10 min of the photopic background of the full-field dome. Photopic responses are cone-driven.

Full-Field ERG Flash Stimulus

The white flash ERG stimulus is delivered in a white full-field dome. The maximal flash is called the *standard flash* with a recommended intensity of $1.5–4.5\,\mathrm{cd\,s\,m^{-2}}$. However, a brighter flash in the range of $10–12\,\mathrm{cd\,s\,m^{-2}}$ elicits a larger better-defined a-wave for assessing photoreceptor activity. The flash is brief lasting usually well under 1 msec. For scotopic rod responses, the flash is dimmed with built-in filters. During photopic cone response recordings, the background of the full-field dome is lit with an even and steady white luminance of $17–34\,\mathrm{cd\,m^{-2}}$ to maintain light adaptation and to suppress rod activity. A centrally located built-in small dim red light is typically used as a fixation target. Proper calibration and periodic re-calibration with a photometer ensure that appropriate light intensities are utilized and no substantial changes occur over time. International guidelines for calibration of stimulus are available on the ISCEV Internet site (3). Periodic calibration of the amplifier by passing a known square wave or sine wave signal through each recording channel ensures that the amplifiers are working accurately and the output of each channel is identical.

Although the flash ERG stimulus is defined by the luminance emitted from the reflecting surface of the full-field dome and the stimulus duration (candela-second per square meter, $\mathrm{cd\,s\,m^{-2}}$), a more precise measure of the effective light stimulus received by the retina is retinal illuminance expressed in *troland*. For clinical ERG, stimulus luminance is usually a more readily available measure than retinal illuminance, but some recording systems can automatically calculate retinal illuminance. The troland (td) is the stimulus luminance in $\mathrm{cd\,m^{-2}}$ multiplied by the pupillary area in $\mathrm{mm^2}$, and the retinal illuminance from a flash is expressed as troland multiplied by the stimulus duration (td s). Photopic troland differs from scotopic troland because the sensitivity of the eye to light wavelengths is different under light and dark adaptation, and the spectral distribution of the stimulus needs to be taken into account. The standard spectral sensitivity function of the eye under photopic condition (V_λ) is a function with peak sensitivity at a wavelength of 555 mm, which is closely approximated by the sum of sensitivities of the long- and middle-wavelength-sensitive cones. In contrast, the standard spectral sensitivity function under scotopic condition (V_λ') is a function with peak sensitivity at a wavelength of 507 mm in part to account for the peak sensitivity of the rods. Photopic troland (td) and scotopic troland (td') are calculated based on the spectral distribution of the stimulus based on V_λ and V_λ'.

ERG Electrodes

Several ERG recording electrodes are available (Fig. 1.2), and their advantages and disadvantages are summarized in Table 1.2. The Burian–Allen and the Dawson–Trick–Litzkow (DTL) electrodes are probably the most popular. Proper placement of the electrodes is critical to obtain accurate and consistent ERG responses, and proper cleaning protocols as recommended by the manufacturer must be followed.

To record an electrophysiologic signal, the signal from the active recording electrode is compared with the signal

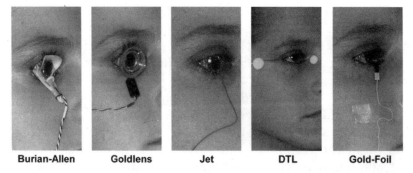

Burian-Allen   Goldlens   Jet   DTL   Gold-Foil

Figure 1.2 ERG recording electrodes. The characteristics of the electrodes are summarized in Table 1.2. Burian–Allen and Dawson–Trick–Litzkow (DTL) electrodes are probably the most commonly used electrodes for the full-field ERG. Proper placement of the electrodes, as described in the text and Table 1.2, is critical to obtain accurate, consistent recordings. (Refer to the color insert.)

from a reference electrode which may be placed on several possible locations including the forehead or lateral regions of the orbital rim. A ground electrode is typically placed on an ear lobe or the forehead.

The Burian–Allen electrode is a contact-lens type electrode with a lid speculum to reduce the effect of blink and eyelid closure (4). Topical anesthesia with eye drops is required, and patient tolerance to the Burian–Allen electrode is less than that to the DTL electrode. The Burian–Allen electrode is available in several sizes. The bipolar version has a conductive coating on the outer surface of the lid speculum that serves as the built-in reference electrode eliminating the need for a separate reference electrode (5). The ERG responses obtained with the bipolar version are slightly smaller than the monopolar version, but the recording is more stable. However, the bipolar version is more vulnerable to recording artifact from light-induced reflexive contraction of the orbicularis called the *photomyoclonic reflex* (6). The view through the Burian–Allen electrode is blurred but this will not affect the full-field ERG. Newer modified versions provide clearer optics and are suitable for multifocal ERG.

The DTL electrode is a conductive Mylar thread typically placed in the lower fornix where the thread contacts the inferior bulbar conjunctiva or the corneal limbal region (7). This preferred position stabilizes the position of the thread (8). Topical anesthesia is not warranted, and patient tolerance is superior compare to contact-lens type electrodes such as the Burian–Allen and Jet electodes (9). Reproducibility of ERG recordings is favorable (10). Eyelid closure and blink artifacts with the DTL electrode are more pronounced than the Burian–Allen electrode, and the recorded ERG amplitudes are lower (11). Compared to the Jet electrode, the DTL electrode recordings have greater variability and recorded amplitudes are lower (12).

Skin electrodes are not recommended for routine ERG recording but may be useful in infants and young children intolerant to other electrodes. The ERG responses from skin electrodes are considerably smaller and more variable than conjunctival or corneal contacting electrodes.

Table 1.2 ERG Recording Electrodes

Electrode	Type	Advantages	Disadvantages
Burian–Allen	Contact-lens electrode with lid speculum	Lid speculum limits effects of blinking and lid closure; bipolar version has built-in reference electrode; numerous sizes for premature infants to adults	Poor tolerance in some patients; image is blurred and not suitable for pattern ERG— image clearer in newer modified versions
DTL (Dawson–Trick–Litzkow)	Conductive Mylar thread placed in inferior fornix contacting bulbar conjunctiva	Higher patient tolerance; low variance of signal amplitude; provide clear imagery, suitable for pattern ERG	Thread can be displaced, more prone to blink and eye movement artifacts; 10% lower recorded amplitude than contact-lens electrode
Gold–foil	Vertical gold foil strip under lower eyelid contacting bulbar conjunctiva curving downward; foil portion should not touch skin	Higher patient tolerance; provide clear imagery, suitable for pattern ERG	Greater than 30% lower recorded amplitude than contact-lens electrode; foil easily displaced, more prone to blink and eye movement artifacts

Jet	Contact-lens electrode	Disposable, packed sterile, easy insertion	Lens movement and lack of lid speculum increase recording variability; easy to fall out; image is blurred, not suitable for pattern ERG; may not be readily available commercially
Goldlens	Contact-lens electrode with lid speculum	Lid speculum limits effects of blinking and lid closure; has built-in reference electrode; pediatric size available; provide clear imagery, suitable for focal foveal ERG	Newer electrode, limited clinical experience; slightly less comfortable in some patients compared to Burian- Allen electrode

System and Patient Set-Up

The pupils should be fully dilated with pharmacologic eye drops, because small pupils reduce retinal illuminance and ERG responses. To avoid electrical interference, the recording environment should be physically and electrically isolated from electrically noisy devices such as appliances, electrical equipment, and fluorescent lighting. The recording room should be light sealed and suitable for dark adaptation.

After electrode placement, impedance and baseline signals are evaluated to assess electrical noise interference and artifacts from eye movement and blink. If problems occur, electrode positions and connections are checked, and the patient is encouraged further to cooperate. The ERG signal is small compared to the electrical noise from power current and from the heart, muscles, and brain. Differential amplifiers amplify the difference in input between the recording and reference electrodes and reject signals common to both inputs. The impedance of the recording and reference electrodes should be matched for noise rejection to work properly. Impedance is the ratio of the measured voltage between the electrode and the ground electrode with respect to the input current: impedance $= V/I$ where $V =$ voltage and $I =$ input current. Most systems have built-in impedance meters that input a current from the active electrode towards the ground electrode allowing rapid check of impedance. A low impedance reading is desirable.

By adjusting the frequency filtering characteristics of the amplifier, the ERG recording is modified to reduce electrical noises and blink and eye movement artifacts. The low and high frequency cut-off's of the amplifier are set to exclude recording of signals with frequencies that are below the low frequency cut-off or above the high frequency cut-off. For full-field ERG, the low and high frequency cut-off's are typically set at 0.3 and 300 Hz, respectively, with the recording frequency range or bandpass being from 0.3 to 300 Hz. The exception is the recording of oscillatory potentials which require the bandpass to be adjusted from 75 to 300 Hz to exclude low frequency ERG components.

Recording Sequence

Binocular full-field ERG responses are usually simultaneously recorded. Whether scotopic or photopic recordings are recorded first is not critical as long as adequate adaptation periods are performed. If photopic responses are recorded first, the number and intensity of the photopic flash stimuli should not be excessive. Otherwise the subsequent dark adaptation will need to be longer to allow for retinal recovery. When contact-lens type electrodes are used, the scotopic responses may be performed first to minimize patient discomfort. The electrodes are placed at the end of the dark-adaptation period under dim red illumination to avoid altering rod sensitivity but this light exposure must be minimized. The patient then continues to wear the electrodes for the rest of the test through the subsequent shorter photopic recordings.

Five Standard Full-Field ERG Responses

Three standard scotopic responses are recommended (Fig. 1.3). First, a rod response is elicited by a dim white flash of 2.5 log units (25 dB) weaker the standard flash. Next, a maximal combined rod and cone response is elicited by the white standard flash. Third, the oscillatory potentials are elicited by the standard flash. The time interval between repeat flashes must be long enough to maintain dark adaptation and to allow retinal recovery. An interval of at least 2 sec between flashes is recommended for the rod response, and longer intervals of at least 10 and 15 sec are necessary for the combined rod–cone response and the oscillatory potentials, respectively.

Two standard photopic cone responses are recommended (Fig. 1.4). The single-flash and 30-Hz flicker cone responses are elicited with the standard flash and are recorded with the lit white photopic background of the full-field dome. The time interval between flashes for the single-flash cone response is not critical and can be as short as 0.5 sec. The stimulus flicker rate for eliciting the 30-Hz flicker cone response is close to but not exactly at 30 Hz (e.g., 30.3 Hz). This is because a flicker rate of exactly 30 Hz will produce a recording that is prone to electrical noise from the power supply which

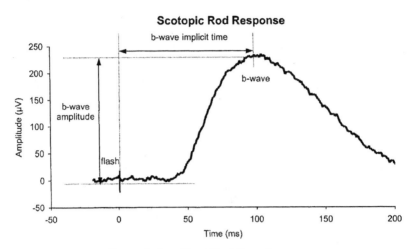

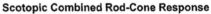

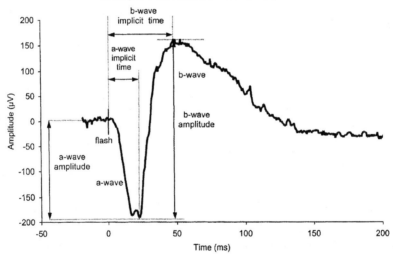

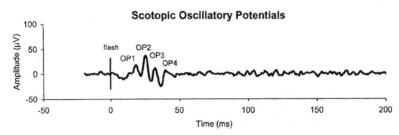

Figure 1.3 (*Caption on facing page*)

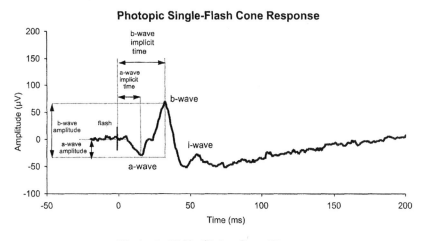

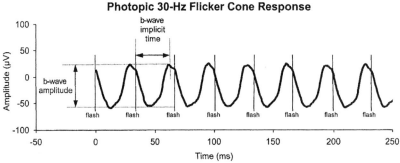

Figure 1.4 (*above*) Standard photopic full-field ERG responses of a normal subject. The definitions of amplitudes and implicit times of the a- and b-waves are shown. Available computer programs allow automated calculation of the amplitude and implicit time for the 30-Hz flicker response.

Figure 1.3 (*Facing page*) Standard scotopic full-field ERG responses of a normal subject. The definitions of amplitudes and implicit times of the a- and b-waves are shown. The waveforms are all plotted to the same scale to demonstrate the relative size of the responses. Available computer programs allow accurate placement of cursors and rapid calculations. The a-wave of the standard scotopic combined rod–cone response for normal subjects may have a single negative peak or double negative peaks.

often has an oscillating rate in multiples of 30 (e.g., 60 Hz in the United States). The recording of the flicker response is not initiated until a few seconds after the start of the flicker since the first response to the flickering stimulus is a single-flash response rather than a flicker response.

At least two repeatable responses should be obtained for each of the five recommended responses. Averaging of multiple responses to the same stimulus produces an averaged waveform that has a smoother contour because random electrical noises cancel each other. The random noise level is decreased by the square-root of the number of responses averaged. Averaging helps to identify very weak responses buried by background electrical noise, but responses should not be averaged blindly, and poor quality responses with artifacts from blinks and eye movements should be excluded. Averaging of flash responses is not required as long as repeated recordings are reproducible and without artifacts. Flicker responses such as the 30-Hz cone response are routinely averaged from multiple flickers or sweeps because the responses are too rapidly for manual rejection.

Evaluating ERG Responses and Measuring Amplitudes and Implicit Times

Electrophysiologic responses are evaluated based on appearance or morphology as well as measurable parameters such as amplitudes and implicit times of waveform components. The measurement of the amplitude and implicit time of each component is demonstrated in Figs. 1.3 and 1.4. The first negative component is called the *a-wave* and the ensuing positive component is called *b-wave*. The amplitude of the a-wave is measured from the baseline to the a-wave negative peak, and the amplitude of the b-wave is measured from the a-wave negative peak to the b-wave positive peak. The implicit time of each wave is the time from stimulus onset to its peak. The recording duration is usually in the range of 250 msec.

The scotopic rod response has a prominent b-wave but no a-wave because the electrical activity of the rod photoreceptors to the dim stimulus is very small, but this signal is amplified tremendously by cells of the inner retina. The scotopic combined rod–cone response has distinct a- and b-waves. The a-wave may demonstrate double negative peaks likely due to the first wavelet of the oscillatory potential. In such cases, the a-wave amplitude may be measured from the baseline to the lower negative peak. Flashes brighter than the recommended standard flash elicit a larger better-defined a-wave.

The oscillatory potentials usually consist of three larger wavelets followed by a smaller one during the ascending phase of the b-wave. The wavelets are designated in order of occurrence as OP1, OP2, OP3, and so on. Several methods of measuring the oscillatory potentials have been proposed. In the peak-to-trough method, the amplitude of each wavelet is measured from the preceding trough to its peak. In the caliper-square method, the line connecting the troughs before and after each peak of the wavelet is calculated, and the amplitude is measured perpendicularly from the peak to the line. Alternatively, an index of the oscillatory potentials is provided by the sum of the amplitudes of all four major wavelets. The summed amplitude is similar regardless of which of two measuring methods is employed (13).

The photopic single-flash cone response has distinct a- and b-waves. The 30-Hz flicker cone response consists of only b-waves and provides a consistent measure of the cone response.

Recognizing Recording Noise and Artifacts

The electrical noise from the power supply and appliances is much larger than ERG signals and may interfere with ERG recording. Electrical noise often oscillates at a frequency related to that of the power supply (e.g., 60 Hz in the United States) (Fig. 1.5). Electrical noise may be reduced by checking the connections of the electrodes as well as unplugging appliances that are plugged into the local circuit. Electrical activities of the heart, muscles, and brain may also be a source of electrical noise.

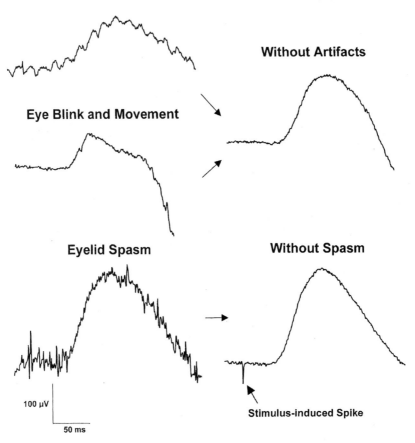

Figure 1.5 Examples of electrical noise and recording artifacts. The responses are from normal adults. The response with the 60-Hz noise and the response with the eye blink and movement are from the same individual; the response without the artifacts is shown for comparison. The responses of another normal adult, with and without eyelid spasm, are also shown.

Several commonly occurring ERG recording artifacts are recognized (Fig. 1.5). A voltage artifact spike coinciding with the flash stimulus is usually not significant in standard clinical recording because it is brief and does not affect the rest of the recording. However, recording artifacts from blinks, eyelid spasm, and eye movement are common obstacles to a clean ERG recording. Checking the baseline electrical tracing before recording helps to predict the occurrence of these artifacts. These artifacts are usually reduced by proper electrode placement with adequate topical anesthesia (when contact-lens electrodes are used) as well as encouraging the patient to remain calm and to keep fixation steady. Eccentric fixation has only modest effect on full-field ERG responses. Although reduced full-field ERG responses may be produced by severe eccentric fixation, this effect is typically not clinical significant (Fig. 1.6).

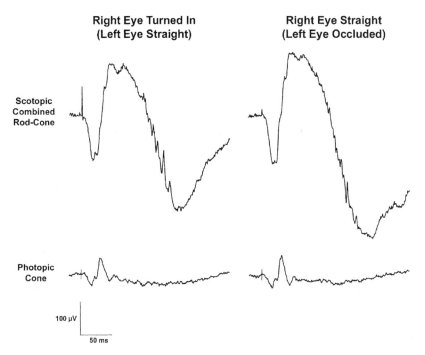

Figure 1.6 Reduced full-field ERG responses due to eccentric fixation. The responses of the right eye of a patient with normal retinal function and large esotropia (approximately 40 diopters) are shown. The responses are reduced when the right eye is turned in as compared to those recorded when the eye is straight. In general, eccentric fixation has only a modest effect on full-field ERG responses except when the eccentricity is extremely large.

Reporting ERG Results and Establishing Normative Data

The full-field ERG report, at the least, should display the recorded waveforms of all five recommended international standard responses along with the amplitudes and implicit times of the ERG components. Because ERG responses are variable among normal persons, a comparison of amplitudes and implicit times between the patient and a group of age-matched normal subjects is required. Collection of normative ERG values by each facility is critical because of differences in recording equipment and technique (e.g., electrode type and position). The values from normal subjects are not distributed in a normal bell-shaped curve. Therefore, calculating the median and the 95% confidence limits are more appropriate than the mean and standard deviation. The normal lower and upper limits also aid interpretation. The effects of maturation and aging on the full-field ERG are discussed in Chapter 6. In addition to a comparison against normal values, an assessment of the interocular difference in ERG amplitudes and implicit times is also important to determine unilateral or asymmetric abnormality. The interocular percentage differences in ERG b-wave amplitude are usually 10% or less for most normal subjects with a difference of greater than 20% being highly unusual.

PHYSIOLOGIC ORIGIN OF THE FULL-FIELD ERG

The ERG waveform represents a summation of the electrical activities of all cells of the retina. The physiologic origin of an ERG response is dependent on the adaptive state of the retina (scotopic vs. photopic), stimulus intensity and duration (flash vs. long-duration), stimulus type (flash vs. flicker), and stimulus color (white vs. chromatic). Knowledge of the physiologic origin of ERG components is derived primarily from animal studies by intraretinal microelectrode recordings and ERG changes in response to chemicals with known retinal cellular effects. This section discusses the physiologic origin of the standard clinical ERG, assuming an understanding of basic retinal physiology detailed at the end of the chapter.

PI, PII, and PIII Potentials

Granit and Riddell (14) demonstrated that the ERG waveform is a summation of three processes or potentials called PI, PII, and PIII (Fig. 1.7). PI is a slow positive potential from the retinal pigment epithelium that contributes to the ERG c-wave which is not ordinarily measured in the clinic. PII is a positive inner retinal potential related mostly to bipolar cell activity and makes a major contribution to the ERG b-wave. PIII is a negative potential composed of two phases. The first phase called *fast* PIII is due to the closure of sodium ion channels of the photoreceptors and is responsible for the onset and

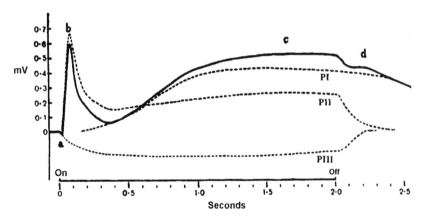

Figure 1.7 PI, PII, and PII potentials. The ERG waveform (a = a-wave; b = b-wave; c = c-wave; d = d-wave) is a summation of three potentials. PI is a slow positive potential from the retinal pigment epithelium that contributes primarily to the c-wave. PII is a positive inner retinal potential related mostly to bipolar cell activity and makes a major contribution to the ERG b-wave. PIII is composed of two phases. The first phase called "fast PIII" is related to photoreceptor activity and is responsible for the onset and descending phase of the a-wave. The second phase called "slow PIII" is related to Müller cell activity. (From Ref. 93 with permission.)

descending phase of the a-wave, that is, the *leading edge* of a-wave. The second phase called *slow* PIII is due to hyperpolarization of the distal portion of the Müller cells related to a decrease in extracellular potassium ions at the photoreceptor inner segments. The slow PIII contributes to the b- and c-waves.

Scotopic Rod Response—Physiologic Origin

The scotopic rod response has a prominent b-wave but no a-wave because the electrical activity of the rod photoreceptors to the dim stimulus is too small to be detected as an a-wave but this rod signal is amplified in the range of 100-fold by the rod-specific depolarizing ON-bipolar cells in the inner retina (15). In addition to this high retinal gain, the b-wave extracellular cellular current involves Müller cells and is more extensive than the a-wave current of the rod photoreceptors (16).

Scotopic Combined Rod–Cone Response: Physiologic Origin

The scotopic bright-flash combined rod–cone response has prominent a- and b-waves. The onset and descending phase of the a-wave are due to photoreceptor activity, that is, the fast PIII potential before PII arises (17,18). This leading edge of the a-wave, as shown by computational models, is directly related to the electrical activity generated by the phototransduction cascade (17,19). Therefore, the initial 14–20 msec of the response is essentially entirely due to photoreceptor activity with virtually no contribution from the inner retina (20). The shape and peak of the b-wave is determined by the interaction between the fast PIII potential of the photoreceptors and PII potential of the inner retina. The b-wave is primarily due to depolarizing ON-bipolar cell activity which produces a light-induced release of potassium that causes depolarization of the Müller cells resulting in a corneal positive potential (21–24). Other cells of the inner retinal layers also contribute to the b-wave.

Photopic Single-Flash Cone Response: Physiologic Origin

The photopic single-flash cone response has discernible a- and b-waves. The initial descending phase of the a-wave is due to the electrical activity generated by the phototransduction of the cones as demonstrated by computational models (25–28). However, the photopic a-wave receives a significant contribution from retinal activity postsynaptic to cone photoreceptors particularly for stimuli typically used for clinical standard ERG (29). The a-wave trough is influenced by inner retinal activity including those of hyperpolarizing OFF-bipolar cells. The photopic b-wave is not only due to the activity of depolarizing ON-bipolar cells affecting perhaps Müller cells but is also shaped by the activities of hyperpolarizing OFF-bipolar cells and horizontal cells (30). The photopic b-wave can be explained by a push–pull model with the depolarizing ON-bipolar cells pulling the ascending phase of the b-wave up and the OFF-hyperpolarizing cells limiting b-wave amplitude by pulling the depolarization toward baseline (30).

Photopic 30-Hz Flicker Cone Response: Physiologic Origin

The photopic 30-Hz flicker cone response consists of b-waves due to inner retinal post-photoreceptoral activity in response to cone activity but the direct contribution from cone photoreceptors is very small. The b-waves of flicker stimuli are made of ON- and OFF-ERG components with large phase differences so that these components partially cancel each other (31,32).

Oscillatory Potentials: Physiologic Origin

The oscillatory potentials consist of about 4–6 wavelets during the ascending phase of the b-wave and have physiologic origin that differs from the a- and b-waves (33,34). The oscillatory potentials are due to both rod- and cone-generated activities and can be recorded in scotopic as well as photopic conditions (35,36). Activity of inhibitory feedback circuits in the inner plexiform layer as the origin of oscillatory potentials has been proposed, but the same retinal mechanisms may not apply to all oscillatory potentials. OP1 and OP2 appear to be more cone-mediated and OP3 and OP4 rod-mediated, but this notion does not explain oscillatory potentials from all recorded conditions (37,38). The oscillatory potentials are likely generated by amacrine and bipolar cells, and the early wavelets are likely related to the ON-pathway while the later wavelets are related to the OFF-pathway (39).

ERG FLUCTUATION RELATED TO CIRCADIAN RHYTHM

The outer segments of the photoreceptors are continuously regenerated, shed, and phagocytized by the retinal pigment epithelium. The greatest rate of shedding occurs diurnally when the photoreceptors are functionally less active—at about 1–3 hr following onset of daylight for rods and in the early darkness hours for cones. Small diurnal changes in ERG responses are found but are unlikely to be clinical significant (40–42). In one study of normal subjects, the scotopic a-wave showed no circadian rhythm, but the b-wave was greatest at noon and lowest at 6 AM in some subjects (43).

NEGATIVE ERG—SELECTIVE REDUCTION OF b-WAVE

The *negative ERG* refers to selective reduction of the b-wave to the extent that the peak of the b-wave fails to reach baseline, and the b-wave to a-wave amplitude ratio is less than 1 (Fig. 1.8). In normal subjects, the peak of the b-wave is well above baseline, and the b-wave amplitude is at least nearly twice the a-wave amplitude. A selective reduction of the b-wave implies a selective dysfunction of the inner retina with a relative preservation of photoreceptor function. A number of conditions can cause a negative full-field ERG (Table 1.3). Although a selective impairment of both photopic and scotopic b-waves may occur, the selective b-wave

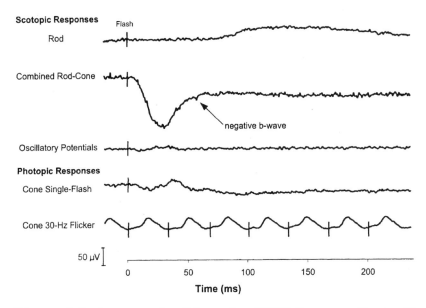

Figure 1.8 An example of "negative ERG" from a patient with retinal ischemia. The standard full-field ERG responses demonstrate reduced and prolonged rod and cone responses. Note the relatively selective reduction of b-wave on the scotopic combined rod–cone response such that the peak of the b-wave is below baseline and the b-wave amplitude is less than the a-wave amplitude. A selective b-wave reduction indicates greater inner retinal dysfunction. A number of conditions can cause a negative ERG (see Table 1.3).

reduction in the negative ERG is most notable for the scotopic combined rod–cone bright flash response.

ADVANCED CLINICAL FULL-FIELD ERG TOPICS

Chromatic Stimulus ERG—Isolated Rod, Cone, and S-Cone Responses and x-Wave

The light-sensitive rod pigment rhodopsin has a spectral absorption peak at 496 nm, and each of the three types of color-sensitive cone pigments has peak sensitivity to long-wavelength (558 nm), mid-wavelength (531 nm), or short-wavelength (419 nm) regions of the visible light spectrum.

Table 1.3 Disorders Associated with Selective b-Wave Reduction Large Enough to Produce a Negative b-Wave (Negative ERG)[a]

Frequently	Rarely
Hereditary retinal disorders	Hereditary retinal disorders
Congenital stationary night blindness (CSNB)	Retinitis pigmentosa
Oguchi disease	Refsum disease
X-linked retinoschisis	Neuronal ceroid lipofuscinosis
Fleck retina of Kandori	Cone–rod dystrophy
Familial internal limiting membrane dystrophy	Cone dystrophy
Bull's eye maculopathy with negative ERG	Enhanced s-cone syndrome
Hereditary systemic disorders	Bietti crystalline dystrophy
Muscular dystrophy	Autosomal dominant
(Duchenne type, Becker type, Oregon eye disease)	neovascular inflammatory vitreoretinopathy (ADNIV)
Myotonic dystrophy	Dominant optic atrophy
Mucolipidosis IV	Vascular condition
Vascular occlusions	Retinopathy of prematurity
Central retinal artery occlusion	Inflammatory conditions
Central retinal vein occlusion	Behcet disease
Inflammatory conditions	Birdshot retinochoroidopathy
Melanoma-associated retinopathy (MAR)	Toxic condition
Toxic conditions	
Metallic intraocular foreign bodies/siderosis	Methanol
Quinine	
Cisplatin	

[a]Typically noted on the scotopic combined rod–cone response.

With selective color stimuli, more specific ERG responses of the rod or cone subtype are elicited.

An essentially pure rod response is elicited scotopically by a dim blue flash stimulus. The short-wavelength ($< 460\,\text{nm}$) characteristic of the blue flash minimizes stimulation of the long-wavelength and mid-wavelength sensitive cones while maximizing stimulation of the rods, and the short-wavelength sensitive cones are minimally active under this recording condition. For instance, a blue flash 1 log unit

(10 dB) dimmer than the international standard flash scotopically elicits a prominent rod response consisting of a large b-wave reflecting inner retinal activity due to rod activity (Fig. 1.9). Similarly, a 10-dB 10-Hz blue flicker scotopic

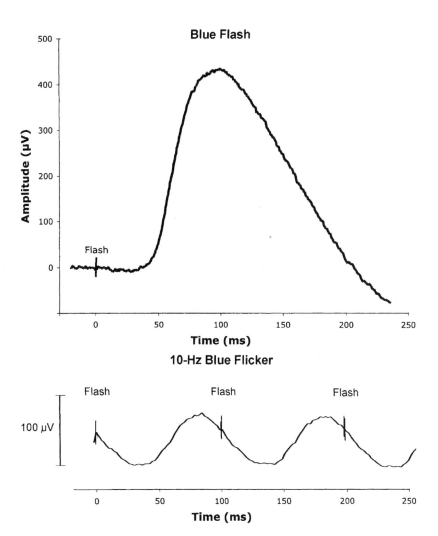

Figure 1.9 Scotopic blue flash and 10-Hz blue flicker rod ERG responses. A blue flash at 1 log unit (10 dB) dimmer than the standard flash elicits a relatively pure rod response under scotopic condition. A 10-Hz blue flicker stimulus elicits b-waves related to rod activity.

stimulus elicits b-waves that are related to rod activity (Fig. 1.9).

Isolated cone responses are obtained with the aid of a red stimulus. A scotopic combined cone–rod response is elicited by a red flash stimulus with a spectral peak of 600 nm and has a distinct ERG component located on the ascending phase of the b-wave called the *x-wave* that is attributable to cone activity (Fig. 1.10) (44). By matching red and blue flash stimuli based on retinal illuminance in scotopic troland, an isolated scotopic cone response can be obtained by subtracting the blue flash rod response from the red cone–rod response. A 30-Hz red flicker scotopic response is also a cone response because cones but not rods respond well to a 30-Hz flicker.

The ERG response of short-wavelength sensitive cones (S-cones) can be elicited photopically with a blue flash stimulus (45–50). Although S-cone ERG is detectable with a strong white background, the response is more robust with a

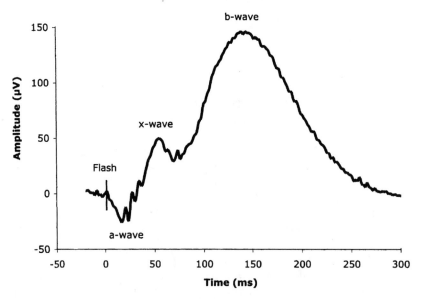

Figure 1.10 Scotopic red flash full-field ERG response (flash intensity $0.2\,cd\,s/m^2$). The red flash elicits a combined cone–rod response under scotopic condition. The x-wave visible on the ascending phase of the b-wave is related to cone activity.

strong yellow background that suppresses the long- and medium-wavelength sensitive cones (L- and M-cones). The S-cone response can be further isolated by recording matched red and blue flash responses with a yellow background, and then subtracting the red flash L- and M-cone response from the blue flash response (Fig. 1.11). The amplitude of the S-cone response is small in the range of 5 μV in part because S-cones comprise only about 10% of the cones. The S-cones have the highest density in a small donut-shaped region

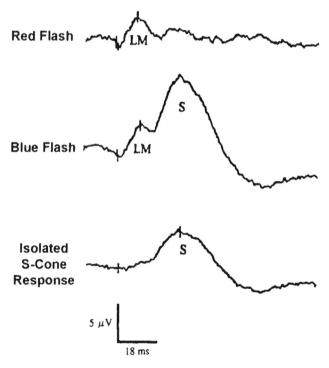

Figure 1.11 Isolation of the full-field ERG response from short-wavelength sensitive cones (S-cones). Photopic full-field ERG responses are recorded with yellow background. The ERG response of the long- and medium-wavelength sensitive cones (LM) to a red flash adjusted to match the LM response elicited by the blue flash is shown. The S-cone ERG response (S) is isolated by subtracting the LM response to the red flash from the response to blue flash. (From Ref. 48 with permission from Kluwer and author.)

within 1–2° surrounding the foveal center but are virtually absent at the center of the fovea. The implicit time of the S-cone ERG response is approximately 40 msec, which is longer than that of the L- and M-cones. Early selectively reduced S-cone ERG responses are found in conditions such as central serous retinopathy, glaucoma, and retinitis pigmentosa. Conversely, the ERGs of L- and M-cones are elicited with a red flash stimulus and a blue background that suppresses the S-cones. Recording photopic chromatic ERG responses helps to distinguish blue-cone monochromatism from rod monochromatism, which is difficult with standard ERG.

Intensity–Response Function: Naka–Rushton Function and Photopic Hill

The intensity–response function, also called luminance-response or stimulus-response function, provides a measure of retinal sensitivity and maximal b-wave amplitude. Theoretically, in disorder with reduced number of photoreceptors and normal functioning of the remaining photoreceptors, the maximal b-wave amplitude is reduced but retinal sensitivity is preserved. In contrast, for conditions with impaired photoreceptor function and no reduction in photoreceptor number, the retinal sensitivity is decreased, and a brighter stimulus is required to elicit a relatively preserved maximal b-wave amplitude.

After recording a series of full-field ERG responses over a range of stimulus intensities, the luminances of the flash stimuli are plotted against the respective ERG b-wave amplitudes to calculate the intensity–response function. The characteristics of the intensity–response curves are different for scotopic and photopic recordings.

Under scotopic condition at low luminance flash levels, the full-field ERG responses demonstrate rod responses with b-waves only. With increasing brighter flashes, the a-wave emerging at a flash luminance level at least 1 log unit brighter than the dimmest flash capable of eliciting a b-wave (Fig. 1.12). With even brighter flashes, the response also receives contributions from cone activity. The amplitudes of

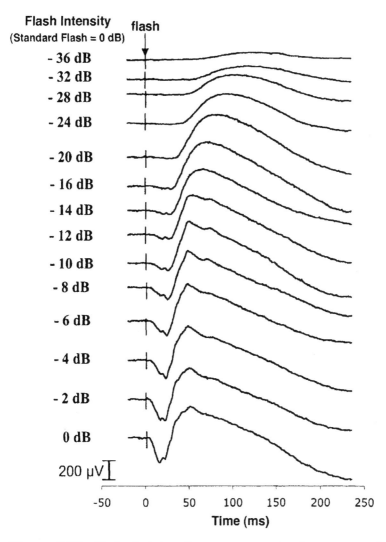

Figure 1.12 Scotopic intensity response series from a normal subject up to the luminance of the international standard white flash. The full-field ERG responses with increasing flash luminance demonstrate initial rod responses with b-waves only with low luminance flashes. With brighter flashes, the a-wave emerges and the responses also receive contributions from cone activity. The b-wave amplitudes obtained from such a series may be plotted against the corresponding flash luminances to calculate an index of retinal sensitivity as shown in Fig. 1.13.

both a- and b-waves increase, implicit times shorten, and oscillatory potentials emerge on the ascending phase of the b-wave. For flash luminances up to the international standard flash, an S-shaped curve results when the flash luminances are plotted against the corresponding b-wave amplitudes (Fig. 1.13). The curve is best described by the Naka–Rushton function:

$$R/R \max = I^n/(I^n + K^n)$$

where R is the b-wave amplitude produced by a flash of intensity I, $R_{\max}$ is the maximal b-wave amplitude, K is the flash intensity that produces half of the maximal response $R_{\max}$, and n is the slope of the function at $I = K$. The slope n is approximately 1 for normal retina, and K is an index of retinal sensitivity (51,52).

In reality, the scotopic intensity–response function is more complex due to interactions between the fast PIII photoreceptors potential and PII potential of the inner retina. The $R_{\max}$ plateau reached with the international standard flash represents only the first portion of the intensity–response function. With even brighter flashes, the b-wave amplitude dips slightly and rises again to a second final plateau (Fig. 1.13). The Naka–Rushton function describes only the first limb of the scotopic intensity-response, and more complex equations are required to describe both limbs of the function. Hood and Birch point out that Naka–Rushton fits are better understood in the context of a dynamic model and should be interpreted with care (53). The b-wave may be a very poor reflection of inner retinal activity when the inner retina is affected by disease, and the b-wave implicit time provides a measure of photoreceptor sensitivity.

Under photopic condition, the full-field flash ERG consists of cone responses with distinct a- and b-waves. With brighter flash stimuli, the amplitudes of the a- and b-waves increase, and the implicit time of the b-wave increases slightly rather than decreases (Fig. 1.14). While the photopic a-wave continues to grow with brighter stimuli, the b-wave amplitude reaches a peak and decreases rapidly with further

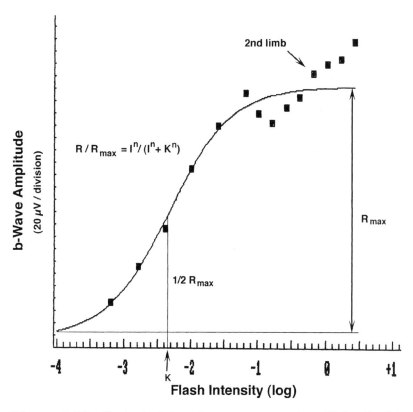

Figure 1.13 Scotopic intensity response series—Naka–Rushton function. The b-wave amplitudes of a series of full-field ERG responses with increasingly brighter stimuli up to the international standard flash ($0 \log = 2.5 \, \mathrm{cd\,s\,m}^{-2}$) of a normal subject are shown. The s-shaped plot may be described by the Naka–Rushton function, $R/R_{max} = I^n/(I^n + K^n)$, where R is the b-wave amplitude produced by flash intensity I, R_{max} is the maximal b-wave amplitude, K is the flash intensity that produces half of R_{max}, and n is the slope at $I = K$. The slope n is approximately 1 for normal retina, and K is an index of retinal sensitivity. A second limb of the scotopic intensity–response occurs with brighter flashes and is due to interactions between the fast PIII photoreceptors potential and PII potential of the inner retina. The Naka–Rushton function describes only the first limb of the scotopic intensity–response, and more complex equations are required to describe both limbs of the function. The plateau of the second limb is reached with stimuli brighter than the standard flash.

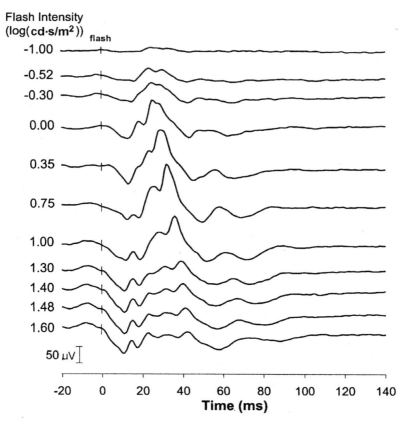

Figure 1.14 Photopic intensity–response series from a normal subject. The a-wave amplitudes of the full-field ERG responses increase with brighter stimuli under photopic condition. The b-wave amplitude increases initially with brighter stimuli then reaches a peak and decreases rapidly with further increments in flash luminance until a final plateau is reached. This paradoxical phenomenon is called the "photopic hill" and is demonstrated in Fig. 1.15 where the b-wave amplitudes are plotted against the corresponding flash luminances. The implicit time of the b-waves increases rather than decreases with brighter stimuli.

increments in flash luminance until a final plateau is reached (54,55). This unique photopic b-wave intensity–response phenomenon is called the *photopic hill* (Fig. 1.15). The paradoxical decrease of photopic b-wave amplitudes with higher

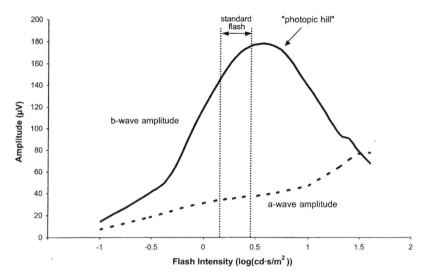

Figure 1.15 Photopic flash intensity vs. amplitude response curve. The plot is from white-flash responses of a normal subject. With brighter flash stimuli, the amplitude of the a-wave grows steadily, but the b-wave amplitude reaches a peak and decreases rapidly with further increments in flash luminance. This phenomenon is called the "photopic hill." The luminance range of the recommended standard flash as indicated by the dash lines is below the peak of the photopic hill.

luminance flashes is caused by interactions of the ON- and OFF-pathways (56,57). At higher flash intensities, the decrease of the photopic b-wave amplitudes is the result of reduced ON-component amplitude and delayed positive peak of the OFF-component (58). Clinically, the international standard flash is too dim to reach the peak of the photopic hill.

Leading Edge of a-Wave as a Measure of Phototransduction in Photoreceptors

The leading edge of the a-wave of the full-field ERG is a measure of the sum of the electrical activity of the photoreceptors. Under scotopic condition, this initial downward phase of the human a-wave behaves similarly to isolated rod responses of other vertebrates to changes in stimulus intensity and wavelength. A computational model based on biochemical stages of phototransduction has been developed to calculate rod sensitivity and maximal response using a series of scotopic full-field ERG responses to increasing flash intensity (Fig. 1.16) (17,19,59–62). Subsequently, a comparable computational model for the cones was also developed using photopic ERG responses (26,27).

A clinical protocol utilizing these computational models to assess rod and cone phototransduction activity has been proposed (63). This protocol utilizes brighter flashes than the international standard flash and adds approximately

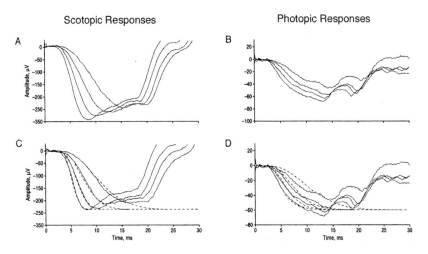

Figure 1.16 Leading edge of a-wave as a measure of phototransduction in photoreceptors. (A) Scotopic a-wave responses from a 65-year-old normal subject to intensities ranging from 3.2 to 4.4 log scotopic troland-seconds (log sc td s). (B) Photopic responses from the same four intensities presented against a 3.2 log td background. (C) Computational model (dashed lines) of the response (R) as a function of time (t) and flash intensity (i) as described in text is applied to the rod-isolated responses obtained by subtracting (B) from (A) where log rod-only sensitivity (S) is $0.89\,s^{-2}[td\,s]^{-2}$ and log rod-only maximum amplitude (Rm_{P3}) is 2.37 log μV. (D). Computational model (dashed lines) as described in text applied to cone responses from (B) where log cone sensitivity (S) is $1.48\,s^{-2}[td\,s]^{-2}$ and cone maximum amplitude is 1.7 log μV. (From Ref. 64 with permission from the American Medical Association.)

10 min to the standard protocol although sophisticated software is necessary for analysis. Scotopic combined rod–cone responses to bright white flashes for four increasing intensities ranging from approximately 3.2 to 4.4 log scotopic troland-seconds are recorded with at least 30 sec between flashes to preserve dark adaptation. Light-adapted cone responses using the same four flash intensities and a rod-saturating background of 3.2 log troland are also recorded with 5 sec between flashes. The photopic cone a-waves are then subtracted from the corresponding scotopic a-waves to yield rod-only a-waves. The four rod-only a-waves from the four light intensities are fitted into a computational model describing the response (R) as a function of time (t) and flash intensity (i):

$$R(i,t) = \{1 - \exp[-iS(t - t_d)^2]\}Rm_{P3}$$

where Rm_{P3} is the maximal rod-only a-wave amplitude, S is a rod sensitivity variable, and t_d is a brief time delay constant of 3.2 msec before the onset of the response. Similarly the four photopic cone a-waves from the four light intensities are fitted into a cone computational model with an additional time constant to reflect the capacitance of the cone outer segment:

$$R(i,t) = \{[iS(t - t_d)^3]/[iS(t - t_d)^3 + 1]\}Rm_{P3}$$

where Rm_{P3} is the maximal cone-only a-wave amplitude, S is a cone sensitivity variable, and t_d is a brief time delay constant of 1.7 msec before the onset of the response.

The sensitivity variable (S) is an index of phototransduction efficiency and decreases with age for cone and rod responses while the maximal cone and rod responses (Rm_{P3}) remain constant and is the measure of choice in following photoreceptor function (64). Several studies have utilized this paradigm in assessing photoreceptor diseases such as retinitis pigmentosa (64,65).

Long-Duration Flash ERG: ON and OFF Pathways, d-Wave and i-Wave

The retina responds not only to the onset of light but also to the cessation of light, and these responses are called

ON-*response* and OFF-*response*, respectively. The clinical ERG utilizes a brief flash of less than a millisecond, and the recorded response is a combination of the ON- and OFF-pathways. The activities of the ON- and OFF-pathways can be separated in time by using bright long-duration flash stimuli of 150 msec (66). Using this method, selective impairment of the OFF-pathway has been demonstrated in conditions such as congenital stationary night blindness and retinoschisis.

The long-duration flash ERG responses are quite different for scotopic and photopic conditions. Differences in scotopic and photopic OFF-components are in part due to the differences in intraretinal synapses. The rods synapse with one type of ON-bipolar cell and connect to OFF-bipolar cells via intermediary AII amacrine cells. On the other hand, the cones synapse directly with a number of ON- and OFF-bipolar cell types. The scotopic rod-driven long-duration flash ERG consists of a large b-wave representing the ON-response followed by a small slow negative dip representing the OFF-component corresponding to the cessation of the stimulus. In contrast, the photopic cone-driven long-duration flash ERG has a prominent OFF-component and is clinically utilized more frequently (Fig. 1.17). The photopic cone-driven long-duration flash ERG consists of a- and b-waves related to the ON-pathway followed by a slight upward plateau and a corneal positive *d-wave* and a small *i-wave* representing the OFF-pathway. The photopic b-wave is smaller with long-duration stimuli than with brief flashes, because the positive d-wave OFF-component is summated into the b-wave with brief flashes.

SPECIALIZED ERG RECORDINGS AND WAVEFORMS

Early Receptor Potential (ERP)

The early receptor potential (ERP) is a rapid short-lived ERG response occurring immediately after stimulus onset and before onset of a-wave (67). The ERP reflects changes

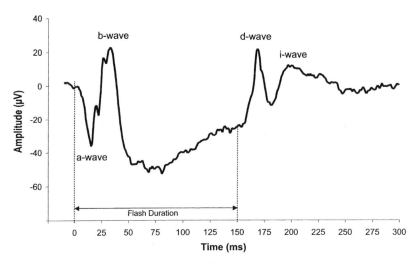

Figure 1.17 Photopic cone-driven long-duration flash ON–OFF ERG response. Note the a- and b-waves related to the ON-pathway followed by a slight upward plateau. A corneal positive *d-wave* and a small *i-wave* occur with the cessation of the flash and represent the activities of the OFF-pathway. The photopic b-wave is smaller with long-duration stimuli than with brief flashes, because the positive d-wave OFF-component is no longer summated into the b-wave. The recording was obtained with a white-flash intensity of $125\,\mathrm{cd/m^2}$ and a duration of 150 msec. The photopic white background was $42\,\mathrm{cd/m^2}$.

in membrane potential at the outer segments of the photoreceptors due to transition of rhodopsin to its activated form. The ERP is not visible on routine clinical ERG recordings because high-intensity flash stimulus is required and isolation of the recording electrode from the flash stimulus is needed to avoid the brief stimulus-induced voltage artifact common in most clinical ERG recordings. The ERP has an initial positive phase R_1 followed by a negative phase R_2 (Fig. 1.18) (67). The R_1 component is related to the conversion of lumirhodopsin to metarhodopsin I, and R_2 is associated with the conversion of metarhodopsin I to metarhodopsin II. The implicit times of R_1 and R_2 are about 0.1 and 0.9 msec, respectively, with completion of the entire ERP by about 1.5 msec. The ERP is derived from both rods and cones with the cones generating about 70% of ERP

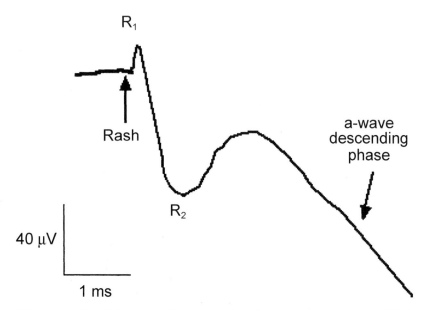

Figure 1.18 Schematic drawing of early receptor potential (ERP). Note the initial positive phase R_1 followed by a negative phase R_2 with implicit times of only 0.2 and 0.75 msec, respectively. The ERP reflects changes in membrane potential at the outer segments of the photoreceptors due to transition of rhodopsin to its activated form. The ERP is not visible on routine ERG recordings because ERP is brief and buried in the stimulus-induced voltage artifact and optimal recordings of ERP require brief flashes much brighter than the standard flash.

(68–70). The ERP is abnormal in disorders involving photoreceptors such as retinitis pigmentosa (71,72). Because of large intra- and inter-individual variability, the clinical value of ERP is not established and ERP abnormality is not specific for a condition (73).

Scotopic Threshold Response (STR)

The scotopic threshold response (STR) is a negative ERG waveform detectable by very dim flash stimuli after full dark adaptation (Fig. 1.19) (74). The STR is the only ERG component detectable by dim stimuli near the minimal light threshold required for rod activation. With progressively brighter stimuli, the STR grows until it is buried by the emerging b-wave. The STR has a maximal amplitude of 12–20 μV and a latency ranging 100–185 msec. The STR is a rod-driven, inner retinal post-photoreceptoral response distinct from the PII potential and the scotopic a-wave; both of which are elicited with brighter stimuli (75). Microelectrode recordings in cat indicate that STR is most prominent at or near the inner plexiform layer, and amacrine cells are likely the generators of STR. Impairment STR is associated with incomplete congenital stationary night blindness and other retinal disorders (76,77).

Photopic Negative Response (PhNR)

The photopic negative response is an ERG component attributed to activities of the retinal ganglion cells and may have potential use in optic neuropathies such as glaucoma (78–80). The PhNR immediately follows the single-flash photopic b-wave, and if long-duration stimulus is used, PhNR appears after the b-wave (ON-pathway PhNR) and again after the d-wave (OFF-pathway PhNR) (Fig. 1.20). The amplitude of the PhNR is measured from the baseline amplitude to the PhNR negative trough. The implicit time of the PhNR is determined from stimulus onset to the negative trough and may be difficult to determine because the trough is relatively broad. The PhNR is best recorded with chromatic conditions that are toned to ganglion cell responses such as with red flash stimulus on a rod saturating blue background.

c-Wave

The c-wave is a slow positive ERG component with a latency of 1.5–4 sec. The c-wave is considered as a reflection of retinal pigment epithelium function but actually receives contributions from both PI and the slow PIII potentials (Fig. 1.21). The PI potential is a corneal positive potential produced by hyperpolarization of the apical membrane of the retinal pigment epithelium. The slow PIII potential is

Flash Intensity

(log q(507) / d^2)

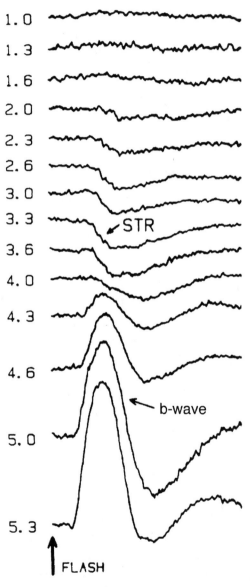

Figure 1.19   *(Caption on facing page)*

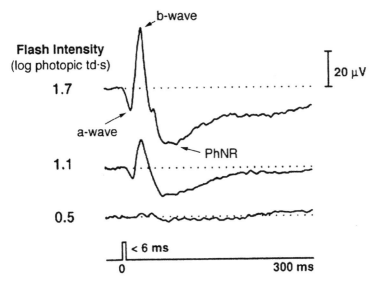

Figure 1.20 (*above*) Photopic negative response (PhNR). Photopic full-field ERG intensity series to brief (<6 msec) red stimuli on a rod saturating (3.7 log scotopic troland) blue background of a normal adult subject is shown. The PhNR immediately follows the b-wave and is related to activities of the retinal ganglion cells. The amplitude of PhNR is measured from the baseline amplitude to the PhNR negative trough. The implicit time may be difficult to determine in some cases as the negative trough is relatively broad. (From Ref. 78, with permission of *Investigative Ophthalmology and Visual Science.*)

Figure 1.19 (*Facing page*) Scotopic threshold response (STR). Scotopic full-field ERG intensity series to brief (10 μsec) stimuli from a normal adult subject is shown. The STR is an inner retinal response recorded as a negative waveform at the cornea and is elicited by very dim stimuli near the minimal light threshold required for rod activation. The stimulus intensities are expressed in integrated energy per flash as 507 nm equivalent quanta per square visual degree $(\log q(507)/\text{deg}^2)$ (1 scotopic troland $= 5.649\log$ q$(507)/\text{deg}^2$sec). The psychophysical threshold for this subject was $1.0\log q(507)/d^2$ and the waveforms were obtained by averaging approximately 20 responses. (From Ref. 74, with permission of *Investigative Ophthalmology and Visual Science.*)

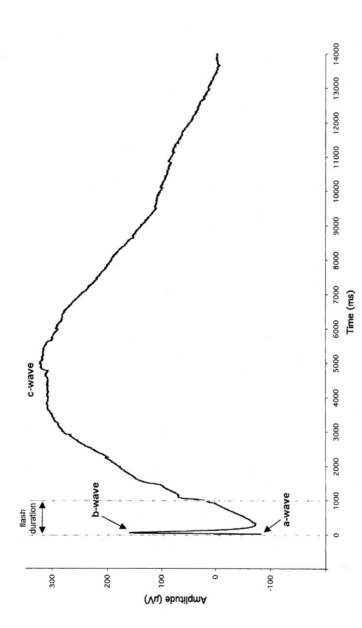

Figure 1.21   The c-wave from a normal subject. Note the recording duration is long at 5 sec. The c-wave is a reflection of retinal pigment epithelium function but actually receives contributions from both PI and the slow PIII potentials. The recording was obtained scotopically using a direct-coupling (DC) system. The flash intensity was 250 cd/m with a duration of 1000 msec. The bandpass was set at 0–1000 Hz.

a corneal negative created by the hyperpolarization of the distal portion of Müller cells occurring in response to a decrease in extracellular potassium ions at the photoreceptor inner segments.

The c-wave is not ordinarily recorded clinically because a recording setup stable enough over several seconds is required (81). The c-wave is optimally recorded with long-duration, high luminance stimuli using a direct-coupling (DC) rather than an alternate-coupling (AC) system. The c-wave has high intra-subject and inter-subject variability, and this has limited its clinical use. Other electrophy siologic measures of retinal pigment epithelium function include the fast and slow oscillations of the electro-oculogram.

Pair-Flash or Double-Flash Response

The pair-flash ERG also called double-flash ERG is a method for studying retinal recovery after light exposure (82–86). A test flash (also called the conditioning flash) is followed shortly by a second flash (also called the probe stimulus), and the retinal recovery to the test flash is reflected by the magnitude of the ERG response to a second flash. The dynamics of retina recovery can be studied by varying the time interval between the test and second flashes and by comparing the ERG responses of the flashes. For example, the recovering kinetics of the rod phototransduction process can be evaluated by analyzing the leading edge of the a-wave of the second flash, which grows and returns to normal with increased elapsed time (Fig. 1.22). Based on similar principle as the pair-flash ERG, a series of flashes at high frequency or flash trains can also be utilized to further study retinal recovery.

ERG Responses During Dark and Light Adaptation

The function of the retina may be studied by the same stimulus to elicit ERG responses during dark or light adaptation. For example, the rate of growth of the a- and b-waves during dark-adaptation can be used as measures of retina function.

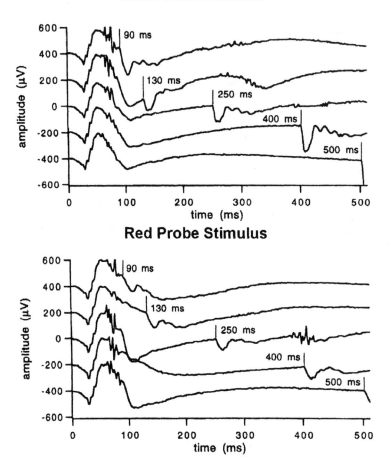

Figure 1.22 Paired-flash ERG. The test stimulus in each trial was a blue flash of intensity 20 scot td s presented at time zero. The probe stimulus was a blue flash of intensity 1.6×10^4 scot td s s or a photopically matched red flash. The vertical line superimposed on each trace indicates the time presentation of the probe flash. Noisy segments of the ERG tracing reflect blinks or other reflexive eye movements. The response to the probe flash grows with increased elapsed time after the test flash and is an indicator of the rate of retinal recovery after the test stimulus. (From Ref. 83 with permission from Cambridge University Press and the author.)

BASIC RETINAL ANATOMY AND PHYSIOLOGY AS RELATED TO ERG

Photoreceptors

Events leading to the full-field ERG response begin at the photoreceptors, the light-detecting cells in the retinal outer layer. The retina contains two classes of photoreceptors, the rods and the cones. The rods contain the light-sensitive pigment rhodopsin with a spectral absorption peak at 496 nm. Each cone contains one of three types of color-sensitive pigments with peak sensitivity to long-wavelength (558 nm), mid-wavelength (531 nm), and short-wavelength (419 nm) regions of the visible light spectrum. The three types of cones are called L-cone, M-cone, and S-cone, respectively, and were previously designated as red-, green-, and blue-sensitive cones.

Photoreceptor Distribution

The retina contains approximately 4–5 million cones and 80–120 million rods. The density of cones is maximal at the fovea reaching over 140,000 cones per mm^2. The cone density decreases rapidly away from the fovea, and beyond 10° of visual angle from the fovea, the density is well below 10,000 per mm^2. Nevertheless, cones are present even in the far peripheral retinal regions. Both L-cones and M-cones have maximal density at the foveal center. However, the S-cones reach highest density in a small donut-shaped region within 1–2° surrounding the foveal center but are virtually absent at the very center of the fovea. S-cones are scarce and make up only about 9% of all cones. Despite the high density of cones at the fovea, a foveal lesion affects only 10% of the total cones and has only a small effect on the full-field cone ERG response.

In contrast, the density of rods is highest from 15° to 40° from the fovea. With the fovea at the center, this high-density rod zone is a donut-shaped, slightly elliptical retinal region with a long horizontal axis. Within this zone, the rod density reaches over 100,000 per mm^2. The rods are found throughout the retina but are absent at the foveal center. The rods, cones, and ganglion cells are slightly denser in the superonasal retina than the inferotemporal retina. This asymmetric distribution reflects the asymmetry of the visual field and accounts in part for the relatively shortened nasal field.

Dark and Light Adaptation

The sensitivity of the photoreceptors adapts dramatically over a wide range of light levels. The cones dark-adapt more rapidly than the rods and reach maximal light sensitivity after 10–12 min. The rods dark-adapt at a slower rate but reach a plateau of much higher light sensitivity after 30–40 min (Fig. 1.23). Under scotopic conditions, the rods are 100- to 1000-fold more sensitive to light than the cones, and a dim flash stimulus activates only rods.

In a lit environment, the sensitivity of the photoreceptors falls rapidly but full light adaptation is not reached until after 15–20 min of light exposure. Under photopic conditions, the cones are very responsive and the rods are suppressed, and a flash stimulus activates only cones. At least 10 min of light adaptation are needed to stabilize photopic ERG responses (2).

Photoreceptor Structure and Renewal

Each photoreceptor cell consists of an inner and an outer segment. The inner segments of the photoreceptors contain the cell nuclei and make up the outer nuclear layer of the retina. The outer segments are cellular extensions contacting the retinal pigment epithelium. The outer segments contain intracellular membranes where initial light activation of the retina takes place. The intracellular membranes of the rods are disc-shaped and are separate from the plasma membrane while the internal membranes of the cones are formed by infoldings of the plasma membrane. The outer segments are continuously regenerated, shed, and phagocytized by the retinal pigment epithelium. The greatest rate of shedding occurs when the photoreceptors are diurnally the least active—at about one to three hours following onset of daylight for rods and in the early darkness hours for cones.

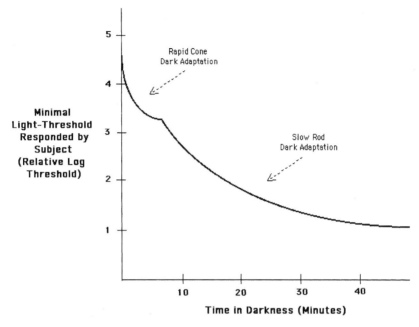

Figure 1.23 A schematic diagram of a dark adaptation curve from a normal subject. The shape of the dark adaptation curve varies with the retinal region tested. In the Goldmann–Weekers dark adaptometer, the light threshold is repeatedly tested in darkness by a 11° circular white test light of gradual-increasing intensity presented at 7° above the fovea. The difference between the dark-adaptive properties of the rods and cones explains the biphasic nature of the curve. The first 10 min of the curve is dominated by the more rapid dark adaptation of the cones which reach their maximal light sensitivity after about 10–12 min. The rods dark-adapt at a slower rate but reach a much lower final light threshold after about 40 min in darkness. The fully dark-adapted retina is in the range of 1000-fold more sensitive to light than the light-adapted retina.

Initial Photoreceptor Response to Light

Light activates the light-sensitive visual pigments in the outer segment of the photoreceptors and trigger events leading to the ERG response. The rod system is better understood because rods are present in all mammals as well as many non-mammals and are therefore easier to study while primates are the only mammals known to have three types of cones. Cone visual pigments are also much less abundant and less stable than the rod visual pigment.

All human rod and cone visual pigments consist of opsin, an intergral intracellular membrane protein of the photoreceptor outer segment, attached to 11-*cis*-retinaldehyde (11-*cis*-retinal), a light-sensitive chromophore molecule derived from vitamin A. The amino acid sequences of rod opsin and the three types of cone opsins are similar, and the chromophore is the same for all four types of visual pigments. The rod visual pigment is called rhodopsin. Light initiates visual excitation by isomerizing the chromophore from 11-*cis*-retinal to 11-*trans*-retinal producing an unfolding of the attached opsin. During this light bleaching process, rhodopsin transforms into several transient intermediaries such as metarhodopsin I and metarhodopsin II before fully activated. A single rod photoreceptor cell contains 10^8–10^9 rhodopsin molecules and the likelihood of passing photons being detected is high.

The Visual Cycle

The recycling or regeneration of the chromophore is called the *visual cycle* (87). This process involves the photoreceptors and the retinal pigment epithelium (Fig. 1.24). Genetic mutations of several proteins of the visual cycle are associated with retinal dystrophies. For example, heterozygous recessive mutations of the gene encoding adenosine triphosphate (ATP)-binding transporter protein called ABCA4 are associated with Stargardt macular dystrophy. Recessive mutations of RPE65 protein cause Leber congenital amaurosis and retinitis pigmentosa.

Phototransduction

The phototransduction cascade is the series of biochemical reactions initiated by the light-activated visual pigment that decreases sodium and calcium ion permeability of the photoreceptor plasma membrane leading to a lower rate of

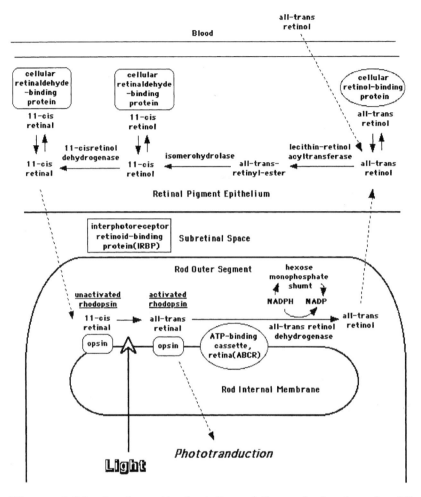

Figure 1.24 A schematic depiction of the rod visual cycle. All visual cycle enzymes are associated with intracellular membranes of the photoreceptor or the retinal pigment epithelium (87). The site of attachment of the chromophore 11-*cis*-retinal to opsin is actually on the intradiscal side of the internal membrane. The interphotoreceptor retinoid-binding protein (IRBP) has a role in the diffusion of retinoids between the photoreceptor and the retinal pigment epithelium. (From Ref. 87 with permission of *Investigative Ophthalmology and Visual Science.*)

release of the photoreceptor neurotransmitter, glutamate (Fig. 1.25).

In darkness, the sodium ion (Na^+) and calcium ion (Ca^{2+}) channels of the outer segment of the rod are open, allowing Na^+ and Ca^{2+} into the cell. The $Na^+/Ca^{2+}-K^+$ exchange pumps at the outer segment cellular membrane and a compensatory extrusion of potassium ion (K^+) at the inner segment maintain the intracellular and extracellular cation concentration. This circulating *dark current* maintains the rod in a relatively depolarized state, and the release of its neurotransmitter, glutamate, continuous at a relatively high rate.

With light, phototransduction causes the closure of the outer segment Na^+ and Ca^{2+} channels, and the release of glutamate is diminished (Fig. 1.25). Light-activated rhodopsin activates transducin that in turn activates phosphodiesterase which subsequently hydrolyzes cyclic guanosine monophosphate (cGMP). Amplification occurs so that one activated rhodopsin produces more than 100 activated transducin molecules and one activated phosphodiesterase can hydrolyze thousands of cGMP. Therefore, one activated rhodopsin can lead to the hydrolysis of 100,000 cGMP. With a decrease in intracellular cGMP, the cellular membrane Na^+ and Ca^{2+} channels close and the rate of release of glutamate is decreased. This hyperpolarization of the photoreceptor causes an increase of predominantly extracellular Na^+ as well as Ca^{2+}. This relative increase in outer retina positivity is measured indirectly at the cornea as the initial negative portion of the ERG a-wave. The modulation of the phototransduction process is complex and involves Ca^{2+} as well as Ca^{2+}-binding proteins.

Transmission and Processing of Visual Signals from the Photoreceptors

Different characteristics of the light signal such as brightness and color are processed by the bipolar, amacrine, and horizontal cells of the inner retina before reaching the retinal ganglion cells. The cone and rod systems are not independent.

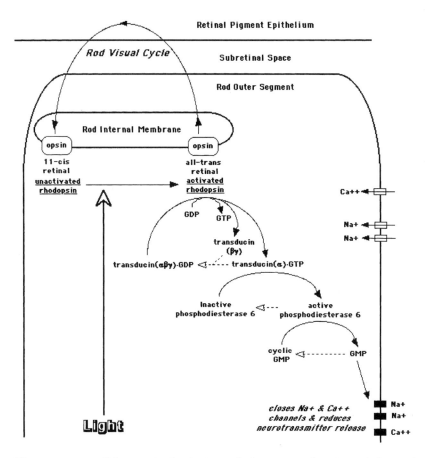

Figure 1.25 Schematic depiction of phototransduction of the rod photoreceptor. In darkness, the Na^+ and Ca^{2+} channels of the outer segment of the rod are open, allowing Na^+ and Ca^{2+} into the cell. With light, a series of biochemical reactions reduces the intracellular concentration of cGMP. The Na^+ and Ca^{2+} channels close, and the rate of release of neurotransmitter glutamate by the photoreceptor is decreased.

The cones and rods are connected by electrical synapses, and a multitude of synapses connects the photoreceptors and to these inner retinal neuronal cells.

The optic nerve consists of approximately 1.2 million axons from the retinal ganglion cells and delivers the visual signal as electrical action potentials to the brain. The axons are eventually separated into tracts that terminate in different areas such as the suprachiasmal nucleus, the lateral geniculate nucleus, the pretectum, the superior colliculus, and the accessory optic nuclei. Each of the 10–20 types of retinal ganglion cells carries specific information of the light stimulus (e.g., brightness, movement, etc.). Each ganglion cell type receives dendritic inputs from the entire retina and a light stimulus, regardless of its retinal location, is detected by all ganglion cell types. In this way, different aspects of the visual signal are initially processed together in parallel within the retina.

Receptive Fields and ON- and OFF-Responses

The receptive field of a neuronal cell is the visual field area where a change in light will alter the cell's activity. This physiologic concept is applicable to any cell at any level of visual processing. For example, each bipolar cell has its own receptive field, and a considerable overlapping of receptive fields occurs for bipolar cells that are near one another. The receptive field can be divided into *center* and *surround* regions, and the cellular response is different for a spot of light positioned at the center vs. surround regions. The specific cellular response is dependent on the size, shape, orientation, intensity, contrast, color, motion, direction, and duration of the light stimulus. In general, the cells can be divided into *"on"* and *"off"* pathways. Neurons that depolarize in response to increased light in their receptive fields are called ON-cells, and neurons that depolarize in response to reduced light are called OFF-cells. Therefore, bipolar cells that depolarize to light are ON-bipolar cells and those that hyperpolarize to light are OFF-bipolar cells. This concept may be applied to other levels of visual processing, and ganglion cells may be classified as ON- and OFF-ganglion cells. By definition, all photoreceptors are "OFF" cells, because they hyperpolarize with light and depolarize in darkness.

Processing of Photoreceptor Signals in the Inner Retina

The bipolar cells are the primary receivers of the visual signals from the photoreceptors. Approximately 10 different types of mammalian bipolar cells can be differentiated anatomically based on shape and axonal position in the inner plexiform layer where the axons of a specific bipolar cell type terminate in a specific sub-layer. This stratification also applies to the dendrites of ganglion cells, and dendrites of OFF-ganglion cells generally originate from the outer half of the inner plexiform layer and those of ON-ganglion cells originate from the inner half of the layer (88,89). Of the 10 types of bipolar cells, nine have cone photoreceptor contacts while only one type has rod contacts. Physiologically, the cone bipolar cell types can be classified into ON- and OFF-cells.

In the outer plexiform layer, the photoreceptors synapse with bipolar and horizontal cells. Dendrites of the rod-specific bipolar cell type make invaginated contacts with rod spherules, the structural endings of the rod photoreceptor. The axons of the rod-specific bipolar cells terminate in the inner region of the inner plexiform layer and synapse with a specific amacrine cell type called *AII amacrine cells*. The AII amacrine cells have narrow receptive fields and make inhibitory chemical synapses with OFF-cone bipolar and OFF-ganglion cells, and electrical synapse though gap junctions with ON-cone bipolar cells (Fig. 1.26) (90).

In contrast, the structural endings of the cone photoreceptors—the cone pedicles—have three kinds of synaptic specializations (91). First, each pedicle has gap junctions for electrical contacts with other cone pedicles and rod spherules. Second, the pedicle has invaginations with synaptic arrangement called *triad*; each consisting of two lateral elements contacting horizontal cells and at least one central element contacting an ON-bipolar cell dendrite. Third, the cone pedicle makes flat contacts with OFF-bipolar cells. Therefore, the cone pedicles generally make invaginated contacts with ON-bipolar cells and flat contacts with OFF-bipolar cells. The number and characteristic of the connections are complex and dependent

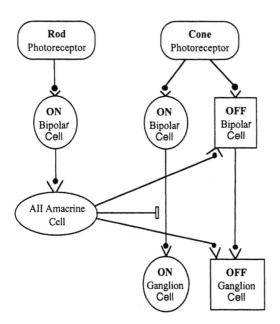

Figure 1.26 Rod and cone photoreceptor ON and OFF connections. The rod-specific ON-bipolar cell uses an intermediary (AII amacrine cell) to connect to the ON- and OFF-ganglion cells. The AII amacrine cells have inhibitory chemical synapses with OFF-cone bipolar and OFF-ganglion cells, and electrical synapse though gap junctions with ON-cone bipolar cells.

on bipolar cell type and cone location. The number of cone contacts for a bipolar cell is highly variable. For instance, bipolar cells providing high spatial resolution information convey signals from only a few cones, whereas those bipolar cells with high contrast sensitivity receive input from many cones.

The inner retinal ERG signal is a summation of all of the cells of the inner retina with primary contributions from depolarizing ON-bipolar cells and hyperpolarizing OFF-bipolar cells (92). The predominantly depolarization process results in an outflow of intracellular potassium ion (K^+) resulting in increased extracellular K^+ in the outer plexiform layer. This produces a depolarization of the Müller cells generating a transretinal potential that is measured as the corneal positive ERG b-wave.

REFERENCES

1. Marmor MF, Zrenner E. Standard for clinical electroretinogrpahy (1999 update). Doc Ophthalmologica 1999; 97:143–156.

2. Peachey NS, Alexander KR, Derlacki DJ, Fishman GA. Light adaptation, rods, and the human cone flicker ERG. Vis Neurosci 1992; 8:145–150.

3. Brigell M, Bach M, Moskowitz A, Robson J. Guidelines for calibration of stimulus and recording parameters used in clinical electrophysiology of vision. Calibration Standard Committee of the International Society for Clinical Electrophysiology of Vision (ISCEV). Doc Ophthalmol 2003; 107:185–193.

4. Burian HM, Allen L. A speculum contact lens electrode for electroretinography. Electroencephalogr Clin Neurophysiol 1954; 6:509–511.

5. Lawwill T, Burian HM. A modification of the Burian–Allen contact-lens electrode for human electroretinography. Am J Ophthalmol 1966; 6:1506–1509.

6. Johnson MA, Massof RW. The photomyoclonic reflex: an artifact in clinical electroretinogram. Br J Ophthalmol 1982; 66:368–378.

7. Dawson WW, Trick GL, Litzkow CA. Improved electrode for electroretinography. Invest Ophthalmol Vis Sci 1979; 18:988–991.

8. Lachapelle P, Benoit J, Little JM, Lachapelle B. Recording the oscillatory potentials of the electroretinogram with the DTL electrode. Doc Ophthalmol 1993; 83:119–130.

9. Dawson WW, Trick GL, Maida TM. Evaluation of the DTL corneal electrode. Doc Ophthalmol Proc Ser 1982; 31:81–88.

10. Hébert M, Vaegan, Lachapelle P. Reproducibility of ERG responses obtained with the DTL electrode. Vision Res 1999; 39:1069–1070.

11. Kuze M, Uji Y. Comparison between Dawson, Trick, and Litzkow electrode and contact lens electrodes used in clinical electroretinography. Jpn J Ophthalmol 2000; 44:374–380.

12. Yin H, Pardue MT. Performance of the DTL electrode compared to the jet contact lens electrode in clinical testing. Doc Ophthalmol 2004; 108:77–86.

13. Severns ML, Johnson MA, Bresnick GH. Methodologic dependence of electroretinogram oscillatory potential amplitudes. Doc Ophthalmol 1994; 86:23–31.

14. Granit R, Riddell LA. The electrical responses of light- and dark-adapted frogs' eyes to rhythmic and continuous stimuli. J Physiol 1934; 81:1–28.

15. Falk G. Signal transmission from rods to bipolar and horizontal cells: a synthesis. In: Osborne N, Chader G, eds. Progressive in Retinal Research. Vol. 8. New York. Pergamon, 1988: 255–279.

16. Steinberg RH, Frishman LJ, Sieving PA. Negative components of the electroretinogram from proximal retina and photoreceptor. In: Osborne N, Chader G, eds. Progress in Retinal Research. Vol. 10. New York: Pergamon, 1991:121–160.

17. Penn RD, Hagins WA. Signal transmission along retinal rods and the origin of the electroretinographic a-wave. Nature 1969; 223:201–205.

18. Qiu H, Fujiwara E, Liu M, Lam BL, Hamasaki DI. Evidence that a-wave latency of the electroretinogram is deter mined solely by photoreceptors. Jpn J Ophthalmol 2002; 46:426–432.

19. Pugh EN Jr, Lamb TD. Amplification and kinetics of the activation steps in phototransduction. Biochim Biophys Acta 1993; 1141:111–149.

20. Jamison JA, Bush RA, Lei B, Sieving PA. Characterization of the rod photoresponse isolated from dark-adapted primate ERG. Vis Neurosci 2001; 18:445–455.

21. Guervich L, Slaughter MM. Comparison of the waveforms of the ON bipolar neuron and the b-wave of the electroretinogram. Vision Res 1993; 33:2431–2435.

22. Müller RF, Dowling JE. Intracellular responses of Müller (glial) cells of mudpuppy retina: their relation to the b-wave of the electroretinogram. J Neurophysiol 1970; 33:323–341.

23. Newman RA, Odette LL. Model of electroretinogram b-wave: a test of the K^+ hypothesis. J Neurophysiol 1984; 51:164–182.

24. Stockton RA, Slaughter MM. B-wave of the electroretinogram: a reflection of ON bipolar cell activity. J Gen Physiol 1989; 93:101–122.

25. Brown GC, Eagle RC, Shakin EP, Gruber M, Arbizio VV. Retinal toxicity of intravitreal gentamicin. Arch Ophthalmol 1990; 108:1740–1744.

26. Hood DC, Birch DG. Phototransduction in human cones measured using the a-wave of the ERG. Vision Res 1995; 35:2801–2810.

27. Hood DC, Birch DG. Human cone receptor activity: the leading edge of the a-wave and models of receptor activity. Vis Neurosci 1993; 10:857–871.

28. Whitten DN, Brown KT. The timecourse of the late receptor potential from the monkey cones and rods. Vision Res 1973; 13:107–135.

29. Bush RA, Sieving PA. A proximal retinal component in the primate photopic ERG a-wave. Invest Ophthalmol Vis Sci 1994; 35:635–645.

30. Sieving PA, Murayama K, Naarendorp F. Push–pull model of the primate photopic electroretinogram: a role for hyperpolarizing neurons in shaping the b-wave. Vis Neurosci 1994; 11:519–532.

31. Kondo M, Sieving PA. Primate photopic sine-wave flicker ERG: vector modeling analysis of component origins using glutamate analogs. Invest Ophthalmol Vis Sci 2001; 42:305–312.

32. Kondo M, Sieving PA. Post-photoreceptoral activity dominates primate photpic 32-Hz ERG for sine-square-, and pulsed stimuli. Invest Ophthalmol Vis Sci 2002; 43:2500–2507.

33. Wachmeister L. Further studies of the chemical sensitivity of the oscillatory potentials of the electroretinogram (ERG), I: GABA and glycine antagonists. Acta Ophthalmol 1980; 58:712–725.

34. Wachmeister L. Further studies of the chemical sensitivity of the oscillatory potentials of the electroretinogram (ERG), II: glutamate, aspartate, and dopamine antagonists. Acta Ophthalmol 1981; 59:247–258.

35. Li X, Yuan N. Measurement of the oscillatory potential of the electroretinogram in the domains of frequency and time. Doc Ophthalmol 1990; 76:65–71.

36. Speros P, Price J. Oscillatory potentials: history, techniques, and potential use in the evaluation of disturbances of retinal circulation. Surv Ophthalmol 1981; 25:237–252.

37. Janaky M, Coupland SG, Benedek G. Human oscillatory potentials: components of rod origin. Ophthalmologica 1996; 210:315–318.

38. Rousseau S, Lachapelle P. The electroretinogram recorded at the onset of dark-adaptation: understanding the origin of the scotopic oscillatory potentials. Doc Ophthalmol 1999; 99:135–150.

39. Wachmeister L. Oscillatory potentials in the retina: what do they reveal. Prog Retin Eye Res 1998; 17:485–521.

40. Birch DG, Berson EL, Sandberg MA. Diurnal rhythm in the human rod ERG. Invest Ophthalmol Vis Sci 1984; 25:236–238.

41. Birch DG, Sandberg MA, Berson EL. Diurnal rhythm in the human rod ERG. Invest Ophthalmol Vis Sci 1986; 27:268–270.

42. Sandberg MA, Baruzzi CM, Hanson AHI, Berson EL. Rod ERG diurnal rhythm in some patients with dominant retinitis pigmentosa. Invest Ophthalmol Vis Sci 1988; 29:494–498.

43. Nozaki S, Wakakura M, Ishikawa S. Circadian rhythm of human electroretinogram. Jpn J Ophthalmol 1983; 27:346–352.

44. François J, Verriest G, de Rouck A. Pathology of the x-wave of the human electroretinogram. Br J Ophthalmol 1956; 40:439–443.

45. Arden G, Wolf J, Berninger T, Hogg CR, Tzekov R, Holder GE. S-cone ERGs elicited by a simple technique in normals and in tritanopes. Vis Neurosci 1999; 39:641–650.

46. Gouras P, MacKay CJ. Electroretinographic responses of the short-wavelength-sensitive cones. Invest Ophthalmol Vis Sci 1990; 31:1203–1209.

47. Gouras P, Mackay CJ, Yamamoto S. The human S-cone electroretinogram and its variation among subjects with and with-

out L and M-cone function. Invest Ophthalmol Vis Sci 1993; 34:437–442.

48. Gouras P. The role of S-cones in human vision. Doc Ophthalmol 2003; 106:5–11.

49. Simonsen SE, Rosenberg T. Reappraisal of a short-wavelength-sensitive (S-cone) recording technique in routine clinical electroretinography. Doc Ophthalmol 1996; 91:323–332.

50. Swanson WH, Birch DG, Anderson JL. S-cone function in patients with retinitis pigmentosa. Invest Ophthalmol Vis Sci 1993; 34:3045–3055.

51. Fulton AB, Rushton WAH. The human rod ERG: correlation with psychophysical responses in light and dark adaptation. Vision Res 1978; 18:793–800.

52. Naka KI, Rushton WAH. S-potentials from colour units in the retina of fish (Cyprimidae). J Physiol 1966; 185:536–555.

53. Hood DC, Birch DG. A computational model of the amplitude and implicit time of the b-wave of the human ERG. Vis Neurosci 1992; 8:107–126.

54. Wali N, Leguire LE. The photopic hill: a new phenomenon of the light adapted electroretinogram. Doc Ophthalmol 1992; 80:335–342.

55. Peachey NS, Alexander KR, Derlacki D, Fishman GA. Light adaptation and the luminance-response function of the cone electroretinogram. Doc Ophthalmol 1992; 79:363–369.

56. Rufiange M, Rousseau S, Dembinska O, Lachapelle P. Cone-dominated ERG luminance-response function: the photopic hill revisited. Doc Ophthalmol 2002; 104:231–248.

57. Rufiange M, Dassa J, Dembinska O, Koenekoop RK, Little JM, Polomeno RL, Dumont M, Chemtob S, Lachapelle P. The photopic ERG luminance-response function (photopic hill): method of analysis and clinical application. Vision Res 2003; 43:1405–1412.

58. Ueno S, Kondo M, Niwa Y, Terasaki H, Miyake Y. Luminance dependence of neural components that underlies the primate photopic electroretinogram. Invest Ophthalmol Vis Sci 2004; 45:1033–1040.

59. Hood DC, Birch DG. A quantitative measure of the electrical activity of human rod photoreceptors using electroretinography. Vis Neurosci 1990; 5:379–387.

60. Hood DC, Birch DG. The relationship between models of receptor activity and the a-wave of the human ERG. Clin Vis Sci 1990; 5:292–297.

61. Hood DC, Birch DG. The a-wave of the human electroretinogram and rod receptor function. Invest Ophthalmol Vis Sci 1990; 31:2070–2081.

62. Breton M, Schueller A, Lamb T, Pugh EN. Analysis of ERG a-wave amplification and kinetics in terms of the G-protein cascade of phototransduction. Invest Ophthalmol Vis Sci 1994; 35:295–309.

63. Hood DC, Birch DG. Assessing abnormal rod photoreceptor activity with the a-wave of the ERG: applications and methods. Doc Ophthalmol 1997; 92:253–267.

64. Birch DG, Hood DC, Locke KG, Hoffman DR, Tzekov RT. Quantitative electroretinogram measures of phototransduction in cone and rod photoreceptors: normal aging, pregression with disease, and test–retest variability. Arch Ophthalmol 2002; 120:1045–1051.

65. Cideciyan AV, Jacobson SG. An alternative phototransduction model for human rod and cone ERG a-waves: normal parameters and variation with age. Vision Res 1996; 36: 2609–2621.

66. Sieving PA. Photopic ON- and OFF-pathway abnormalities in retinal dystrophies. Trans Am Ophthalmol Soc 1993; 91: 701–703.

67. Brown KT, Murakami M. A new receptor potential of the monkey retina with no detectable latency. Nature 1964; 201:626–628.

68. Goldstein EB, Berson EL. Rod and cone contributions to the human early receptor potential. Vision Res 1970; 10:207–218.

69. Okamoto M, Okajima O, Tanino T. The early receptor potential in the human eye. III. ERP in dichromats. Jpn J Ophthalmol 1982; 26:23–28.

70. Zanen A, Debecker J. Wavelength sensitivity of the two components of the early receptor potential (ERP) of the human eye. Vision Res 1975; 15:107–112.

71. Berson EL, Goldstein BE. Early receptor potential in dominantly inherited retinitis pigmentosa. Arch Ophthalmol 1970; 83:412–420.

72. Fioretto M, Lotti R, Rela S, Fava GP, Sannita WG. Retinal early receptor potential in retinitis pigmentosa: correlations with visual field and fluorangiography estimates. Ophthalmologica 1991; 203:82–88.

73. Müller W, Töpke H. The early receptor potential (ERP). Doc Ophthalmol 1987; 66:35–74.

74. Sieving PA, Nino C. Scotopic threshold response (STR) of the human electroretinogram. Invest Ophthalmol Vis Sci 1988; 29:1608–1614.

75. Frishman LJ, Sieving PA, Steinberg RH. Contributions to the electroretinogram of currents originating in proximal retina. Visu Neurosci 1988; 1:307–315.

76. Miyake Y, Horiguchi M, Terasuki H, Kondo M. Scotopic threshold response in complete and incomplete types of congenital stationary night blindness. Invest Ophthalmol Vis Sci 1994; 35:3770–3775.

77. Graham SL, Vaegan. High correlation between absolute psychophysical threshold and the scotopic threshold response to the same stimulus. Br J Ophthalmol 1991; 75:603–607.

78. Viswanathan S, Frishman LJ, Robson JG, Walters JW. The photopic negative response of the flash electroretinogram in primary open angle glaucoma. Invest Ophthalmol Vis Sci 2001; 42:514–522.

79. Viswanathan S, Frishman LJ, Robson JG. The uniform field and pattern ERG in macaques with experimental glaucoma: removal of spiking activity. Invest Ophthalmol Vis Sci 2000; 41:2797–2810.

80. Colotto A, Falsini B, Salgarello T, Iarossi G, Galan ME, Scullica L. Photopic negative response of the human ERG: losses associated with glaucomatous damage. Invest Ophthalmol Vis Sci 2000; 41:2205–2211.

81. Marmor MF, Hock PA. A practical method for c-wave recording in man. Doc Ophthalmol Proc Ser 1982; 31:67–72.

82. Kooijiman AC, Zwarts J, Damhof A. Double-flash electroretinography in human eyes. Doc Ophthalmol 1989; 73:377–385.

83. Pepperberg DR, Birch DG, Hood DC. Photoresponses of human rods in vivo derived from paired-flash electroretinogram. Vis Neurosci 1997; 14:73–82.

84. Saeki M, Gouras P. Cone ERGs to flash trains: the antagonism of a later flash. Vision Res 1996; 36:3229–3235.

85. Schneider T, Zrenner E. Double-flash responses in different retinal layers. Ophthalmic Res 1987; 19:193–199.

86. Wagman IH, Waldman J, Naidoff D, Feinschil LB, Cahan R. The recording of the electroretinogram in humans and in animals. Investigation of retinal sensitivity following brief flashes of light. Am J Ophthalmol 1954; 38:60–69.

87. Saari JC. Biochemistry of visual pigment regeneration. Invest Ophthalmol Vis Sci 2000; 41:337–348.

88. Nelson R, Famiglietti EV Jr, Kolb H. Intracellular staining reveals different levels of stratification for on- and off-center ganglion cells in cat retina. J Neurophysiol 1978; 41:472–483.

89. Peichi L, Wässle H. Morphological identification of on- and off-centre brisk transient (Y) cells in the cat retina. Proc R Soc Lond B 1981; 212:139–156.

90. Wässle H, Grünert U, Chun M, Boycott BB. The rod pathway of the macaque monkey retina: identification of AII-amacrine cells with antibodies against calretinin. J Comp Neurol 1995; 361:537–551.

91. Boycott B, Wässle H. Parallel processing in the mammalian retina. Invest Ophthalmol Vis Sci 1999; 40:1313–1327.

92. Stell WK, Ishida AT, Lightfoot DO. Structural basis for on- and off-center responses in retinal bipolar cells. Science 1977; 198:1269–1271.

93. Granit R. The components of the retinal action potential and their relation to the discharge in the optic nerve. J Physiol 1933; 77:207–240.

2

Focal and Multifocal Electroretinogram

Conventional full-field electroretinogram (ERG) records the summed electrical responses from the entire retina elicited by full-field "ganzfeld" flash stimulation. Under different test conditions, the full-field ERG can assess general rod and cone function separately but cannot adequately detect local retinal dysfunction. For instance, an isolated macular lesion is unlikely to decrease the overall ERG response enough to be detectable by the full-field ERG. On the other hand, a large localized retinal lesion may be detectable by the full-field ERG as a non-specific reduction but no topographical information will be available.

Focal ERG and multifocal ERG are two techniques that have been developed to detect local retinal dysfunction. The focal ERG uses a focal light stimulus to elicit a local ERG response and is used primarily to assess foveal function. The multifocal ERG measures topographical retinal function by providing a visual field map of mathematically calculated local ERG signals (1). Focal ERG and multifocal ERG generally assess only light-adapted retinal activity generated by the cone photoreceptors because dark adaptation is difficult to maintain with these techniques. With recent rapid advances, multifocal ERG is now more commonly utilized than focal ERG. This chapter discusses these two techniques assuming an understanding of ERG basics provided in Chapter 1.

4-degree foveal flicker stimulus with suppressive light ring

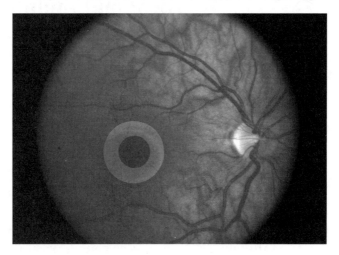

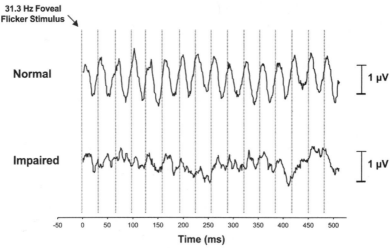

Figure 2.1   (*Caption on facing page*)

FOCAL ELECTRORETINOGRAM

In focal ERG, a focal light stimulus is used to record a local ERG response (2–5). Clinically, the test is usually performed to assess foveal cone response. Because the local cone response is small in the range of a few microvolts or less, the typical focal ERG stimulus consists of a 30–42 Hz white circular flicker stimulus, and numerous responses up to hundreds are averaged to improve the signal-to-noise ratio. To eliminate any rod or cone response from scattered light of the test stimulus that falls outside of the test area, the circular flicker test stimulus is encircled by a concentric annulus ring of steady background light that is typically brighter than the test stimulus (Fig. 2.1). A hand-held device that combines focal ERG stimulator with a direct ophthalmoscope allows the direct visualization of the retinal test area to ensure adequate fixation (6). A built-in start–stop switch activates data acquisition only when the stimulus is on the retinal area being tested. The patient is instructed to look directly on the center of the stimulus for foveal testing or a reference point so that the examiner can place the test stimulus on the fovea. The electrodes are connected the same way as for the full-field ERG, and the pupil is dilated with eye drops. Bipolar recording contact-lens electrodes such as the Burian–Allen and the Goldlens electrodes are typically

Figure 2.1 (*Facing page*) Example of focal foveal ERG. The responses were recorded with a direct ophthalmoscope device that delivers a 31.3 Hz white flicker stimulus to the central 4–5° of the fovea. A ring of photopic background illumination surrounding the stimulated area suppresses any unwanted response from the adjacent retina. The fovea is directly visualized during testing to assess fixation and to ensure that the stimulus is centered on the fovea. The size of the stimulated retinal area is small, and the normal response has an amplitude in the range of only one microvolt (μV). Because the response is small, averaging of multiple responses is necessary. A normal response (average amplitude 1.226 μV, implicit time 38.1 msec) and an impaired response (average amplitude 0.28 μV, implicit time 41.6 msec) are shown.

used. Aside from stimulator-ophthalmoscope devices, full-field domes or fundus cameras may also be modified for focal ERG recording.

Foveal cone responses obtained from focal ERG are mini cone flicker responses that resemble the photopic full-field ERG cone flicker response. Collecting a group of age-related normal values is critical in the clinical inter pretation of focal foveal ERG as response amplitudes and timings are related not only to age but also to the stimulus diameter, flickering rate, and retinal illuminance (7). Because of the numerous focal ERG methodologies, international standard or guidelines have not been established. Focal ERG responses are particularly unreliable in patients with poor fixation or media opacity, which may result in falsely impaired foveal responses.

Focal rod ERG responses from a relatively large test spot of 30°–40° may be recorded with specialized techniques but are not commonly performed in the clinic (8,9). To maintain dark adaptation, a concentric annulus ring of steady background light cannot be used. Without the suppressive effect of the surrounding light ring, the scattered light from the test stimulus that falls outside of the test area will result in unwanted response from the surrounding retina. The effect of this stray-light response can be reduced by subtracting response from a dimmer rod-matched full-field flash (8).

MULTIFOCAL ELECTRORETINOGRAM

The multifocal ERG is a technique developed by Sutter and Tran (10) to provide topographical retinal function by simultaneously recording and calculating ERG signals from multiple retinal areas (Fig. 2.2). This technique evolved because sequential recordings from multiple retinal areas using traditional focal ERG are too time-consuming to be practical. The multifocal ERG has emerged as a valuable clinical tool to assess topographical photopic retinal function (11). Experience with quality full-field ERG recordings is beneficial

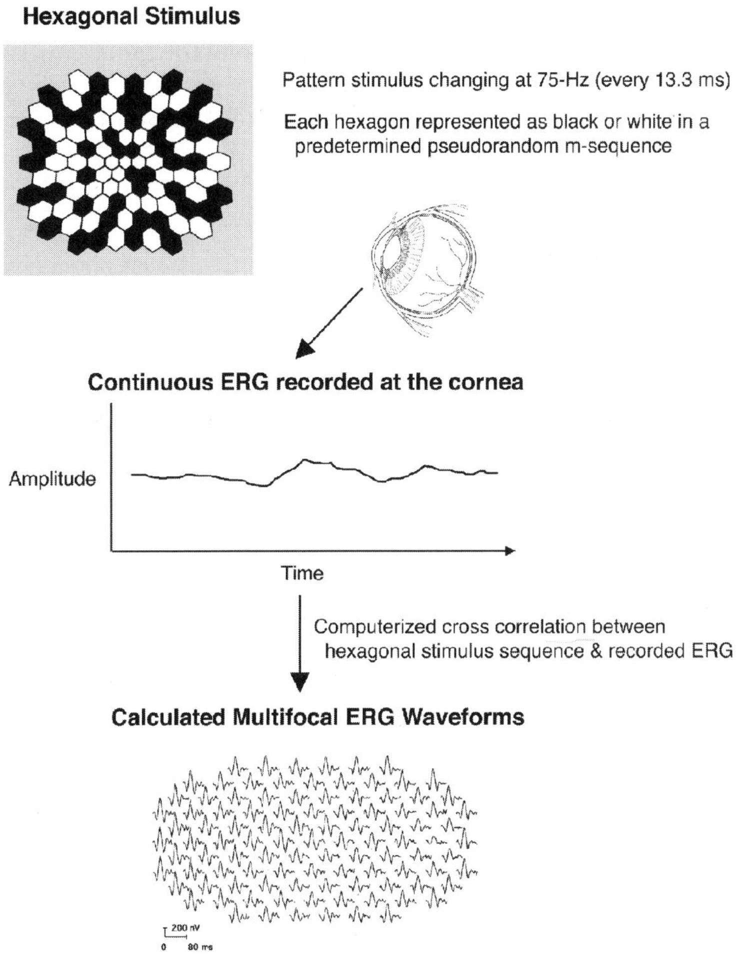

Hexagonal Stimulus

Pattern stimulus changing at 75-Hz (every 13.3 ms)

Each hexagon represented as black or white in a predetermined pseudorandom m-sequence

Continuous ERG recorded at the cornea

Amplitude

Time

Computerized cross correlation between hexagonal stimulus sequence & recorded ERG

Calculated Multifocal ERG Waveforms

200 nV

0   80 ms

Figure 2.2 Schematic diagram showing the basic principles of multifocal ERG.

in dealing with similar recording issues in multifocal ERG. Like all diagnostic tests, the multifocal ERG is not a test without limitations. For instance, the multifocal ERG cannot easily assess scotopic retinal function, and a quality recording may be difficult to obtain from a patient with poor visual acuity due to inadequate steady fixation. Therefore, the multifocal ERG is not a replacement for the full-field ERG but may be considered as a different test that provides important topographical retinal information. Guidelines for basic multifocal ERG have been established by the International Society for Clinical Electrophysiology of Vision (ISCEV) and are available on the ISCEV Internet site (1).

MULTIFOCAL ERG RECORDING ENVIRONMENT AND PATIENT SET-UP

The recording environment and patient set-up for multifocal ERG are similar to those of full-field ERG (see Chapter 1). First, the pupils are dilated fully with eye drops. Several types of recording electrodes may be used. Contact-lens electrodes such as the Burian–Allen electrodes provide stable recordings with less blink artifacts, and the newer version provides clearer view of the stimulus. Contact-lens electrodes are less comfortable than non-contact-lens electrodes; among which the DTL electrode is the most commonly used. As with full-field ERG, some differences in recording results exist when different types of electrodes are employed (12).

Similar to the focal ERG, multifocal ERG is used to assess light-adapted retinal activity generated by the cone photoreceptors. Although multifocal ERG recording of rod function is possible, maintaining dark adaptation during testing is difficult, and the effect of light scatter is greater under dark adaptation. Taken together, these factors make recording multifocal rod ERG responses challenging in clinical settings. Therefore, clinical multifocal ERG recordings are performed under light-adapted condition. Because photopic ERG responses are known to stabilize after 15 min of light adaptation, the patient should have been exposed to ordinary ambient room light for at least 15 min before multifocal ERG testing (13). To maintain full-field light adaptation, the room lights should produce illumination close to that of the stimulus screen during testing. Multifocal ERG recording may follow standard photopic full-field ERG as long as the exposure to the full-field flash stimulus is not excessive.

MULTIFOCAL ERG STIMULUS

The multifocal ERG stimulus is displayed on a video monitor and typically has a diameter of about 50° subtending about 25° radially from fixation. Therefore, the multifocal ERG tests the activity generated by only about 25% of cone photoreceptor cells. The stimulus consists of a pattern of hexagons such that the size of each hexagon is scaled to produce approximately equal ERG responses from the normal retina (Fig. 2.3). For example, in a 103-hexagon display, each central hexagon is about 3° wide while each outermost hexagon is more than 7° wide. During recording, each hexagon reverses from white-to-black or white-to-black in a predetermined fixed pseudo-random maximum-length sequence called the "m-sequence" and has a probability of 0.5 of reversing on any frame change. The sequence is the same for each hexagon but the starting point is different for each hexagon. To maintain overall isoluminance and thus the same level of retinal light adaptation through the test, approximately half of the total hexagons are white and half are black. The area of the display outside of the hexagons should have a luminance equal to the mean luminance of the stimulus array. For example, the luminance of a hexagon when it is white could be $100 \, cd/m^2$ compared to $2 \, cd/m^2$ when it is dark with a brightness of $50 \, cd/m^2$ for the part of display outside of the stimulus. The rate of frame change is rapid in the order of 75 Hz with a frame change occurring every 13.3 msec. The number of hexagons for the multifocal stimulus array ranges from 61 to 241, and tradeoffs are made when choosing the number of hexagons. A lower number of hexagons requires shorter recording time, produces larger responses and lower noise-to-signal ratio but decreases spatial resolution. Conversely, a higher number of hexagons requires longer recording time, produces smaller responses and higher noise-to-signal ratio but increases resolution. An array of 103 hexagons is commonly used.

RECORDING MULTIFOCAL ERG

Stable central fixation during multifocal ERG recording is critical to ensure accuracy of the topographical ERG

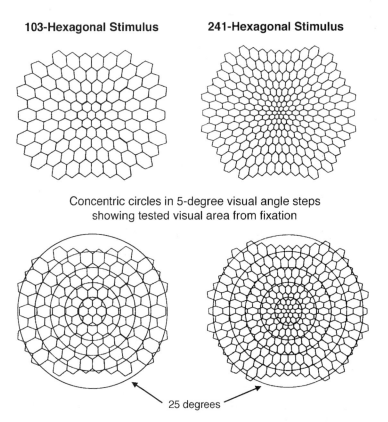

103-Hexagonal Stimulus   **241-Hexagonal Stimulus**

Concentric circles in 5-degree visual angle steps
showing tested visual area from fixation

25 degrees

Figure 2.3 Multifocal ERG stimulus. The hexagons of the multi-focal ERG stimulus are smaller centrally and larger peripherally and are scaled to produce approximately equal ERG response for each hexagon from the normal retina. The 103-hexagon and 241-hexagon stimuli are shown with concentric circles indicating the distance from the fovea in 5° steps. The stimulus typically subtends approximately 25° radially from the fovea. The number of hexagons usually ranges from 61 to 241. A high number of hexagons increases topographical resolution of the calculated responses but produces smaller responses with higher noise-to-signal ratio and requires longer recording time.

information (14). Poor fixation will lead to falsely impaired responses and erroneous clinical interpretation. A central fixation target such as a dot, "X", or cross is provided by the system, and the target size should be increased accordingly based on reduced visual acuity. Fixation can be monitored during testing with simultaneous viewing of the test eye by using an infrared external video camera or a fundus video camera. Because a steady fixation does not necessary imply an accurate fixation, the use of a fundus video camera helps to monitor the location of the stimulus array on the retina and thus the accuracy of the fixation (15).

Sequential monocular recordings are usually performed. During monocular recording, the fellow eye is occluded with a patch or the patient may feel more comfortable holding the eyelid closed with his hand. Sufficient period of light adaptation should be allowed before the testing of the second eye. Binocular recording is possible but simultaneous monitoring of decentration of the stimulus in each eye is required.

Best-corrected vision is recommended for recording especially for persons with high refractive errors. Corrective lens may be placed in front of the eye but an adjustment of the viewing distance to account for change in magnification of the stimulus is needed based on the manufacturer's recommendations (16). This problem is reduced in newer recording systems with a compact stimulus display mounted on a swing-arm so that the display is brought close in front of the eye being tested. A built-in focusing knob on the display allows the patient to self-adjust the focus for optimal viewing clarity without the use of corrective lens. Regardless of the system used, periodic calibration of the system should be performed as recommended by the manufacturer and based on international calibration standard (17).

Multifocal ERG may be recorded in a single continuous recording lasting several minutes or in a series of shorter recording runs lasting less than 1 min. Recording in segments reduces patient fatigue and allows discarding and repeating low quality recording segments without re-running the entire test. Regardless, the sequence of white-to-black or black-to-white reversal of each hexagon follows a fixed m-sequence predetermined by the computer. Programs are available to remove recording artifacts from blinks and eye movements and should not be applied multiple times.

Similar to other electrophysiologic tests, multifocal ERG results vary depending on the protocol and the recording system (16,18,19). Therefore, collection of age-matched normative data by each facility is recommended. Age-related changes of multifocal ERG are discussed in Chapter 6. For each ERG parameter, the median normal value along with 5% and 95% percentile normal values should be reported and used for interpretation.

FIRST-ORDER "RESPONSE" OF MULTIFOCAL ERG

In multifocal ERG, local retinal signals are calculated by correlating the continuous recorded ERG signal with the on–off phases of each hexagon. Multifocal waveforms are not true direct, recorded responses but mathematical calculations (20). The first-order "response," known as first-order kernel (K_1), of each hexagon is calculated by adding all ERG recordings following a white frame and then subtracting all ERG recordings following a black frame (Figs. 2.4 and 2.5). In this way, the response of the hexagon is summed and isolated while the responses from other hexagons are eliminated. The calculated first-order response lasts much longer than the duration of one frame (13.3 msec at 75 Hz).

The calculated first-order response consists of an initial negative component (N1) followed by a positive component (P1) and then a second negative component (N2) (Fig. 2.4). The N1 amplitude is measured from baseline to the N1 trough, and the P1 amplitude is measured from the N1 trough to the P1 peak. The implicit time of N1 is measured from the onset of the stimulus to the N1 trough, and the implicit time of P1 is measured from stimulus onset to the P1 peak. Programs to reduce background electrical noise and to smooth waveforms are available. These programs average the response from each hexagon with a percentage of the signals from adjacent hexagons and should be used with caution such that no more 50% of the waveform are contributed from neighbor hexagons.

Normal Trace Array from 103-Hexagonal Stimulus (right eye)

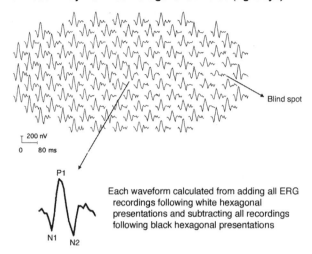

Each waveform calculated from adding all ERG recordings following white hexagonal presentations and subtracting all recordings following black hexagonal presentations

Proposed model of cellular origin of multifocal ERG components

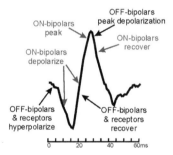

Figure 2.4 First-order calculated responses of the multifocal ERG. A normal trace array and a proposed model of cellular origin of the first-order waveform are shown. (From Ref. 22 with permission of *Investigative Ophthalmology and Visual Science*.)

The clinical utility of the first-order response in evaluating topographical retinal function is well established (Fig. 2.6). The calculated N1 and P1 components of the multifocal ERG correlate with but are not exact equivalents of the a- and b-waves of the recorded responses of the photopic full-field ERG (21). Not all aspects of cellular activity contribution to the multifocal ERG are understood. A detailed

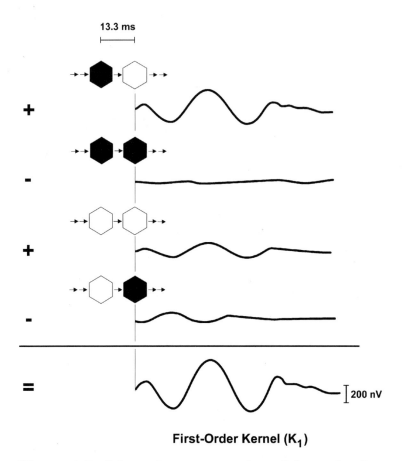

First-Order Kernel (K$_1$)

Figure 2.5 Schematic representation of how the first-order response (first-order kernel, K$_1$) of the multifocal ERG is calculated for a specific hexagon. The first-order response is calculated by adding all of the calculated records following the stimulus, a white frame, and subtracting all calculated records following no stimulus, a black frame. Note that whether the preceding frame is white or black influences the calculation. The calculated first-order response lasts much longer than the duration of one frame (13.3 msec at 75 Hz).

review of retinal physiology is provided in the full-field ERG chapter (Chapter 1). Similar to the full-field ERG, multifocal ERG components are influenced mostly by bipolar cell activity with contributions from photoreceptors and other cells of the

Patient with Previously Unexplained Visual Loss

Humphrey 24-2 SITA Visual Field - Left Eye

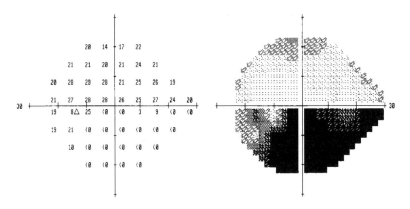

Multifocal ERG First-Order Trace Array

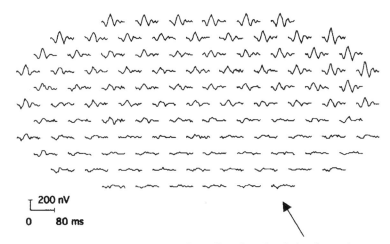

**localized retinal dysfunction
corresponding to visual deficit**

Figure 2.6 The multifocal ERG trace array of a patient with previously unexplained inferior visual field defect. The multifocal ERG shows that the visual deficit is due to localized retinal dysfunction.

inner retina. A proposed model of the cellular origin of the multifocal ERG components is presented in Fig. 2.4. (22). Like the a-wave of the photopic full-field flash response, N1 receives contribution from the hyperpolarization of cone photoreceptors and OFF-bipolar cells. Similar to the photopic b-wave, P1 is influenced mostly by the depolarization of the ON-bipolar cells.

The first-order kernel also contains contributions from ganglion cells and the optic nerve head but these waveforms are small and not readily recognizable with typical clinical recording protocols. The clinical value of these components still warrants further investigation, and they are mentioned under the section on "Specialized Multifocal ERG Techniques and Waveforms."

DISPLAYING MULTIFOCAL ERG RESULTS

The trace array is the true representation of the calculated topographical ERG responses and is the most useful display of multifocal ERG results (Fig. 2.4). Amplitudes and implicit times of each response are readily available. Software can also generate a combined response from a chosen group of hexagons. The size of each hexagon is scaled to produce approximately equal ERG responses. The amplitudes of the N1 and P1 components of each hexagon are similar but falls off somewhat with eccentricity. When response amplitudes are calculated per retinal area, response density is highest in the fovea corresponding to the highest density of cone photoreceptors. Implicit times of P1 are high at the blind spot, the upper and lower borders of the stimulus, and the macula (23). Low P1 implicit times are found in the area encircling the macula.

The three-dimensional (3D) plot is the most colorful eye-catching display of multifocal ERG results but may be misleading. The 3D plot is helpful in visualizing the blind spot and scotomas. However, the 3D plot should always be accompanied by the trace array and should never be the sole display of multifocal ERG data. The 3D plot is obtained by dividing the response amplitude by the area of the hexagon (response density, nV/deg^2) (Fig. 2.7). Because the hexagonal area is the smallest at the center, the amplitude-to-area ratio may be falsely elevated at the center resulting in a small artificial center peak when all responses are markedly reduced. An artificial center peak may also occur with noisy recordings since the 3D plots typically combine the amplitudes of both positive and negative components and cannot distinguish components from electrical noise. Combining amplitudes of positive and negative components causes loss of information. Actual spatial resolution of the responses is also compromised when responses are interpolated to give the appearance of a continuous 3D surface. In addition, the appearance of the 3D plot is dependent on what reference template was used to scale the plot, called the scaler template. A reference template from averaged data of normal control subjects is better than a template from other patients.

Another way of displaying multifocal data involves response density expressed as amplitude per degree area (nV/deg^2) from the center and grouped responses from concentric rings (Fig. 2.7). These response density plots are helpful to evaluate responses with respect to eccentricity from fixation but should be used with caution. Although the highest response density is found in the fovea due to high cone photoreceptor density, the summed response is actually lowest in the fovea and increases with eccentric rings as responses from progressively larger retinal area are summed. This type of data representation obscures isolated scotomas unless the scotoma is in the center. The representation also does not account for asymmetric responses due to disease or the physiologic naso-temporal asymmetry that may occur in normal recordings.

PHYSIOLOGIC BLIND SPOT IN MULTIFOCAL ERG

The physiologic blind spot is not sharply delineated by the multifocal ERG. The optic nerve head reflects more light than

Multifocal ERG - Three-Dimensional (3D) Response Density Plot

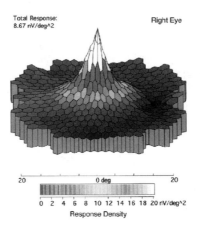

Multifocal ERG - Response Density from Center and Concentric Ring Groups

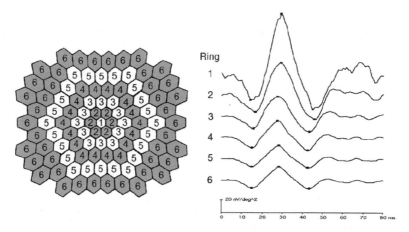

Figure 2.7 Normal response density plots of the multifocal ERG: three-dimensional (3D) plot and center and concentric rings. The multifocal ERG trace array of this normal subject is shown in Fig. 2.4. *Top*: The 3D plot is based on response density (nV/deg^2) obtained by dividing the response amplitude by the area of the hexagon. The fovea has the highest response density consistent with its high cone photoreceptor density. *Bottom*: The response density for the center and concentric rings of grouped hexagon is shown. (Refer to the color insert.)

the retina, and this scattered light produces multifocal ERG responses from adjacent retinal areas that are calculated as small and delayed responses attributed to the region of the blind spot (Fig. 2.4) (24). In addition, the optic nerve head does not completely cover adjacent hexagonal stimulus areas and this could also contribute to an indistinct blind spot. The second-order responses are absent at the blind spot because no short-term adaptation response to a preceding flash in this non-retinal region is possible (Fig. 2.8).

SECOND-ORDER "RESPONSE" OF THE MULTIFOCAL ERG

Like all multifocal waveforms, the second-order response, also known as second-order kernel (K_2), is not a true recorded response but a mathematical derivation. Although the second-order response is perhaps more closely related to the pattern ERG, not all aspects of the physiologic contribution to this mathematical extraction are understood (25). The clinical utility of the second-order response continues to be developed, and whether it is more sensitive and specific than other clinical measures remains to be determined.

While the first-order response is calculated to determine the response of a flash, that is, a hexagonal white frame, the second-order response calculates the effect of successive flashes. The first slice of the second-order kernel calculates the effect of a flash in the immediately preceding frame while the second slice calculates the effect of a flash in the frame before the immediately preceding frame. As most discussions about the second-order kernel deal with the first-slice, the "second-order response" is usually used to refer to be the first slice of the second-order kernel unless specified otherwise.

The second-order response measures the short-term adaptation from a preceding flash. For example, the effect of a flash in the immediately preceding frame causes the normal multifocal ERG flash response to be slightly smaller and faster. The second-order kernel is calculated by adding all of the calculated records following a frame change from either

Second-Order Kernel (K$_2$) - Multifocal ERG

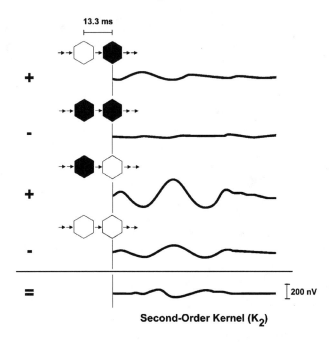

**Normal Second-Order Kernel Trace Array
103-Hexagonal Stimulus (right eye)**

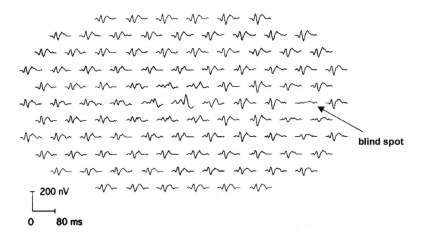

Figure 2.8 (*Caption on facing page*)

white-to-black or black-to-white and subtracting all calculated records following no change (Fig. 2.8). The second-order
response is smaller than the first-order response and, similar
to the first-order response, lasts much longer than the duration of one frame (13.3 msec at 75 Hz). In fact, the first-order
response overlaps with its own induced second-order response
and actually contains an inverted copy of the second-order
kernel referred to as the "induced component" (26).

The second-order response is related to the activity of the
inner retina and ganglion cells. In monkeys, the second-order
response is reduced but not eliminated by tetrodotoxin (TTX)
which abolishes retinal action potentials generated by ganglion cells and perhaps some amacrine cells. The second-order
response is reduced in ganglion cell disorders, and further
investigation of its clinical utility is required.

SPECIALIZED MULTIFOCAL ERG TECHNIQUES
AND WAVEFORMS

Several other multifocal ERG waveforms are recognized. Specialized recordings and algorithms for extracting signals are
required to maximize these waveforms as they are not readily
available with typical clinical recording protocols.

Figure 2.8 (*Facing page*) The second-order response (second-
order kernel, K_2) of the multifocal ERG. *Top*: Schematic representation of how the second-order response (second-order kernel, K_2) of
the multifocal ERG is calculated for a specific hexagon. The first
slice of the second-order kernel calculates the effect of a flash in
the immediately preceding frame. The second-order kernel is calculated by adding all of the calculated records following a frame
change from either white-to-black or black-to-white and subtracting
all calculated records following no change. Similar to the first-order
response, the second-order response lasts much longer than the
duration of one frame (13.3 msec at 75 Hz). *Bottom*: Normal trace
array of the second-order response is shown. The calculated second-order response is smaller than the first-order response, and
in contrast to the first-order response, the second-order response
is not present at the blind spot.

Optic Nerve Head Component

The first-order kernel also contains contributions from ganglion cells and the optic nerve head. The strength of these contributions is related to the distance of the retinal region to the optic nerve head, and generally, the components have higher amplitudes and shorter implicit times in the nasal region of the retina as compared to the temporal region. When retinal action potentials are abolished by TTX which blocks voltage-gated sodium channels in monkeys, the physiologic naso-temporal asymmetry of the first-order responses resolves suggesting that action potentials generated by ganglion cells and perhaps some amacrine cells are likely responsible (27).

The optic nerve head component (ONHC) of the multifocal ERG is thought to originate from the beginning of axonal myelination near the optic nerve head. This component can be better isolated with an interleaved global flash protocol that inserts all-white and all-black frames into the multifocal stimulus presentations (Fig. 2.9) (26). The delay in ONHC is related to the length of the unmyelinated nerve fibers that action potentials must travel between the focal stimulation and the nerve head. The ONHC is reduced in optic neuropathies such as glaucoma, and its clinical utility requires further investigation (28).

The s-Wave

The s-wave ("s" for small) is a positive wavelet on the descending limb of P1 of the first-order response that appears when the stimulus frequency is decreased from 75 to 18 Hz or lower by inserting "blank" frames into the multifocal stimulus presentations. The "blank" frames are all-gray frames that would tend not to elicit a multifocal ERG response (Fig. 2.10) (29). The s-wave is likely to originate from the neural activity of the ganglion cells.

Other Specialized Techniques

The multifocal ERG can provide topographical oscillatory potentials which are best detected by a decreased stimulus

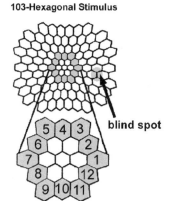

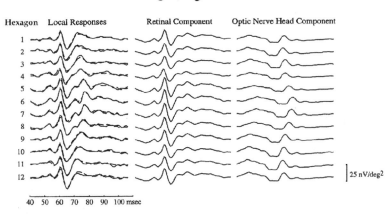

Figure 2.9 The optic nerve head component (ONHC). The ONHC waveforms of a normal subject from each designated hexagon are demonstrated. The first-order traces of the multifocal ERG are obtained with a sequence of all-black, all-white, and all-black stimulus frames inserted between each of the multifocal stimulus presentations. Separation of the retinal component and the ONHC shows increased delay of the ONHC for hexagons further away from the optic nerve head. This corresponds to the distance that action potentials traveled between the focal stimulation and the nerve head before producing the ONHC at the beginning of axonal myelination near the optic nerve head. (From Ref. 28 with permission of *Investigative Ophthalmology and Visual Science*.)

Multifocal ERG s-Wave

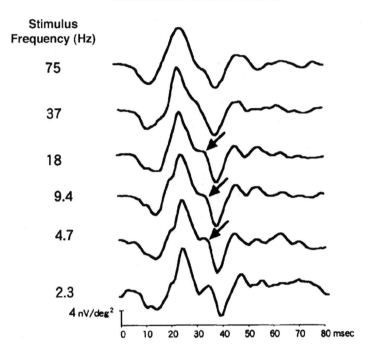

Stimulus Frequency (Hz)

75

37

18

9.4

4.7

2.3

4 nV/deg^2

0 10 20 30 40 50 60 70 80 msec

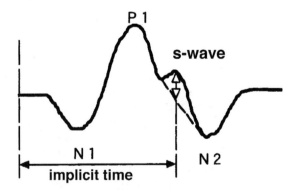

P 1

s-wave

N 1

implicit time

N 2

Figure 2.10   (*Caption on facing page*)

frequency and a higher low-end bandpass to remove other ERG components (30). Both first-order and second-order analysis of the oscillatory potentials are possible, and the topographic distribution of the second-order oscillatory potentials shows combined features of both rod and cone distributions. The oscillatory potentials are generally higher in the temporal retina than corresponding nasal locations (31).

The distribution of ON- and OFF-responses can be studied with the multifocal ERG by a low stimulus frequency of 5 Hz or lower to simulate long duration stimulus (32). A study of a-, b-, and d-wave components shows different spatial distribution across the retina (33). However, with the CRT monitors used for multifocal ERG, the luminance of each white hexagon is optimally maintained only during the first few milliseconds after the frame change and then decreases subsequently; this may hamper the simulation of a long duration stimulus.

Dark-adapted multifocal rod ERG recordings are possible but require the use of blue flashes and modified conditions to allow rod recovery and to reduce the effect of stray light (34). The signal-to-noise ratios of rod ERG recordings are worse than cone recordings.

Figure 2.10 (*Facing page*) The s-wave. The summated waves (all-trace waves) of the individual retinal multifocal ERG first-order kernel for different stimulus frequencies from a normal eye are shown. The s-wave (black arrows) is a positive wavelet on the descending limb of P1 detectable with stimulus frequencies equal to or less than 18 Hz (typical clinical stimulus frequency = 75 Hz). The s-wave is likely related to activities of the ganglion cells. The amplitude of the s-wave (white arrows) may be measured as the height of a vertical line from the peak of the wavelet to where it intersects a line connecting the troughs of successive negative waves on either side of the wavelet. (From Ref. 29, reproduced with permission of *Investigative Ophthalmology & Visual Science* via Copyright Clearance Center.)

REFERENCES

1. Marmor MF, Hood DC, Keating D, Kondo M, Seeliger M, Miyake K. Guidelines for basic multifocal electroretinography (mfERG). Doc Ophthalmol 2003; 106:105–115.

2. Hirose T, Miyake Y, Hara A. Simultaneous recording of electroretinogram and visual evoked response. Focal stimulation under direct observation. Arch Ophthalmol 1977; 95: 1205–1208.

3. Seiple WH, Siegel IM, Carr RE, Mayron C. Evaluating macular function using the focal ERG. Invest Ophthalmol Vis Sci 1986; 27:1123–1130.

4. Arden GB, Banks JL. Foveal electroretinogram as a clinical test. Br J Ophthalmol 1966; 50:740.

5. Jacobson JH, Kawasaki K, Hirose T. The human electroretinogram and occipital potential in response to focal illumination of the retina. Invest Ophthalmol 1969; 106:348–357.

6. Sandberg MA, Ariel M. A hand-held, teo-channel stimulator-ophthalmoscope. Arch Ophthalmol 1977; 95:1881–1882.

7. Brodie SE, Naidu EM, Goncalves J. Combined amplitude and phase criteria for evaluation of macular electroretinograms. Ophthalmology 1992; 99:522–530.

8. Sandberg MA, Pawlyk BS, Berson EL. Isolation of focal rod electroretinograms from the dark-adapted human eye. Invest Ophthalmol Vis Sci 1996; 37:930–934.

9. Nusinowitz S, Hood DC, Birch DG. Tod transduction parameters from the a-wave of local receptor populations. J Opt Soc Am 1995; 12:2259–2266.

10. Sutter EE, Tran D. The field topography of ERG components in man—I. The photopic luminance response. Vision Res 1992; 32:433–446.

11. Hood DC. Assessing retinal function with the multifocal technique. Prog Retin Eye Res 2000; 19:607–646.

12. Mohidin N, Yap MK, Jacobs RJ. The repeatability and variability of the multifocal electroretinogram for four different electrodes. Ophthal Physiol Optics 1997; 17:530–535.

13. Kondo M, Miyake Y, Piao C, Tanikawa A, Horiguchi M, Terasaki H. Amplitude increase of the multifocal electroretinogram during light adaptation. Invest Ophthalmol Vis Sci 1999; 40:2633–2637.

14. Chisholm JA, Keating D, Parks S, Evans AL. The impact of fixation on the multifocal electroretinogram. Doc Ophthalmol 2001; 102:131–139.

15. Kondo M, Miyake Y, Horiguchi M, Suzuki S, Tanikawa A. Recording multifocal electroretinograms with fundus monitoring. Invest Ophthalmol Vis Sci 1997; 38:1049–1052.

16. Palmowski AM, Berninger T, Allgayer R, Andrielis H, Heinemann-Vernaleken B, Rudolph G. Effects of refractive blur on the multifocal electroretinogram. Doc Ophthalmol 1999; 99: 41–54.

17. Brigell M, Bach M, Barber C, Kawasaki K, Koojiman A. Guidelines for calibration of stimulus and recording parameters used in clinical electrophysiology of vision. Calibration Standard Committee of the International Society for Clinical Electrophysiology of Vision (ISCEV). Doc Ophthalmol 1998; 95:1–14.

18. Bock M, Andrassi M, Belitsky L, Lorenz B. A comparison of two multifocal ERG systems. Doc Ophthalmol 1999; 97: 157–178.

19. Keating D, Parks S, Evans A. Technical aspects of multifocal ERG recording. Doc Ophthalmol 2000; 100:77–98.

20. Sutter E. The interpretation of multifocal binary kernels. Doc Ophthalmol 2000; 100:49–75.

21. Hood DC, Seiple W, Holopigian K, Greenstein V. A comparison of the components of the multi-focal and full-field ERGs. Visual Neurosci 1997; 14:533–544.

22. Hood DC, Frishman LJ, Saszik S, Viswanathan S. Retinal origins of the primate multifocal ERG: implications for the human response. Invest Ophthalmol Vis Sci 2002; 43: 1676–1685.

23. Seeliger MW, Kretschmann UH, Apfelstedt-Sylla E, Zrenner E. Implicit time topography of multifocal electroretinograms. Invest Ophthalmol Vis Sci 1998; 39:718–723.

24. Shimada Y, Horiguchi M. Stary light-induced multifocal electroretinograms. Invest Ophthalmol Vis Sci 2003; 44: 1245–1251.

25. Yoshii M, Yanashima K, Wada H, Sakemi F, Enoki T, Okisaka S. Analysis of second-order kernel response components of multifocal electroretinograms elcited form normal subjects. Jpn J Ophthalmol 2001; 45:247–251.

26. Sutter EE, Bearse MA. The optic nerve head component of the human ERG. Vision Res 1999; 39:419–436.

27. Hood DC, Frishman LJ, Viswanathan S, Robson JG, Ahmed J. Evidence for a ganglion cell contribution to the primate electroretinogram (ERG): effects of TTX on the multifocal ERG in macaque. Vis Neurosci 1999; 16:411–416.

28. Fortune B, Bearse MA, Cioffi GA, Johnson CA. Selective loss of an oscillatory component from temporal retinal multifocal ERG responses in glaucoma. Invest Ophthalmol Vis Sci 2002; 43:2638–2647.

29. Sano M, Tazawa Y, Nabeshima T, Mita M. A new wavelet in the multifocal electroretinogram, probably originating from ganglion cells. Invest Ophthalmol Vis Sci 2002; 43:1666–1672.

30. Wu S, Sutter EE. A topographic study of oscillatory potentials in man. Vis Neurosci 1995; 12:1013–1025.

31. Bearse MA Jr, Shimada Y, Sutter EE. Distribution of oscillatory components in the central retina. Doc Ophthalmol 2000; 100:185–205.

32. Kondo M, Miyake Y. Assessment of local cone on- and off-pathway function using multifocal ERG technique. Doc Ophthalmol 2000; 100:139–154.

33. Kondo M, Miyake Y, Horiguchi M, Suzuki S, Tanikawa A. Recording multifocal electroretinogram on and off responses in humans. Invest Ophthalmol Vis Sci 1998; 39:574–580.

34. Hood DC, Wladis EJ, Shady S, Holopigian K, Li J, Seiple W. Multifocal rod electroretinograms. Invest Ophthal Vis Sci 1998; 39:1152–1162.

3

Pattern Electroretinogram

The pattern ERG records the retinal response generated by a checkerboard-like stimulus of alternating black and white square checks that reverses in a regular phase frequency (Fig. 3.1). The pattern ERG is a measure of retinal ganglion cell function and also receives contribution from other intraretinal cellular elements. The pattern ERG is dominated by activity from the macula because of its high density of photoreceptors and high number of retinal ganglion cell projections. Standard for pattern ERG recording has been established by the International Society for Clinical Electrophysiology of Vision (ISCEV) and is available on the ISCEV Internet website. The standard is reviewed every 3 years and published periodically (1). A summary of the standard is provided in Table 3.1.

CLINICAL UTILITY OF PATTERN ERG

The pattern ERG provides a clinical measure of macular and ganglion cell function. Pattern ERG has been used in macular disorders and optic nerve diseases extensively by centers with special clinical and investigative interests in the pattern ERG. However, in general, the pattern ERG is not used as frequently as the multifocal ERG to assess macular

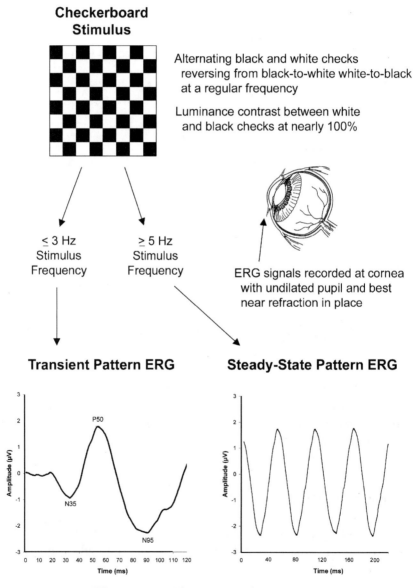

Figure 3.1   (*Caption on facing page*)

dysfunction, because unlike the multifocal ERG, pattern ERG gives no topographical information about localized macular dysfunction. Although the pattern ERG is a more direct and specific measure of retinal ganglion cell function than the VEP, pattern reversal VEP is performed more frequently to detect optic nerve dysfunction perhaps because VEP is a more familiar established test. Like other visual electrophysiologic tests, the pattern ERG should be used in combination with a thorough ocular examination as well as other clinical ancillary tests such as visual field, fluorescein angiography, optical coherence tomography, optic nerve head imaging, and neuroimaging. Aside from maculopathies and optic neuropathies, pattern ERG can also serve as a useful objective measure in non-organic visual loss. However, pattern ERG testing requires good fixation and may not be possible in uncooperative patients or in patients with nystagmus or poor visual acuity.

BASIC CONCEPTS AND PHYSIOLOGIC ORIGINS OF PATTERN ERG

The concept of recording retinal electrical signals in response to a pattern stimulus is attributed to Riggs et al. (2). Whereas conventional full-field ERG measures retinal activity in response to a change in luminance, pattern ERG detects

Figure 3.1 (*Facing page*) Schematic diagram showing the basic principles of pattern ERG. When the pattern stimulus reversal rates are slow enough ($\leq$3 Hz) to allow the retina to recover, a transient pattern ERG response is recorded, and when the stimulus frequency is too fast ($\geq$5 Hz) to allow the retina to reach resting state between stimuli, a steady-state pattern ERG response is elicited. Transient pattern ERG allows the identification of specific pattern ERG waveform components and their amplitudes and latencies. Steady-state ERG responses are sinusoidal, and Fourier analysis is required to determine amplitude and the amount of time phase shift relative to the stimulus. The amplitude of steady-state ERG response is similar to that of the N95 component.

Table 3.1 Summary of International Standard and
Recommendations for Pattern Electroretinography (PERG)

Clinical protocol
Preparation of patient

Pupillry dilation	Undilated
Fixation	Fixation point in center of stimulus screen
Refraction	Optimal visual acuity at testing distance
Monocular and binocular Recording	Simultaneous binocular recording recommended for "Basic PERG"
Noise trials	Determination of noise level by averaging in absence of stimulation (blank trials); these values reported whenever possible
Recording	Averaging continued until a stable waveform is obtained; minimum of 150 responses; at least two replications of each stimulus to confirm responses

PERG reporting

Reporting	Amplitudes and implicit times of P50 and N95
Clinical norms	Each laboratory establishes normal values; age norms essential

Basic technology
Electrode

Recording	Non-contact lens corneal electrodes, thin conductive fibers or foils, usually placed without anesthesia
	Fiber electrodes: placed in lower fornix
	Foil electrodes: placed directly under center of pupil
Reference	Skin reference electrodes placed at ipsilateral lateral canthi. For monocular recording, corneal electrode in the occluded eye may be used
Ground	Skin electrode connected to ground, typically on forehead
Skin electrode characteristics	Skin electrodes for reference or ground, $\leq 5\,k\Omega$ impedance; skin cleansed with alcohol or skin-preparing material; electrode applied with a conductive paste
Cleaning	Cleaned and sterilized after each use

(Continued)

Table 3.1 (*Continued*)

Stimulus parameters	
Field and check size	Black-and-white reversing checkerboard, stimulus field size between 10° and 16°, check size 0.8° (48 min)
Contrast	Maximal contrast near 100% between black and white squares, not <80%
Luminance	Photopic luminance level for white areas of >80 cd m^{-2}; overall screen luminance should not vary during checkerboard reversals
Transient and steady-state recording	Transient PERG helpful for optic nerve and macular diseases Steady-state PERG for glaucoma studies
Reversal rate	Transient PERG: 2–6 reversals per second (1–3 Hz) Steady-state PERG: 16 reversals per second (8 Hz)
Recalibration	Regular stimulus recalibration
Background illumination	Dim or ordinary room light; keep bright lights out of subject's view
Electronic recording equipment	
Amplification	Bandpass of amplifiers and preamplifiers include range from 1 to 100 Hz; no notch filters that remove alternating current line frequency; alternating-current-coupled amplifiers with impedance of 10 MΩ
Averaging and signal analysis	Always necessary due to small amplitude of PERG; analysis period for transient PERG≥150 msec; Fourier analysis needed for steady-state PERG
Artifact rejection	Computerized artifact reject is essential, set no higher than 100 μV peak-to-peak
Display	Adequate resolution for small-amplitude signal; simultaneous display of input signal and average or a rapid alternation between these two displays, so quality and stability of input signal can be adequately monitored

retinal activity in response to a reversing black and white checkerboard stimulus that has the same mean luminance throughout recording. Photoreceptor cells are more responsive to change in luminance, but cells involved in visual signal processing such as retinal ganglion cells and other inner retinal cellular elements generate responses to changing light–dark edges of a pattern stimulus.

Two categories of pattern ERG responses are recognized—transient and steady-state (Fig. 3.1). Transient pattern ERG responses are produced when the pattern stimulus reversal rates are slow enough to allow the retina to recover to its resting state between stimuli. Steady-state pattern ERG responses occur when stimulus rates are too fast to allow the retina to reach resting state between stimuli. Transient pattern ERG responses are elicited with a stimulus reversal rate of six reversals per second or less, equivalent to a phase frequency of 3 Hz or less. Steady-state responses are generated by a reversal rate of 10 reversals per second or greater, equivalent to a frequency of 5 Hz or more. Transient pattern ERG allows the identification of specific pattern ERG waveform components and their amplitudes and latencies. Steady-state ERG responses are sinusoidal, and Fourier analysis program is required to determine amplitude and the amount of time phase shift relative to the stimulus.

The transient pattern ERG waveform consists of a series of negative (N) and positive (P) components designated by their approximate latencies in milliseconds from the onset of the stimulus. Three components are recognized—N35, P50, and N95, but N35 is not always visible (Fig. 3.2). The amplitude of P50 is measured from the negative N35 peak to the positive P50 peak, and in cases of an ill-defined N35, the N35 peak amplitude is substituted by the average of the stimulus onset amplitude and the P50 onset amplitude. The amplitude of N95 is measured from the P50 peak to the N95 peak. The latency of P95 may be difficult to determine because its negative trough may be broad.

In general, P50 is produced by retinal ganglion cells and other retinal cellular elements, and N95 is generated predominantly by retinal ganglion cells (3,4). The P50 component

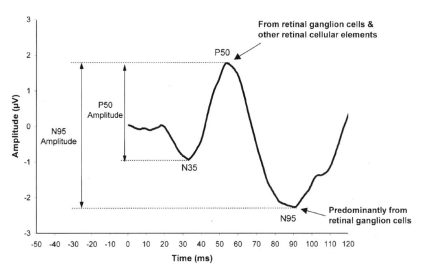

Figure 3.2 Normal transient pattern ERG response. The method of amplitude measurements and physiologic origins of the components are shown. In cases of ill-defined N35, the N35 peak amplitude is substituted by the average of the stimulus onset amplitude and the P50 onset amplitude. The latency of N95 may be difficult to determine due to its broad trough.

is partly reduced and N95 is severely reduced in monkeys treated with tetrodotoxin (TTX) which abolishes retinal action potentials generated by ganglion cells (5). This finding is also consistent with pattern ERG findings in humans after optic nerve resection (6). Luminance and contrast response studies also suggest that P50 receive contributions from cells other than retinal ganglion cells and is responsive at least to luminance. In contrast, N95 is dominated almost exclusively by retinal ganglion cell activity and responds well to contrast.

The different physiologic origins of P50 and N95 allow transient pattern ERG to differentiate between macular and optic nerve conditions (Fig. 3.3). In macular disorders, notable reductions of P50 are encountered with a concomitant reduction of N95 such that the N95 to P50 amplitude ratio is not reduced or in some cases even increased. In contrast, optic nerve diseases are associated with a relatively preserved P50 and a selective reduction of N95.

Normal   **Macular Dysfunction**   **Optic Nerve Dysfunction**

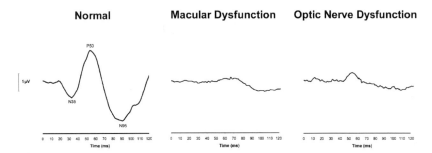

Figure 3.3 Examples of transient pattern ERG responses. The macular dysfunction example shows reduced P50 as well as N95. The example of optic nerve dysfunction from demyelination demonstrates more preserved P50 with a greater selective loss of P95.

Compared to transient pattern ERG responses, steady-state responses have amplitudes that are similar to those of N95, and this makes steady-state responses suitable in assessing optic neuropathies such as glaucoma.

CLINICAL RECORDING OF PATTERN ERG

The pattern ERG response is small and usually less than 10 μV resulting in a high noise-to-signal ratio. Therefore, computer averaging of multiple recordings or sweeps is necessary to isolate this relatively small response. In addition, clarity of the pattern stimulus is critical, and best-corrected near visual acuity and consistent accurate fixation are needed to optimize this small response. Dilation of the pupils and contact-lens electrodes are not recommended because they cause blurring of the pattern stimulus. Instead, non-contact-lens type electrodes that contact the cornea and adjacent bulbar conjunctiva are utilized, and topical anesthesia to the cornea is not necessary. The Dawson–Trick–Litzkow fiber (DTL) electrode, the Arden gold foil electrode, and the Hawlina–Konec (HK) loop electrode are suitable, and proper placement of the electrode is critical in obtaining a high quality pattern ERG signal (see Chapter 1 for more information on ERG recording electrodes) (7–9). The DTL electrode should be placed with the fiber in the lower fornix (Fig. 3.4). The distal end of the gold foil electrode should be placed vertically under the lower lid just below the center of the pupil with the foil curving downward over the lower lashes. No portion of the gold foil should touch the skin. The HK loop electrode should be hooked into the lower fornix, and the contact windows should be positioned on the bulbar conjunctiva. Skin electrodes may be used for those who are intolerant to fiber, foil, and loop electrodes, but they are likely to have high noise-to-signal ratio. The reference electrode may be a skin electrode placed at the ipsilateral lateral canthus. During monocular recording, the recording electrode of the occluded fellow eye may serve as the reference electrode. The ground electrode is typically placed on the forehead.

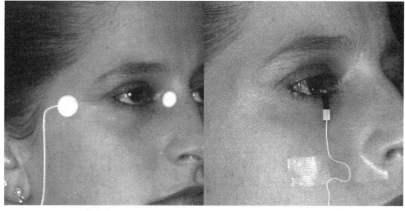

DTL **Gold-Foil**

Figure 3.4 Dawson–Trick–Litzkow (DTL) and gold foil electrodes for pattern ERG recording. Clarity of the pattern stimulus is critical in pattern ERG, and non-contact-lens type electrodes such as the DTL electrode and the Arden gold foil electrode are suitable. The DTL electrode should be placed with the fiber in the fornix of the lower lid. The distal end of the gold foil electrode should be placed vertically under the lower lid just below the center of the pupil with the foil curving downward over the lower lashes. No portion of the gold foil should touch the skin.

The black and white checkerboard stimulus of the pattern ERG is similar but not identical to the stimulus of the pattern reversal VEP. Similar to pattern reversal VEP, the stimulus consists of equal number and size of alternating black and white squares. A fixation point is located at the corner of four checks located at the center of the stimulus. The luminance of the white squares should be at least $80 \, \text{cd/m}^2$. The pattern stimulus is defined by the visual angle subtended by the side length of a single check. To calculate the visual angle, the check side length is divided by the distance from the stimulus center to the tested eye. The result is the tangent of the visual angle subtended by each check, and the visual angle is obtained by taking the inverse tangent.

Several stimulus parameters are critical to the pattern ERG and differ from those of pattern reversal VEP. The pattern ERG amplitude increases with luminance contrast between the white and black checks, and a maximal contrast of as near 100% is desired (10–13). In pattern reversal VEP, the pattern contrast has little effect on the response for contrasts above about 50% (14). While the responses of both pattern ERG and pattern reversal VEP increase with greater stimulus field, the amplitude of pattern reversal VEP is more macular dependent (15,16). The pattern ERG correlates well with static perimetry with 6° and 10° stimulus fields but not with larger 20° stimulus field (17). The international standard for pattern ERG recommends a stimulus size between 10° and 16°, and the standard for pattern reversal VEP recommends a stimulus size of at least 15°.

A check size of 0.8° (48 min) is recommended for clinical pattern ERG, but results of studies into the optimal check size for pattern ERG are mixed and are in part related to the stimulus size (3,4,18). For most clinical recordings, transient pattern ERG responses are elicited with a stimulus reversal rate of six reversals per second or less, equivalent to a phase frequency of 3 Hz or less. For steady-state recordings, a reversal rate of 8 Hz demonstrates the best correlation to check size (i.e., spatial tuning) (10).

During pattern ERG recording, the room light should be at low or medium luminance level, and the luminance of the screen beyond the checkerboard stimulus is not critical (19). Simultaneous binocular or sequential monocular recordings are typically performed. Interocular pattern ERG asymmetry is relatively low in a normal subject. Collection of age-matched normative data by each facility is recommended. The maturation and age-related changes of pattern ERG are discussed in Chapter 6.

REPORTING PATTERN ERG RESULTS

Report of pattern ERG results should include waveforms with values of amplitudes and latencies for P50 and N95. The report should also include normative data from each individual facility. Stimulus parameters such as check sizes should be stated as well as whether international standard was followed. If the response is abnormal, an interpretation of the N95 to P50 amplitude ratio is helpful. For steady-state pattern ERG, amplitude and phase shift derived from Fourier analysis should be available.

REFERENCES

1. Bach M, Hawlina M, Holder GE, Marmor MF, Meigen T, Vaegan, Miyake Y. Standard for pattern electroretinography. Doc Ophthalmol 2000; 101:11–18.

2. Riggs LA, Johnson LP, Schick AM. Electrical responses of the human eye to moving stimulus pattern. Science 1964; 144:567–568.

3. Berminger T, Schuurmans RP. Spatial tuning of the pattern ERG across temporal frequency. Doc Ophthalmol 1985; 61: 17–25.

4. Schuurmans RP, Berminger T. Luminance and contrast responses recorded in man and cat. Doc Ophthalmol 1985; 59:187–197.

5. Viswanathan S, Frishman LJ, Robson JG. The uniform field and pattern ERG in macaques with experimental glaucoma:

removal of spiking activity. Invest Ophthalmol Vis Sci 2000; 41:2797–2810.

6. Harrison JM, O'Connor PS, Young RS, Kincaid M, Bentley R. The pattern ERG in man following surgical resection of the optic nerve. Invest Ophthalmol Vis Sci 1987; 28:492–499.

7. Arden GB, Carter RM, Hogg CR, Siegel IM, Margolis S. A gold foil electrode: extending the horizons for clinical electroretinography. Invest Ophthalmol Vis Sci 1979; 18:421–426.

8. Dawson WW, Trick GL, Litzkow CA. Improved electrode for electroretinography. Invest Ophthalmol Vis Sci 1979; 18:988–991.

9. Hawlina M, Konee B. New noncorneal HK-loop electrode for clinical electroretinography. Doc Ophthalmol 1992; 81: 253–259.

10. Hess RF, Baker C Jr. Human pattern-evoked electroretinogram. J Neurophysiol 1984; 51:939–951.

11. Korth M, Rix R, Sembritzki O. Spatial contrast transfer function of the pattern-evoked electroretinogram. Invest Ophthalmol Vis Sci 1985; 26:303–308.

12. Thompson D, Drasdo N. The effect of stimulus contrast on the latency and amplitude of the pattern electroretinogram. Vision Res 1989; 29:309–313.

13. Zapt HR, Bach M. The contrast characteristic of the pattern electroretinogram depends on temporal frequency. Graefes Arch Clin Exp Ophthalmol 1999; 237:93–99.

14. Tetsuka S, Katsumi O, Mehta M, Tetsuka H, Hirose T. Effect of stimulus contrast on simultaneous steady-state pattern reversal electroretinogram and visual-evoked potential. Ophthalmic Res 1992; 24:110–118.

15. Aylward GW, Billson V, Billson FA. The wide-angle pattern electroretinogram: relation between pattern electroretinogram amplitude and stimulus area using large stimuli. Doc Ophthalmol 1989; 73:275–283.

16. Sakaue H, Katsumi O, Mehta M, Hirose T. Simultaneous pattern reversal ERG and VER recordings: effect of stimulus field and central scotoma. Invest Ophthalmol Vis Sci 1990; 31:506–511.

17. Junghardt A, Wildberger H, Torok B. Pattern electroretinogram, visual evoked potential and psychophysical functions in maculopathy. Doc Ophthalmol 1995; 90:229–245.

18. Bach M, Holder GE. Check size tuning of the pattern electroretinogram: a reappraisal. Doc Ophthalmol 1997; 92:193–202.

19. Bach M, Schumacher M. The influence of ambient room lighting on the pattern electroretinogram (PERG). Doc Ophthalmol 2002; 105:281–289.

4

Electro-oculogram

While the ERG is a transient retinal electrophysiologic response to a brief light stimulus, the electro-oculogram (EOG) is a measure of the continuous resting electrical potential across the retina. This standing potential was discovered by DuBois-Raymond in 1849, and the term "electro-oculogram" was introduced by Marg in 1951 (1,2). The EOG is a clinically useful test in conditions such as Best disease, but its clinical applications are not as extensive as the ERG. Standard for clinical EOG has been established by the International Society for Clinical Electrophysiology of Vision (ISCEV) since 1993 and the most updated version is available on the ISCEV Internet site (3). The clinical EOG standard is reviewed every 3 years, and no significant revision has occurred. A summary of the standard is provided in Table 4.1.

PHYSIOLOGIC ORIGINS AND CHARACTERISTICS OF EOG

The retinal pigment epithelium (RPE) maintains a resting potential of a few millivolts. The RPE cell basal surface is

Table 4.1 Summary of International Standard and
Recommendations for Clinical Electro-oculogram (EOG)

Clinical protocol
Preparation of patient

Pupillary dilation	Undilated if stimulus intensity for light response is 400–600 cd m^{-2}
	Dilated if stimulus intensity for light response is 50–100 cd m^{-2}
Electrode placement	Two skin electrodes for each eye, placed as close to each canthus as possible
Saccades	Eyes alternate direction every 1–2.5 sec (complete back-and-forth cycle every 2–5 sec); minimum of 10 sets of saccades once per minute throughout test
Preadaptation	Room light (35–70 lux looking ahead) for $\geq$15 min before dark phase; sunlight, ophthalmoscopy, or fluorescein angiography avoided within 60 min of EOG testing
Dark phase	Two alternative methods
	1. Ratio of light peak to dark trough (Arden ratio)
	Lights turned off and EOG values recorded for 15 min in darkness; minimum amplitude (dark trough) most often occurs between 11–12 min
	2. Ratio of light peak to dark-adapted baseline
	Dark adaptation for $\geq$40 min and EOG values recorded for $\geq$5 min before light phase to establish dark-adapted baseline amplitude
Light phase	Steady light stimulus turned on and EOG recorded until maximal amplitude (light peak) is reached; if no clear light peak is seen, continue testing for $\geq$20 min
Measurement of EOG	Saccadic amplitudes and calculating ratio of light peak to dark trough or light peak to dark-adapted baseline
Normal values	Each laboratory establishes normal values

(*Continued*)

Table 4.1 (*Continued*)

Reporting of EOG	State which EOG ratio method was used (light peak to dark trough or light peak to dark-adapted baseline); include latency of the light peak and the amplitude of the dark trough or dark baseline
Basic technology	
Light stimulation	
Stimulus field	Full-field (Ganzfeld) stimulation with full-field dome
Fixation targets	Red light-emitting diodes, 30° of visual angle in the horizontal meridian built into full-field dome, sufficiently visible during dark and light phases
Skin electrodes	
Construction	Nonpolarizable material such as silver–silver chloride or gold
Resistance	$\leq 10\,k\Omega$ impedance measured between 30 and 200 Hz
Electrode application	Skin cleansed with alcohol or skin-preparing material; electrode applied with a conductive paste
Cleaning	Cleaned after each use
Light sources	
Luminance and adjustment	Visibly steady white light; stimulus intensity determines whether pupil should be dilated or undilated (see "pupillary dilation" above); stimulus intensity adjustable by filters if variation in stimulus intensity is needed to examine patient with dilated and undilated pupils
Calibration	Luminance of the full-field dome measured by photometer in a non-integrating mode. Frequency of recalibration depending on system used
Recording equipment	
Amplification systems	AC (alternate current) couple amplification with lower frequency cutoff $\leq 1\,Hz$ and high frequency cutoff preferably <50 or 60 Hz
Display system	Original waveforms displayed during recording so stability and quality of recording can be determined
Patient isolation	Electrically isolated

attached to a thin basement membrane forming the inner layer of Bruch's membrane which separates the RPE from the choroid, and the RPE cell apical surface has multiple villous processes that adhere to the photoreceptor outer segments by a mucopolysaccharide matrix (Fig. 4.1). To maintain the RPE standing potential, the integrity of the RPE as well as the contact between the photoreceptors and the RPE must be intact. This explains why the EOG is decreased in retinal detachment as well as degenerative disorders involving the photoreceptors or the RPE or both. In those disorders due primarily to photoreceptor dysfunction, decreases in EOG generally parallel impaired ERG responses.

Physiologic Origin of Electro-Oculogram (EOG)

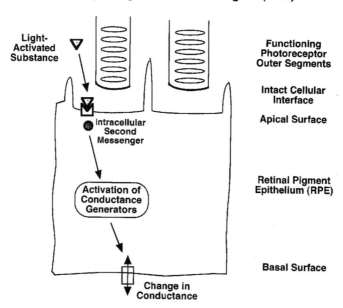

Figure 4.1 Schematic diagram of the physiologic origin of the clinical EOG. Light causes increase of a light-activated substance presumably produced by the photoreceptors, which binds to receptors at the RPE apical membrane surface. This activates an intracellular second messenger causing the basal surface of the RPE to depolarize with increased Cl$^-$ conductance.

The physiologic origin of EOG is not completely understood. Intraretinal microelectrode recordings in animals indicate that light adaptation causes increase of a biochemical agent, presumably produced by the photoreceptors, that bind to the membrane of the RPE apical surface (Fig. 4.1) (4–7). This causes an intracellular second messenger within the RPE to depolarize the basal surface of the RPE by increasing the conductance of negative chloride ions (Cl^-). The result is a transepithelial potential of the RPE that produces, at the basal surface of the RPE, a negative charge which can be measured indirectly as a positive charge change at the cornea. This increase in the transepithelial potential of the RPE in response to light is referred to as the light-sensitive component of the EOG. A lower transepithelial RPE potential unrelated to light-induced photoreceptor activity exists in darkness and is the light-insensitive component of the EOG. Thus, the EOG is a measure of the function of the photoreceptors, subretinal space, and the RPE.

The resting potential of the retina is not a steady potential but a slow oscillating potential that continues to rise and fall even in a stable state of light adaptation. In a light-adapted retina, the rise reaches a higher peak amplitude than a dark-adapted retina in which the rise is minimal or absent. The EOG light rise reaches "light peak" in about 7–12 min from the onset of light adaptation and falls to a "dark trough" in about 12 min with dark adaptation. This *"slow oscillation"* is measured by the clinical EOG.

In reality, the slow oscillations of the EOG is not the only light-induced response of the RPE (Table 4.2) (4). Light absorption by the photoreceptors results in a decrease in extracellular potassium ions (K^+) around its outer segments which causes a transient hyperpolarization at the apical RPE surface that is measured as part of the c-wave of the flash ERG occurring 2–5 sec after the light stimulus. Moreover, a transient rapid initial fall in the RPE standing potential over 60–75 sec follows the onset of light adaptation. This phenomenon is the *"fast oscillation"* and is produced by the hyperpolarization of the basal RPE membrane in response to the decrease in the extracellular K^+ of the photoreceptor

Table 4.2 Light-Related Electrophysiologic Responses of the Retinal Pigment Epithelium

Clinical measure	Origin	Physiologic process	Charge measured at cornea, timing, and characteristics
EOG slow oscillations	RPE basal membrane	Depolarization due to increased Cl^- conductance	Positive standing potential peaking 7–12 min with light adaptation
EOG fast oscillations	RPE basal membrane	Hyperpolarization due to decreased extracellular K^+ from photoreceptor activity	Standing potential decreasing rapidly during 60–75 sec of light period and increasing rapidly with similar period of darkness
ERG c-wave (positive contribution)	RPE apical membrane	Hyperpolarization due to decreased extracellular K^+ from photoreceptor activity	Positive transient potential 2–5 sec after onset of flash stimulus

outer segments. The c-wave and the fast oscillations are not ordinarily recorded clinically. In contrast, the clinical EOG is a measure of the slow oscillations of the resting potential of the RPE which is not related to the decrease in K^+ at the subretinal space nor is it significantly affected by a brief light stimulus (8).

CLINICAL EOG RECORDING—PATIENT SET-UP

In clinical EOG recording, cutaneous electrodes made of silver–silver chloride or gold are placed near the medial and lateral canthal regions of each eye, and the resting potential between the cornea and the retina is indirectly obtained by having the subject look back and forth repetitively at two fixation targets (Fig. 4.2). The fixation targets are located 15° from primary gaze horizontally to the right and the left of primary gaze. The fixation targets are typically red diodes that are built into the full-field stimulus dome of the full-field ERG or flash VEP (Fig. 4.3). To assist in the rapid saccadic eye movements, the fixation targets can be alternately lit and the subject is instructed to look at the lit target. The goal

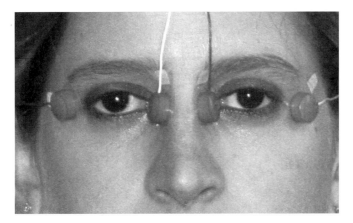

Figure 4.2 Cutaneous electrodes for EOG recording placed near the medial and lateral canthi of each eye.

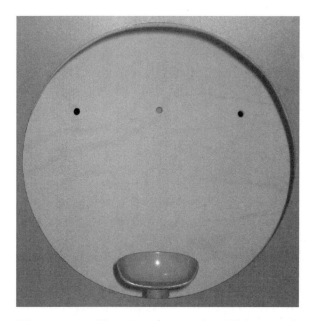

Figure 4.3 Fixation targets for EOG recording. The targets are typically built into the full-field dome and consist of red diodes located 15° to the right and left of the primary gaze fixation target. The targets are alternately lit during EOG recording to assist the subject in making accurate saccades.

is to complete a cycle of right-to-left and left-to-right eye movements every 2–5 sec.

With the recording electrodes near the medial and lateral canthi, the relative position of each eyes with respect to the electrodes changes with the horizontal saccadic eye movements (Fig. 4.4). For instance, when the eyes are looking at the right fixation target, the cornea of the right eye is closer to the lateral canthus electrode and the retina is closer to the medial canthus electrode. The position of the right eye is reversed with fixation to the left target. Therefore, with the lateral canthus electrode serving as the recording electrode and the medical canthus electrode as the reference electrode, the change in the measured potential between right gaze and left gaze is the approximate potential difference between the cornea and the retina. The results of the EOG

Electro-Oculogram (EOG)

Back-and-Forth Horizontal Saccades

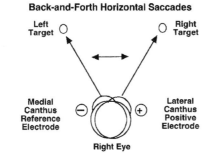

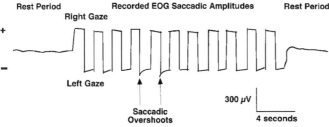

Figure 4.4 Clinical EOG recording. Note the change of the position of the eye relative to the electrodes with horizontal saccadic eye movements. The positive electrode at the lateral canthus of the right eye is closer to the cornea on right gaze and closer to the retina on left gaze. At the beginning of each minute of testing, at least 10 sets of back-and-forth horizontal saccades are obtained simultaneously from both eyes. The averaged amplitude of the saccades is the EOG amplitude for the given minute. The saccadic recording displayed by the recording system should be monitored for inaccurate eye movements such as saccadic overshoots that may adversely affect EOG result.

recording are a square-shaped waveform of the horizontal saccades with the height of the square waves corresponding to the EOG amplitude (Fig. 4.4). In short, the clinical EOG is an indirect measure of the resting potential of the retina by measuring the potential difference between the cornea and the retina. Aside from the transepithelial potential of the RPE, other ocular tissues also make small contributions to the measured EOG potential. Of interest, direct EOG recordings by the use of corneal electrode are possible with specialized technique; indirect and direct EOG recordings have comparable results (9,10).

At the beginning of each minute of EOG testing, at least 10 complete sets of horizontal saccades are obtained. The amplitudes of the 10 sets of saccades are averaged to provide the EOG amplitude for the given minute. The saccadic waveforms displayed by the recording system should be assessed to determine the stability and quality of the eye movements. Saccadic overshoots and imprecise saccades will produce inaccurate EOG amplitude (Fig. 4.4). Patients with eye movement disorders such as nystagmus and large angle strabismus may not be able to perform clinical EOG. Likewise, EOG testing may not be possible for those who are not cooperative enough to perform adequate saccades.

OBTAINING LIGHT PEAK AND DARK TROUGH EOG AMPLITUDES

The goal of EOG testing is to acquire the maximal light-adapted amplitude, the "light peak," and the minimal dark-adapted amplitude, the "dark trough." The light peak is influenced by the light intensity used for light adaptation (11–14). Therefore, whether the pupils should be dilated with eye drops is determined by the available background light intensity of the full-field dome. The international standard for clinical EOG recommends a luminance between 400 and $600\,cd/m^2$ for undilated pupils and a luminance between 50 and $100\,cd/m^2$ for dilated pupils. Further, the wavelength of the light stimulus may also influence the light peak, and white light is typically utilized. Periodic calibration of the recording system should be performed as recommended by the manufacturer and based on international calibration standard (15).

The EOG test session consists of three phases—preadaptation, dark adaptation, and light adaptation (Fig. 4.5). During preadaptation, the patient is exposed to a recommended light level of 35–70 lux for at least 15 min. Dimmer

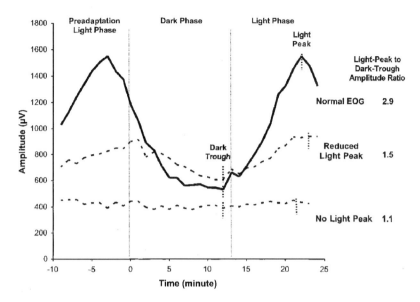

Figure 4.5 Time vs. EOG saccadic amplitude plots. The plots of a normal EOG, reduced light-peak EOG, and no light-peak EOG are shown. The recordings were obtained from a normal subject and two patients with retinitis pigmentosa. The dark and light phases do not always have the same duration and are individualized depending on when dark trough and light peak occur.

preadaptation light levels may fail to suppress rod function and can diminish the size of the subsequent dark trough obtained during the second phase of testing. On the other hand, stronger light levels or sudden changes in illumination may produce excessive light stimulation and more difficulty in reaching a subsequent steady dark trough. Excessive light exposure such as ophthalmoscopy and fundus photography should be avoided prior to EOG testing. Although not required, commencing EOG recording during the preadaptation period has several advantages. First, it minimizes differences of light exposure among subjects by having all subjects exposed to a proper luminance level provided by the full-field dome. Second, it provides the patient with opportunities to practice performing EOG saccades, and it also allows the assessment of the quality of the saccadic recordings.

The second phase of EOG is the dark adaptation phase during which EOG amplitudes are recorded for about 15 min in darkness. As the EOG amplitude gradual decreases, the dark trough is reached after about 11–12 min although it may be reached earlier or later. To ensure that the true minimal EOG amplitude has been reached, testing should continue until the EOG amplitudes have risen above the dark trough for at least 2 min.

The third phase of EOG is the light adaptation phase during which EOG amplitudes are recorded with the steady background light stimulus of the full-field dome. The light peak is usually reached after about 7–10 min, and testing is continued until the EOG amplitude has fallen below the light peak for at least 2 min. If no light peak can be identified, testing should be continued for a total of 20 min to exclude the presence of a late light peak.

The results of the EOG are typically plotted as a graph of time vs. saccadic amplitude by the recording system (Fig. 4.5). The dark trough and the light peak amplitudes are identified visually or mathematically by smoothing the plot. Unusually high or low points due to eye movement or blink artifacts should be excluded from analysis.

EOG AMPLITUDE RATIO—ARDEN RATIO

In 1962, Arden and Fojas (16) discovered that the ratio of the EOG light-peak to dark-trough amplitude ratio provides a more consistent measure and is clinically more useful than the actual value of the amplitudes which may vary widely among individuals. The large interindividual differences in EOG amplitudes are due not only to the normal physiologic variation of the resting retinal potential but also due to anatomical variation of the location of the globe to the canthi. For instance, persons with shallow orbits or proptosis have higher absolute EOG amplitude because the canthal electrodes are located more posteriorly to the globe during saccades (17). Differences in recording techniques also contribute to the interindividual differences in EOG amplitudes. In contrast, interocular amplitude differences in normal individual are usually small.

The light-peak to dark-trough amplitude ratio is commonly called the Arden ratio. The Arden ratio is typically 1.8 or greater in normal subjects, and is considered abnormal below 1.6. In rare cases, recorded EOG amplitudes may be so low that a minor upward drift of amplitude during the light adaptation phase could result in a falsely elevated Arden ratio. Re-test variability has less effect on the Arden ratio than on the actual EOG amplitudes. Collection of age-matched normative data by each facility is recommended. The maturation and age-related changes of EOG are discussed in Chapter 6.

ALTERNATIVE EOG METHOD: LIGHT-PEAK TO DARK-ADAPTED BASELINE AMPLITUDE RATIO

As an alternative EOG measure to the light-peak to dark-trough amplitude ratio, the light-peak to dark-adapted baseline amplitude ratio can also be acquired. In this method, during the preadaptation phase, excessive light exposure should be similarly avoided but exposure to dimmer than recommended light levels has little effect on the ensuing extended dark adaptation phase. After at least 40 min of dark adaptation, the EOG is recorded for 5 min or longer until a stable baseline is reached. A light adaptation phase is then performed to establish the light peak, and the ratio of the light-peak to dark-adapted baseline amplitude is calculated.

REPORTING THE EOG RESULT

The EOG report should mention whether the procedure meets the international standard and whether the calculated light-peak to darkness amplitude ratio is based on the dark-trough or the dark-adapted baseline. Amplitudes and latencies of the light peak and dark trough should be available, and the time vs. saccadic amplitude plot is helpful. An evaluation of the quality and accuracy of the saccades is also useful.

NON-PHOTIC EOG RESPONSES

Changes in EOG are not always induced by light. A reduction in EOG amplitude occurs with intravenous infusion of hyperosmolar agents such as mannitol, and this is called the hyperosmolarity-induced response (18). Carbonic anhydrase inhibitors such as acetazolamide inhibit the conversion of carbon dioxide to bicarbonate and reduce EOG amplitude by interfering with RPE function (19). Infusion of bicarbonate ions also reduces EOG amplitude most likely because of an increase in bicarbonate concentration on the basal RPE membrane which produces depolarization of the apical RPE membrane (20). In contrast, ingestion of ethyl alcohol increases the dark-adapted EOG amplitude in the absence of light (21). Similar to the effect of light, the alcohol-induced response is due to an increased in the Cl^- conductance in the basal and lateral surfaces of the RPE.

These non-photic EOG responses have been proposed as possible objective provocative tests of RPE function, and several reports have demonstrated abnormal non-photic EOG responses in various retinal conditions such as retinitis pigmentosa, Stargardt macular dystrophy, fundus albipunctatus, and Best macular dystrophy (22–24). Further investigations are needed to determine whether the non-photic EOG responses are clinically useful.

FAST OSCILLATIONS OF THE EOG

The fast oscillation of the EOG occurs over 60–75 sec after the onset of light adaptation (3,25,26). The fast oscillation is produced by hyperpolarization of the basal RPE membrane in response to the decrease in extracellular K^+ of the photoreceptor outer segments. The clinical utility of EOG fast oscillations is unclear and specialized recording techniques are required. Brief alternating light and dark periods of 60–80 sec each are recommended for recording the fast oscillation and a period of preadaptation is not essential. Continuous recording of the saccades is done over at least six completed light–dark cycles. The fast oscillations decrease with light and increase with darkness and are delayed by approximately 50% of the stimulus cycle.

REFERENCES

1. Dubois-Reymond EH. Chapter 3. Von dem ruhen Nervenstrome. Untersuchungen Uber Thierische Electricität. Vol. 2. Berlin: G Reimer, 1849:251–288.

2. Marg E. Development of electro-oculography. Arch Ophthalmol 1951; 45:169–185.

3. Marmor MF, Zrenner E. Standard for clinical electro-oculogram. Arch Ophthalmol 1993; 111:601–604.

4. Steinberg RH, Linsenmeier RA, Griff ER. Three light-evoked responses of the retinal pigment epithelium. Vision Res 1983; 23:1315–1323.

5. Linsemeter RA, Steinberg RH. Origin and sensitivity of the light peak of the intact cat eye. J Physiol 1982; 331:653–673.

6. Miller SS, Edelman DJ. Active ion transport pathways in the bovine retinal pigment epitehlium. J Physiol 1990; 424:283–300.

7. Miller SS, Steinberg RH. Active transport of ions across the frog retinal pigment epithelium. Exp Eye Res 1977; 25:235–248.

8. Steinberg RH, Griff ER, Linsenmeier RA. The cellular origin of the light peak. Doc Ophthalmol Proc Ser 1983; 39:1–11.

9. Röver J, Bach M. C-wave versus electrooculogram in diseases of the retinal pigment epithelium. Doc Ophthalmol 1987; 65:385–391.

10. Skoog K-O. The directly recorded standing potential of the human eye. Acta Ophthalmol (Copenh) 1975; 53:120–132.

11. Arden GB, Kelsey JH. Changes produced by light in the standing potential of the human eye. J Physiol (Lond) 1962; 161:189–204.

12. François J, Szmigielski M, Verriest G, DeRouck A. The influence of changes in illumination on the standing potential of the human eye. Ophthalmologica 1965; 150:83–91.

13. Homer LD, Kolder HE. The oscillation of the human corneoretinal potential at different light intensities. Pflügers Arch Gesamte Physiol 1967; 296:133–142.

14. Krüger C, Baier M. Increment threshold function of the light-induced slow oscillation of the EOG. Doc Ophthalmol Proc Ser 1983; 37:75–80.

15. Brigell M, Bach M, Barber C, Kawasaki K, Koojiman A. Guidelines for calibration of stimulus and recording parameters used in clinical electrophysiology of vision. Calibration standard committee of the international society for clinical electrophysiology of vision (ISCEV). Doc Ophthalmol 1998; 95:1–14.

16. Arden G, Fojas MR. Electrophysiologic abnormalities in pigmentary degenerations of the retina. Arch Ophthalmol 1962; 68:369–389.

17. Alexandridis E, Ariely E, Gronau G. Einfluss der Bulbuslage und der Bulbausalänge auf das EOG. Graefes Arch Ophthalmol 1975; 194:237–241.

18. Madachi-Yamamoto S, Yonemura D, Kawasaki K. Hyperosmolarity response of ocular standing potential as a clinical test for retinal pigment epithelial activity. Normative data. Doc Ophthalmol 1984; 57:153–162.

19. Madachi-Yamamoto S, Yonemura D, Kawasaki K. Diamox response of ocular standing potential as a clinical test for retinal pigment epithelial activity. Acta Soc Ophthalmol Jpn 1984; 88:1267–1272.

20. Segawa Y, Shirao Y, Kawasaki K. Retinal pigment epithelial origin of bicarbonate response. Jpn J Ophthalmol 1997; 41:231–234.

21. Arden GB, Wolf JE. The human electro-oculogram interaction of light and alcohol. Invest Ophthalmol Vis Sci 2000; 41:2722–2729.

22. Arden GB, Wolf JE. The electro-oculographic responses to alcohol and light in a series of patients with retinitis pigmentosa. Invest Ophthalmol Vis Sci 2000; 41:2730–2734.

23. Gupta LY, Marmor MF. Sequential recording of photic and non photic electro-oculogram responses in patients with extensive extramacular drusen. Doc Ophthalmol 1994; 88:49–55.

24. Yonemura D, Kawasaki K, Madachi-Yamamoto S. Hyperosmolarity response of ocular standing potential as a clinical test for retinal pigment epithelial activity. Chorioretinal dystrophies. Doc Ophthalmol 1984; 57:163–173.

25. Kolder H, Brechner GA. Fast oscillations of the corneoretinal potential in man. Arch Ophthalmol 1966; 75:232–237.

26. Weleber RG. Fast and slow oscillations of the electro-oculogram in Best's macular dystrophy and retinitis pigmentosa. Arch Ophthalmol 1989; 107:530–537.

5

Visual Evoked Potential

In visual evoked potential (VEP), the electroencephalographic (EEG) signals of the brain elicited by visual stimuli are recorded with cutaneous electrodes placed on the scalp in the occipital region. Unlike the EOG and different types of ERG which measure activities of the retina or the retinal ganglion cells, VEP is the only electrophysiologic test that assesses visual cortical activity. Standard for VEP recording has been established by the International Society for Clinical Electrophysiology of Vision (ISCEV) and is available on the ISCEV Internet website. The standard is reviewed every 3 years and published periodically. A summary of the standard is provided in Table 5.1.

CLINICAL UTILITY OF VEP

The VEP provides a clinical measure of the function of the visual pathway. In the clinic, VEP is commonly performed to detect visual pathway deficits in patients with no apparent objective signs of ocular dysfunction, in other words, unexplained visual loss. For instance, the utility of VEP in

Table 5.1 Summary of International Standard for Visual Evoked Potential (VEP)

Clinical protocol	
Pupils	Undilated
Fixation	Fixation target in center of stimulus
Refraction	Best-correction for testing distance for pattern reversal VEP and pattern onset/offset VEP
Normal values	Each laboratory to determine age gender, and interocular difference norms from direct tabulation of normal responses with median and 95% confidence limits as minimum outer limits of normal
Recording	At least two replications of each stimulus to confirm responses
Analysis time	$\geq$250 msec; 500 msec if both onset and offset responses are analyzed for pattern onset/offset VEP
Electrode placement	International 10/20 system
Stimulus parameters of the three standard responses	
Pattern reversal VEP	Abrupt alternating black and white checkerboard; white element $> 80 \, cd \, m^{-2}$, contrast between white and black elements $> 75\%$, mean luminance $> 40 \, cd \, m^{-2}$, background $\sim 40 \, cd \, m^{-2}$; reversal rates between 1 and 3 reversals per second (0.5–1.5 Hz); overall screen luminance should not vary during testing (usually requires equal number of light and dark elements); at least two pattern element sizes, 1° and 15 min checks should be tested; visual field stimulated should subtend $\geq$15° visual angle
Pattern onset/offset VEP	Pattern similar to pattern reversal VEP with interspersed abrupt diffuse blank luminance between pattern stimulus; no change in mean luminance as pattern appears or disappears; 100 msec to 200 msec of pattern presentation separated by at least 400 msec diffuse background

Flash VEP	Standard flash ($1.5–3.0\,\mathrm{cd\,s\,m^{-2}}$) as defined in ERG standards; background light $15–30\,\mathrm{cd\,m^{-2}}$, subtend $\geq 20°$ visual angle
Designation of waveform components	
Flash VEP	N_1, P_1, N_2, P_2, N_3, P_3, N_4
Pattern reversal VEP	N_{75}, P_{100}, N_{135}
Pattern onset/offset VEP	C_1, C_2, C_3
Pre-chiasmal, chiasmal, and postchiasmal assessment	Prechiasmal assessment
	Pattern VEP with monocular stimulation recommended; pattern onset/offset VEP has greater inter-subject variability than pattern reversal VEP but has little intra-subject variability. Pattern onset/offset VEP is less prone to deliberate patient defocusing of stimulus and is most effective for estimating visual acuity; flash VEP used for any assessments for patients with poor fixation and/or dense media opacities
	Chiasmal and postchiasmal assessment
	Not part of standard; multiple electrodes at midline and laterally recommended; pattern stimulation
Reporting results	Indicate whether the international standard were met; inclusion of the following are recommended-eye tested, designated electrode position of the recording channel, field size of stimulus, flash intensity, pattern element size, and contrast of pattern stimuli; two replications of waveforms obtained

(Continued)

Table 5.1 Summary of International Standard for Visual Evoked Potential (VEP) (*Continued*)

Basic technology	
Stimulus calibration	Flash stimulus intensity measured by an integrated photometer
	Photometer in non-integrating mode or spot photometer for white stimulus areas, luminance $\geq 80\,cd\,m^{-2}$; field luminance uniform, varying by $< 30\%$ between center and periphery of tested field; contrast maximal (not $<75\%$) between black and white squares or gratings
Electrode	Standard silver–silver chloride or gold disc electroencephalography (EEG) electrodes ($\leq 5\,k\Omega$ impedance); fixed to scalp and maintained as recommended by manufacturer
Recording parameters	
Amplification and averaging systems	Analog high pass and low pass filters set at $\leq 1\,Hz$ and $\geq 100\,Hz$, analogue filter roll-off slopes $\leq 12\,dB$ per octave for low frequencies and $\leq 24\,dB$ per octave for high frequencies
	Amplification of input signal by 20,000–50,000, channel to channel amplification difference $<1\%$; impedance of preamplifiers $\geq 10\,M\Omega$
	Analogue signal digitized ≥ 500 samples per second per channel, 8 bit minimal resolution
	Automatic artifact rejection to exclude signals exceeding ± 50–$100\,\mu V$
	Number of repetition or sweeps for each stimulus, ≥ 64 for each trial
Repetition rate	Low temporal frequency, <2 stimuli per second

identifying occult visual pathway dysfunction in patients with multiple sclerosis has been demonstrated. An impaired VEP can be produced by a deficit large enough anywhere along the visual pathway including the retina, optic nerve, and brain. Therefore, an impaired VEP is anatomically non-specific unless it is used in combination with a thorough ocular examination and other clinical modalities such as visual field, ERG, and neuroimaging. In short, VEP should not be performed in place of a comprehensive ophthalmic examination or neuroimaging. Impaired VEP responses may be produced in some normal persons by deliberate poor fixation, defocusing, or conscious suppression (1–3). Pattern onset/offset and flash VEP are less susceptible to this effect than pattern reversal VEP. The use of VEP in cortical blindness and non-organic visual loss are discussed in Chapters 17 and 16, respectively. The VEP as a measure of visual function in infants and young preverbal children is detailed in Chapter 6.

Physiologic Origins of VEP

The physiologic basis of VEP is predominantly from the activity of the primary visual cortex located at the posterior tip of the occipital lobe (Fig. 5.1). The primary visual cortex, referred to as the striate cortex and anatomically designated as V1, is not a flat surface but folds inward to form the calcarine sulcus. The striate cortex receives visual projections from the lateral geniculate neurons by way of the optic radiations. These projections terminate in alternating eye-specific columns called ocular dominance columns of cortical layer IV of the striate cortex. The signals of the two eyes are combined beyond this cellular layer so that most cortical neurons are binocular with receptive fields that are in the same visual field location in each eye. As a consequence of the semi-decussation of the retinal ganglion cell fibers at the optic chiasm, the right hemifield is represented in the left striate cortex and the left hemifield is represented in the right striate cortex. In addition, the upper visual field is represented below the calcarine sulcus, and the lower visual field is represented above the calcarine sulcus.

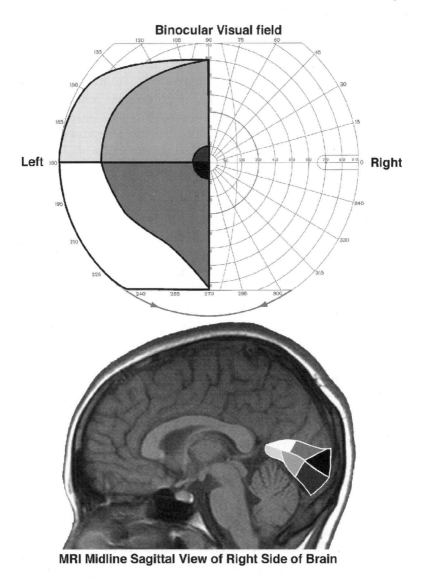

MRI Midline Sagittal View of Right Side of Brain

Figure 5.1   Visual field representation of the striate cortex. The central 10° of the visual field is represented by a disproportionately large caudal part of the striate cortex. This portion of the visual cortex is closest to the electrodes placed at the scalp for VEP recording, and therefore, VEP is dominated by the central visual field. In contrast, peripheral visual field is represented more anteriorly, further away from the VEP recording electrodes.

The clinical VEP is dominated by activity from the central visual field because the topographical representation of visual field in the striate cortex is not evenly distributed (4). The fovea or central vision is represented disproportionately by a large cortical area occupying the posterior portion of the striate cortex, near the scalp where the VEP recording electrodes are placed (Figs. 5.1 and 5.2). This disproportionate representation of central vision reflects the high density of photoreceptors and the high number of retinal ganglion cell projections from the fovea. At least 50% of the cortical neurons of the striate cortex have receptive fields in the central 10° of the visual field. In contrast, the peripheral retina has a lower ganglion cell density with each ganglion cell receiving converging signals from several photoreceptors. The peripheral visual field is represented by smaller cortical area located more anteriorly in the striate cortex. This cortical area lies deep in the calcarine sulcus away from the VEP scalp electrodes and has a limited contribution to the clinical VEP.

Pattern stimulus consisting of alternating black-white checkerboard is commonly used in clinical VEP because it generates the most vigorous cortical response. While the cells of the retina and the lateral geniculate body respond well to a change in luminance in their receptive field, the cortical neurons of the striate cortex respond more actively to light–dark edges and orientation (5,6). Three physiologic categories of retinal ganglion cells are recognized, magnocellular, parvocellular, and koniocellular (7,8). Information derived from magnocellular ganglion cells is related to movement of objects in space, information from parvocellular ganglion cells is related to visual acuity and color perception, and information from koniocellular ganglion cells is related to form. These physiologic-specific ganglion cells project to different layers of the lateral geniculate nucleus. This physiologic segregation continues in the striate cortex, V1, as well as in the projections from V1 to V2.

In addition to the striate cortex, the clinical VEP receives lesser contributions from other extrastriate visual processing areas in the occipital, parietal, and temporal lobes. These areas rely on signals from the striate cortex for their activation.

VEP Electrode Positions

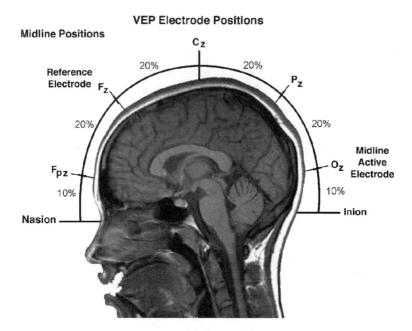

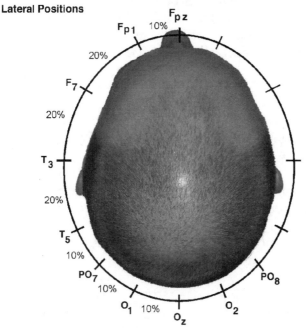

Figure 5.2 (*Caption on facing page*)

These areas may be organized into two broad pathways starting from the striate cortex forward. A ventral pathway to the temporal lobe is involved in object recognition, and a dorsal pathway to the parietal lobe is implicated in spatial vision. Visual processing areas such as V2, V3, V4, VP, MT, and MST are buried in deeper sulci, and each has specific response properties. For instance, V4 responds selectively to color of the stimulus while the middle temporal (MT) area responds selectively to direction. Specialized VEP techniques with different stimulus characteristics and electrode placements may be utilized to activate and record activities from more specific visual processing pathways.

Clinical VEP Recording

The noise-to-signal ratio of VEP recording is high, and computer averaging of multiple recordings or sweeps is necessary to isolate the VEP response. The VEP amplitude from a visual stimulus is usually less than $25\,\mu V$ and significantly smaller than the continuous ongoing EEG that could be up to $100\,\mu V$. For a clinical VEP recording run, an average of at least 64 sweeps is recommended, and at least two similar results are required to confirm reproducibility.

The high noise-to-signal ratio of VEP explains why VEP amplitude has relatively high intra-subject as well as inter-subject variability (9,10). A variability of 25% in VEP amplitude is not too uncommon with repeat flash VEP testing during a single recording session in the same person. The placement of VEP electrodes is guided by surface bony

Figure 5.2 *(Facing page)* Placement of VEP electrodes based on the International 10/20 system. The electrode locations are obtained by percent distances with respect to bony landmarks. The anterior/posterior midline measurements for placement of the reference electrode at F_z and recording electrode O_z are determined by the distance between the nasion (the junction between the nose and the forehead) and the inion (the ridge at the back of the skull just above the neck). The circumferential distance from the frontal pole to O_z (occipital pole) is used to locate lateral electrode positions.

landmarks, therefore, the anatomical differences in folding patterns of gyri and sulci as well as in the relationship between visual cortex and surface landmarks contribute to VEP variability among individuals.

In contrast to VEP amplitude, VEP latency is the more consistent and useful clinical measure (9,10). The reproducibility of VEP latency in a normal subject is usually less than 5%, and variability among subjects is much less than VEP amplitude. Collection of age-matched normative data by each facility is recommended. The maturation and age-related changes of VEP are discussed in Chapter 6.

Pharmacologic dilation of the pupils is generally not needed for VEP testing. Pattern reversal VEP and pattern onset/offset VEP require best-corrected near visual acuity and consistent accurate fixation—both of which may be impaired by pupil dilation. Pupil dilation is typically not necessary for flash VEP. However, marked miosis can cause increased VEP latency, and a large anisocoria may produce falsely asymmetric VEP.

Monocular stimulated VEP should be performed for each eye to detect monocular visual pathway dysfunction. Interocular VEP asymmetry is relatively low in a normal subject. Binocular stimulated VEP is helpful when monocular responses are questionable to determine if any signals are reaching the visual cortex. Periodic calibration of the recording system should be performed as recommended by the manufacturer and based on the international calibration standard (11).

VEP Electrode Placement

Standard silver–silver chloride or gold disc EEG electrodes are placed on the scalp for recording VEP responses. The positions of the electrodes are determined by measurement from identifiable bony landmarks based on a method supported by anatomical studies known as the International 10/20 system (Fig. 5.2) (12). The designated electrode positions take into account brain size and underlying brain area but cannot account for interindividual variations in folding patterns of gyri and sulci. With the reference electrode placed at F_z, VEP may be recorded by a single midline electrode at O_z. If more channels are available, additional electrodes may be placed laterally. Three channels using the midline and two lateral active electrodes are suggested if more specific detection of chiasmal and retrochiasmal dysfunction is desired. A ground electrode is typically placed on the forehead, vertex (position Cz), mastoid, or earlobe.

Three Standard VEP Responses

At least one of three recommended transient VEP responses should be included in clinical VEP testing—pattern reversal VEP, pattern onset/offset VEP, and flash VEP (Fig. 5.3). Transient VEP responses are produced when the stimulus rates are slow enough to allow the brain to recover to its resting state between stimuli. Steady-state VEP responses occur when stimulus rates are too fast to allow the brain to reach resting state between stimuli. Transient VEP responses are usually elicited when the stimulus rate is less than 5 Hz, which permits the identification of specific VEP waveform components and their amplitudes and latencies. Steady-state VEP provides higher frequency response components and is not ordinarily performed in the clinic except with specialized techniques.

The VEP tracing is presented often as positive upward in the ophthalmic literature or positive downward in the neurologic literature. Therefore, any VEP waveform should have its polarity clearly labeled. Positive upward is recommended by the ISCEV standard.

Pattern Reversal VEP

The pattern reversal VEP is elicited by a checkerboard-like stimulus of alternating black and white square checks that reverse in a regular phase frequency (Fig. 5.3). The pattern reversal VEP is the clinical VEP study of choice because it generates relatively consistent and vigorous responses from the visual cortex. The pattern reversal VEP has relatively high reproducibility within a subject and low variability of

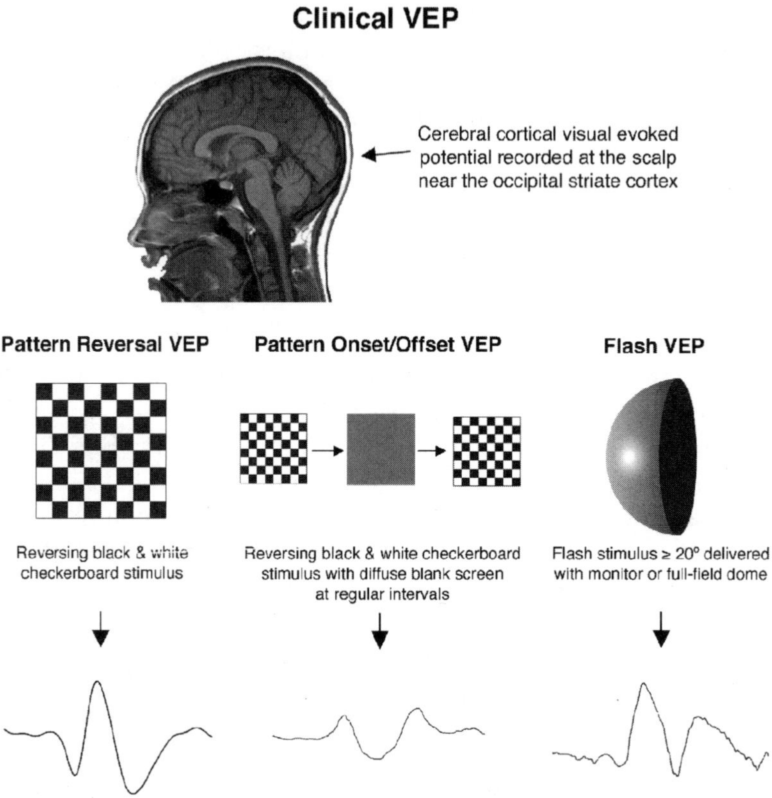

Clinical VEP

Cerebral cortical visual evoked
potential recorded at the scalp
near the occipital striate cortex

Pattern Reversal VEP　　**Pattern Onset/Offset VEP**　　　**Flash VEP**

Reversing black & white
checkerboard stimulus

Reversing black & white checkerboard
stimulus with diffuse blank screen
at regular intervals

Flash stimulus ≥ 20° delivered
with monitor or full-field dome

Figure 5.3 Clinical VEP responses. At least one of the three standard VEP responses should be included in clinical VEP assessment. In most cases, the pattern reversal VEP is the study of choice because it generates relatively consistent and vigorous responses from the visual cortex.

waveform and peak latency across normal subjects. Steady fixation and best-corrected near visual acuity are required during testing.

The black-and-white checkerboard stimulus consists of equal number and size of alternating black and white squares. A fixation point is located at the center of the stimulus at the common corner of the central four checks. The luminance of the white squares should be at least 80 cd/m^2 with a contrast of at least 75% compared to black squares. The pattern stimulus is defined by the visual angle subtended by the side length of a single check. To calculate the visual angle, the check side length is divided by the distance from the stimulus center to the tested eye. The result is the tangent of the visual angle subtended by each check. Inverse tangent is then used to obtain the visual angle. The overall size of the stimulus should be greater than 15° at its narrowest dimension. The overall mean luminance should be uniform and remain stable during pattern reversal. The room is illuminated at a level approximately the same as the illuminance produced by the stimulus at the patient position.

Responses from two check sizes, 15 and 60 min (min = minutes, 1° = 60 min), are recommended. The large 60-min check stimulus will elicit more parafoveal response while the small 15-min check stimulus will elicit mostly foveal response. The reversal rate should be between 1 and 4 reversals per second, equivalent to a phase frequency of 0.5–2 Hz.

The pattern reversal VEP waveform consists of a series of negative (N) and positive (P) components designated by approximate latency (Fig. 5.4). Components N75, P100, and N135 are recognized. The amplitude of P100 is measured from the preceding negative peak N75 to the peak of P100. The latency is the time from stimulus onset to the peak of each component. The P100 peak has a latency of near 100 msec in normal subjects but its value depends on check size, check contrast, overall stimulus size, and pattern mean luminance.

Pattern Onset/Offset VEP

The pattern onset/offset VEP is elicited by a reversing checkerboard stimulus separated by regular periods of diffuse blank screen (Fig. 5.3). The checkerboard stimulus is the same as pattern reversal VEP, but the stimulus is periodically interrupted by a diffuse blank screen with the same luminance as the mean luminance of the checkerboard. For example, 200 msec of pattern reversal presentations are separated by 400 msec of isoluminant blank screen.

Pattern onset/offset VEP has greater variability across subjects than pattern reversal VEP and is less frequently

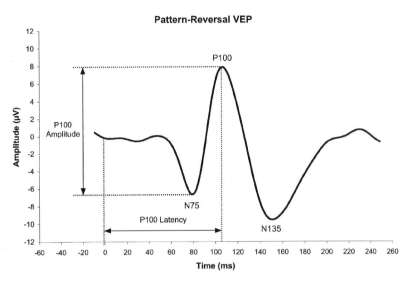

Figure 5.4 Normal standard pattern reversal VEP response. The pattern reversal VEP waveform consists of a series of negative (N) and positive (P) components designated by approximate latency. The amplitude of P100 is measured from the preceding negative peak N75 to the peak of P100. The latency is the time from stimulus onset to the peak of each component. The P100 peak has a latency of near 100 msec in normal subjects but its value depends on check size, check contrast, overall stimulus size, and pattern mean luminance.

performed. Pattern onset/offset VEP responses are less affected by poor fixation, and clinical applications include estimating potential visual acuity in preverbal children and VEP assessment in patients with nystagmus or poor fixation. Pattern onset/offset VEP is less susceptible than pattern reversal VEP to deliberate poor fixation, defocusing, or conscious suppression that may occur in patients with non-organic visual loss.

The pattern onset/offset VEP waveform consists of a series of positive and negative components designated by order of appearance (Fig. 5.5). Component C1, C2, and C3 are recognized. Positive peak C1 has a latency of approximately 75 msec, negative peak C2 has a latency of approximately 125 msec, and

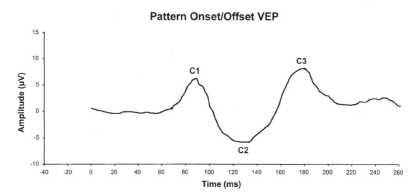

Figure 5.5 Normal standard pattern onset/offset VEP. Positive C1, negative C2, and positive C3 have latencies of approximately 75, 125, and 150 msec, respectively, measured from stimulus onset. The amplitude of each component is measured from the preceding peak to the peak of the component. Only the pattern onset response is recorded with a recording time of 260 msec.

positive peak C3 has a latency of approximately 150 msec. The amplitude is measured from the preceding peak to the peak of the component, and latency is the time from stimulus onset to the peak of each component.

Flash VEP

The flash VEP is elicited by a flash stimulus as defined by the standard flash of the international ERG standard (see Chapter 1) (Fig. 5.3). The white flash stimulus can be delivered in a full-field dome in the presence of the light adapting (photopic) background from the ERG standard. The stimulus rate should not be high enough to elicit a steady-state response, and a typical rate of 2–3 Hz is commonly used to attain a transient response. Flash VEP is highly variable among subjects and are usually tested in persons who are unable to perform pattern VEP because of poor fixation due to poor visual acuity, nystagmus, or inability (Fig. 5.6).

The flash VEP waveform consists of a series of negative (N) and positive (P) components designated by numerical order based on the timing sequence (Fig. 5.5). The most prominent

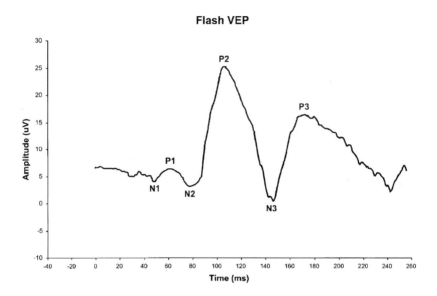

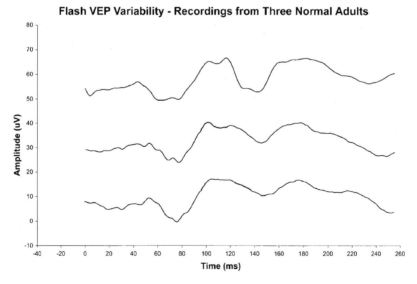

Figure 5.6 Standard flash VEP and its variability. The flash VEP waveform consists of a series of negative (N) and positive (P) components. The most prominent response is P2 with a normal peak of near 100–120 msec measured from stimulus onset. Variations of size and shape of flash VEP components across normal subjects are commonly encountered.

response is P2, and its amplitude is measured from the preceding negative peak N2 to the peak of P2. Latency of P2 is the time from stimulus onset to its peak and is near 100–120 msec in normal subjects. This nomenclature is recommended to automatically differentiate flash VEP components from pattern reversal and onset/offset components but is not universally followed. For example, P2 has been called P100 based on its approximate latency. Variations of size, timing, and shape of flash VEP components across normal subjects are commonly encountered.

Reporting VEP Results

Report of VEP results should specify which three standard responses were performed and whether the international standard was followed. Stimulus parameters such as check sizes should be stated. The polarity of the presentation of the waveform should be clearly labeled. Positive upward used commonly in ophthalmic literature is recommended rather than positive downward as used in neurologic literature. Amplitude and latency values should be available along with normative data.

SPECIALIZED VEP TECHNIQUES

Sweep VEP

The sweep VEP technique involves the recording of steady-state VEP activity to a high-frequency stimulus that lasts several seconds (13,14). The stimulus changes slowly with either increasing spatial or contrast frequency. In the sweep spatial frequency stimulus, the spatial frequency of a reversing stimulus is increased in steps while the rate of the reversal, that is, temporal frequency, remains unchanged. This type of stimulus usually consists of vertically oriented alternating black-and-white stripes whose width decreases in linear or logarithmic steps during recording. As the gratings go from coarse to fine, that is, increasing spatial frequency, a quasi-sinusoidal response is generated at the visual cortex, and the resultant VEP is recorded (Fig. 5.7). With this type of

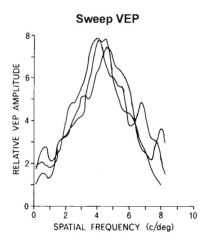

Figure 5.7 Sweep VEP. The steady-state VEP response from a spatial linearly swept stimulus is shown. The stimulus consists of reversing vertically oriented alternating black-and-white stripes whose width decreases in linear steps during recording. As the gratings go from coarse to fine, that is, increasing spatial frequency, a quasi-sinusoidal steady-state VEP response is generated by the visual cortex. Three tracings are shown to demonstrate reproducibility. (From Ref. 14 with permission of *Investigative Ophthalmology and Visual Science.*)

rapid response retrieval, the steady VEP voltage is recorded without signal averaging. In the sweep contrast stimulus, the contrast of a reversing pattern is increased while the spatial and temporal frequencies remain unchanged. As the stimulus goes from faint to distinct, the VEP activity is recorded.

Sweep VEP is analyzed by measuring the VEP activity at the actual and harmonic temporal frequencies of the stimulus. In sweep spatial frequency VEP, the results are graphed by plotting the width of the gratings in cycles per degree against the corresponding VEP amplitudes to obtain the stimulus–response function (Fig. 5.7). Several studies have demonstrated that visual acuity can be estimated in infants and preverbal children based on extrapolating the graph to obtain the highest spatial frequency that produces noise level amplitude (see Chapter 6) (15,16). Similarly, in sweep contrast frequency VEP, a stimulus–response function is generated by plotting the VEP amplitudes against the corresponding stimulus contrast.

Multifocal VEP

In multifocal VEP, VEP responses from multiple localized visual field areas are recorded simultaneously by using the same principle as the multifocal ERG (see Chapter 2). The result is a visual field map of VEP responses. The stimulus typically consists of an alternating black-and-white checkerboard pattern organized in sectors, which are scaled to account for cortical magnification (Fig. 5.8). During recording, the checkerboard elements of each visual field sector reverse in a pseudorandom maximum-length sequence (m-sequence) and have a probability of 0.5 of reversing on any frame change. To maintain overall isoluminance, at any given moment, about half of the total elements are white and half are black. The rate of frame change is in the order of 75 Hz. The VEP responses within each visual field sector are calculated and combined as the overall response for that visual field area. Although multifocal VEP may be recorded with one midline occipital electrode, recordings from multiple electrodes or channels reduce signal-to-noise ratio and improve the quality of multifocal VEP (17).

Summed multifocal VEPs are not equivalent to the conventional pattern-reversal VEP response (18). In contrast to conventional VEP, multifocal VEP from the upper visual field is reversed compared to multifocal VEP of the lower visual field (Fig. 5.8). This difference may be due to the fast multifocal VEP sequence that produces less contribution from the extrastriate cortex. When multifocal VEP responses from the lower visual field are summed, an initial negative component (C1) occurs at about 65 msec followed by a positive component (C2) at about 95 msec. The C1 and C2 components of the multifocal VEP are analogous to the N75 and P100 components of the conventional pattern VEP, but the C2

Multifocal VEP

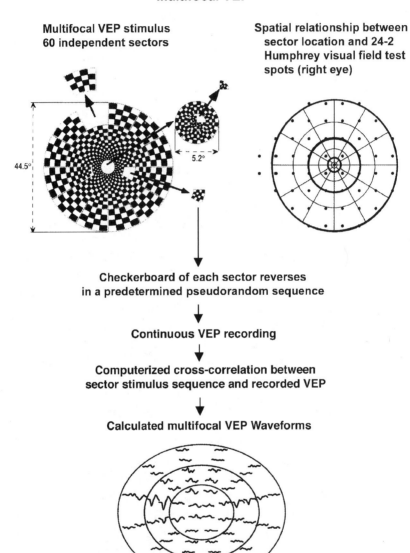

Figure 5.8 Schematic diagram showing the basic principles of multifocal VEP. (From Ref. 42 with permission from the American Medical Association.)

component is smaller and slightly faster than the conventional P100 component.

Multifocal VEP responses are variable among normal subjects due to anatomical differences of the cerebral cortex as well as the location of the external cranial bony landmarks that guide placement of the VEP electrodes (19). On the other hand, multifocal VEP responses from the two eyes of normal subjects are essentially identical except for small interocular difference in timing attributable to nasotemporal retinal differences so that interocular comparison of multifocal VEP may be helpful in identifying local monocular dysfunction (20).

Several authors have demonstrated a direct correlation between multifocal VEP responses and visual field defects such as those occurring in glaucoma (17,21–24). Whether multifocal VEP is more useful than conventional tests such as visual field remains to be determined. Because a majority of patients, who are poor visual field performers, are able to perform multifocal VEP, multifocal VEP may be helpful in patients who cannot perform reliable visual fields such as in those with non-organic visual loss. However, a few patients with normal automated visual fields cannot produce usable multifocal VEP recordings because of high noise level presumably due to a large EEG alpha contribution or scalp muscle tension or both.

Binocular Beat VEP

The binocular beat VEP technique assesses binocularity of the visual cortex by dichoptic luminance stimulation in which stimuli of different luminance frequencies are presented simultaneously to each eye (25). The stimulus consists of two uniform fields of equal average luminance but whose luminances are modulating sinusoidally at different temporal frequencies. During testing, the two eyes of the subject are stimulated simultaneously with each eye being stimulated by one of the two fields. As the two monocular stimulus fields fade in and out at two different rates, the two stimulus fields will come in and out of phase with each

other. The combined monocular signals at the normal binocular visual cortex will summate and cancel each other at
a frequency known as the beat frequency, which is equal
to the difference of the two luminance frequencies of the
monocular stimuli (Fig. 5.9). The binocular response of the
visual cortex is recordable as a VEP steady-state response
at the selected binocular beat frequency. In subjects with
impaired binocularity such as amblyopia, the cells of the
visual cortex are predominantly monocular, and the binocular beat VEP is impaired (26–28).

Motion VEP

Several authors have reported VEP responses generated by a
variety of motion stimuli consisting mostly of moving gratings
or dot patterns. For example, the stimulus may alternate
between moving in one direction and staying
stationary to elicit a motion-onset response. Alternatively, a
steady-state motion VEP response may be produced by a ran-
dom-dot pattern which oscillates between phases of perceiva-
ble motion (coherent motion) and snowstorm (incoherent
motion) (29). Motion VEP may also be generated by a stimulus which moves in alternating directions.
Similar to conventional pattern reversal VEP, motion VEP
typically has a positive peak (P1) at 100–120 msec followed
by a negative peak (N2) at 160–200 msec, but the motion
VEP waveform is more complex and variable. The motion
VEP response is highly dependent on the characteristics of
the stimulus such as stimulus type, contrast, and spatial frequency as well as the location of the recording and reference
electrodes (30). In general, the motion response is represented
by N2 while form processing is represented mostly by P1, and
the motion response signals are located more laterally anatomically as compared to conventional VEP responses (31–35).
Several authors have proposed that magnocellular pathway
projecting to the cortical region V5 is involved (36); but other
influences such as color sensitive motion mechanisms have
also been implicated (37,38). The clinical utility of motion
VEP still warrants further study. Motion VEP may be helpful

Principle of Binocular Beat VEP

18 Hz

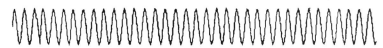

20 Hz

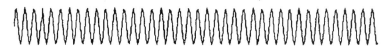

18 + 20 Hz Linear Addition

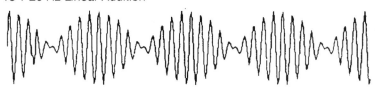

|← ——————————— 2 Seconds ——————————— →|

Figure 5.9 Principle of binocular beat VEP. Binocular beat VEP assesses binocularity of the visual cortex by dichoptic luminance stimulation in which stimuli of different luminance frequencies are presented simultaneously to each eye. The stimulus consists of two uniform fields of equal average luminance but whose luminances are modulating sinusoidally at different temporal frequencies. When two dichoptic uniform fields are sinusoidally modulated in luminance at frequencies f_R in the right eye and f_L in the left eye, the beat is manifested only after integration of the two separate monocular signals in binocular neural channels. This figure illustrates the simple linear combination of the two carrier frequencies, f_R (18 Hz) and f_L (20 Hz) to show a beat at the difference frequency, $f_R - f_L$ (2 Hz). Because the neural mechanisms evoking the actual beat perception are non-linear, the difference frequency (beat) is also accompanied in varying magnitudes by the sum of the two monocular frequencies $(f_R + f_L)$, as well as by harmonic combinations of the beat, sum and carrier frequencies. (From Ref. 25 with permission from Elsevier.)

in detecting defective binocularity in patients with infantile esotropia by demonstrating directional asymmetries of monocular VEP responses in which a nasalward vs. temporalward response bias occurs (39–41).

REFERENCES

1. Bumgartner J, Epstein CM. Voluntary alteration of visual evoked potentials. Ann Neurol 1982; 12:475–478.

2. Morgan RK, Niugent B, Harrison JM, O'Connor PS. Voluntary alteration of pattern visual evoked responses. Ophthalmology 1985; 92:1356–1363.

3. Uren SM, Stewart P, Crosby PA. Subject cooperation and the visual evoked response. Invest Ophthalmol Vis Sci 1979; 18:648–652.

4. Horton JC, Hoyt WF. The representation of the visual field in human striate cortex: a revision of the classic Holmes map. Arch Ophthalmol 1991; 109:816–824.

5. Hubel DH, Wiesel TN. Receptive fields, binocular interaction and functional architecture in the cat's visual cortex. J Physiol (Lond) 1962; 160:106–154.

6. Hubel DH, Wiesel TN. Receptive fields and functional architecture of monkey striate cortex. J Physiol (Lond) 1968; 195:215–243.

7. Hendry SH, Reid RC. The koniocellular pathway in primate vision. Annu Rev Neurosci 2000; 23:127–153.

8. Rodieck RW, Watanabe M. Survey of the morphology of macaque retinal ganglion cells that project to the pretectum, superior colliculus, and parvicellular laminae of the lateral geniculate nucleus. J Comp Neurol 1993; 338:289–303.

9. DeVoe RC, Ripps H, Vaughan HG. Cortical responses to stimulation of the human fovea. Vision Res 1968; 8:135–147.

10. Okens BS, Chiappa KH, Gill E. Normal temporal variability of the P100. Electroencephalogr Clin Neurophysiol 1987; 68:153–156.

11. Brigell M, Bach M, Barber C, Kawasaki K, Koojiman A. Guidelines for calibration of stimulus and recording parameters used

in clinical electrophysiology of vision. Calibration Standard Committee of the International Society for Clinical Electrophysiology of Vision (ISCEV). Doc Ophthalmol 1998; 95:1–14.

12. American Encephalographic Society. Guideline thirteen: guidelines for standard electrode position nomenclature. J Clin Neurophysiol 1994; 11:111–113.

13. Nelson JI, Seiple WH, Kupersmith M, Carr R. Lock-in techniques for the swept stimulus evoked potential. J Clin Neurophysiol 1984; 1:409–436.

14. Tyler CW, Apkarian P, Levi DM, Nakayama K. Rapid assessment of visual function: and electronic sweep technique for the pattern visual evoked potential. Invest Ophthalmol Vis Sci 1979; 18:703–713.

15. Gottlob I, Fendick MG, Guo S, Zubcov AA, Odom JV, Reinecke RD. Visual acuity measurements by swept spatial frequency visual-evoked-cortical potentials (VECPs): clinical application in children with various visual disorders. J Pediatr Ophthalmol Strabismus 1990; 27:40–47.

16. Riddell PM, Ladenheim B, Mast J, Catalano T, Rita N, Hainline L. Comparison of measures of visual acuity in infants: Teller acuity cards and sweep visual evoked potentials. Optom Vis Sci 1997; 74:702–707.

17. Hood DC, Zhang X, Hong JE, Chen CS. Quantifying the benefits of additional channels of multifocal VEP recording. Doc Ophthalmol 2002; 104:303–320.

18. Fortune B, Hood DC. Conventional pattern-reversal VEPs are not equivalent to summed multifocal VEP. Invest Ophthalmol Vis Sci 2003; 44:1364–1375.

19. Baseler HA, Sutter EE, Klein SA, Carney T. The topography of visual evoked response properties across the visual field. Electroencephalogr Clin Neurophysiol 1994; 90:65–81.

20. Hood DC, Zhang X, Greenstein VC, Kangovi S, Odel JG, Liebmann JM, Ritch R. An interocular comparison of the multifocal VEP; a possible technique for detecting local damage to the optic nerve. Invest Ophthalmol Vis Sci 2000; 41:1580–1587.

21. Klistorner AI, Graham SL, Grigg JR, Billson FA. Multifocal topographic visual evoked potential: improving objective

detection of local visual field defects. Invest Ophthalmol Vis Sci 1998; 39:937–950.

22. Klistorner AI, Graham SL. Multifocal pattern VEP perimetry: analysis of sectoral waveforms. Doc Ophthalmol 1999; 98: 183–196.

23. Seiple W, Clemens C, Greenstein VC, Holopigian K, Zhang X. The spatial distribution of selective attention assessed using the multifocal visual evoked potential. Vision Res 2002; 42:1513–1521.

24. Goldberg I, Graham SL, Klistorner AI. Multifocal objective perimetry in the detection of glaucomatous field loss. Am J Ophthalmol 2002; 133:29–39.

25. Baitch LW, Levi DM. Binocular beats: psychophysical studies of binocular interaction in normal and stereoblind humans. Vision Res 1989; 29:27–35.

26. Sloper JJ, Garnham C, Gous P, Dyason R, Plunkett D. Reduced binocular beat visual evoked responses and stereoacuity in patients with Duane syndrome. Invest Ophthalmol Vis Sci 2001; 42:2826–2830.

27. Struck MC, Ver Hoeve JN, France TD. Binocular cortical interactions in the monofixation syndrome. J Pediatr Ophthalmol Strabismus 1996; 33:291–297.

28. Stevens JL, Berman JL, Schmeisser ET, Baker RS. Dichoptic luminance beat visual evoked potentials in the assessment of binocularity in children. J Pediatr Ophthalmol Strabismus 1994; 31:368–373.

29. Snowden RJ, Ulrich D, Bach M. Isolation and characteristics of a steady-state visually evoked potential in humans related to the motion of a stimulus. Vision Res 1995; 35:1365–1373.

30. Odom JV, De Smedt E, Van Malderen L, Spileers W. Visual evoked potentials evoked by moving unidimensional noise stimuli: effects of contrast, spatial frequency, active electrode location, reference electrode location, stimulus type. Doc Ophthalmol 1998–1999; 95:315–333.

31. Bach M, Ullrich D. Motion adaptation governs the shape of motion-evoked cortical potentials. Vision Res 1994; 34: 1541–1547.

32. Bach M, Ullrich D. Contrast dependency of motion-onset and pattern-reversal VEPs: interaction of stimulus type, recording site and response component. Vision Res 1997; 37:1845–1849.

33. Gopfert E, Muller R, Breuer D, Greenlee MW. Similarities and dissimilarities between pattern VEPs and motion VEPs. Doc Ophthalmol 1998–1999; 97:67–79.

34. Hoffmann MB, Unsold AS, Bach M. Directional tuning of human motion adaptation as reflected by the motion VEP. Vision Res 2001; 41:2187–2194.

35. Niedeggen M, Wist ER. Characterstics of visual evoked potentials generated by motion coherence onset. Brain Res Cogn Brain Res 1999; 8:95–105.

36. Kubova Z, Kuba M, Spekreijse H, Blakemore C. Contrast dependence of motion-onset and pattern-reversal evoked potential. Vision Res 1995; 35:197–205.

37. McKeefry DJ. The influence of stimulus chromaticity on the isoluminant motion-onset VEP. Vision Res 2002; 42:909–922.

38. Tobimatsu S, Timoda H, Kato M. Parvocellular and magnocellular contributions to visual evoked potentials in humans: stimulation with chromatic and achromatic gratings and apparent motion. J Neurol Sci 1995; 134:73–82.

39. Norcia AM. Abnormal motion processing and binocularity: infantile esotropia as a model system for effects of early interruptions of binocularity. Eye 1996; 10:259–265.

40. Shea SJ, Chandna A, Norcia AM. Oscillatory motion but not pattern reversal elicits monocular motion VEP biases in infantile esotropia. Vision Res 1999; 39:1803–1811.

41. Brosnahan D, Norcia AM, Schor CM, Taylor DG. OKN, perceptual and VEP direction biases in strabismus. Vision Res 1998; 38:2833–2840.

42. Hood DC, Greenstein VC, Odel JG, Zhang X, Ritch R, Liebmann JM, Chen CS, Thienprasiddhi P. Visual field defects and multifocal visual evoked potentials: evidence of a linear relationship. Arch Ophthalmol 2002; 120:1672–1681.

6

Maturation, Aging, and Testing in Infants

The physiologic effects of maturation and aging on visual electrophysiologic responses are numerous. These influences need to be considered when interpreting electrophysiologic results. Electrophysiologic recording in infants presents unique challenges, and techniques for estimating visual acuity in preverbal children are available. This chapter covers these topics as well as gender and amblyopia. The outline of the chapter is as follows:

- Maturation
- Delayed visual maturation
- Electrophysiologic testing in infants
- Estimating visual acuity in infants
- Amblyopia
- Aging
- Gender

MATURATION

The visual system is not fully developed at birth. The foveal pit is incomplete, and the foveal cone photoreceptors are immature. Myelination of the optic nerve is unfinished, and synapses at the lateral geniculate nucleus and the occipital lobe are underdeveloped. Subsequent development and maturation of the visual system require physiologic maturation and environmental visual stimulation. While studies of maturation of VEP and full-field ERG responses are readily available, similar investigations of focal ERG, multifocal ERG, and pattern ERG are more limited in young patients because of difficulty in maintaining required fixation. Obtaining EOG is also difficult in young patients because of the cooperation needed to perform voluntary eye movements.

Maturation of ERG

Full-field cone and rod ERG responses are small and prolonged but detectable after birth for term newborns as well as for preterm infants as young as 30 weeks after conception (Fig. 6.1) (1–11). However, the retinal luminance of the standard ERG as recommended by the International Society for Clinical Electrophysiology of Vision (ISCEV) is too low to reliably elicit responses at birth (12). A quarter of normal infants 5 weeks and younger have no detectable ISCEV standard rod response, and the lower limits of normal b-wave amplitudes for the ISCEV standard rod response as well as for the combined rod–cone response and the cone response include zero until age 15 weeks (7). Therefore, higher intensity stimuli are required to elicit responses reliably in young infants. A retinal illuminance of approximately 2.0 log units higher than the recommended standard flash is necessary to elicit a rod response in virtually all infants at 36 weeks after conception to produce a mean amplitude of $14\,\mu V$ (1).

Full-field ERG amplitudes and implicit times improve most rapidly during the first 4 months of life followed by slower development thereafter (Fig. 6.1). In general, mean ERG parameters enter the low range of adult values by age

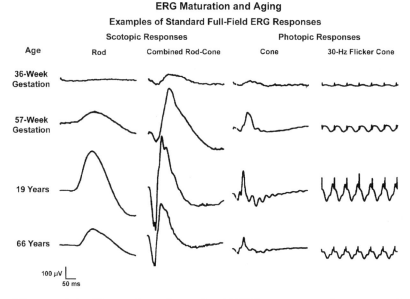

Figure 6.1 Examples of standard ERG responses demonstrating the effects of maturation and aging. (From Ref. 12 with permission from the American Medical Association.)

6 months and approach mean adult values by age 1 year (7,13). However, the ERG components develop at different rates (14). Cone photoreceptors mature earlier than rod photoreceptors. At age 3 months, the maximal scotopic b-wave response (V_{max}) and the semisaturation sensitivity constant, $\log K$ (the light intensity which elicits half of the maximal response) are about half those of adults (13,15). Likewise, phototransduction of the rod photoreceptors as studied by scotopic high-intensity stimuli and analyses of the leading edge of the a-wave demonstrate sensitivity (S) and maximum responses (Rm_{p3}) reaching half of adult values at about age 9 and 14 weeks, respectively (16). In contrast, rod-mediated parafoveal visual sensitivity does not reach 50% adult value until about 19 weeks (13). However, by age 26 weeks, sensitivity (S) reaches adult value, and rod sensitivity is the same for parafoveal and peripheral retinal regions as in adults (17). Under standard ISCEV conditions, the implicit times of the

combined rod–cone response and cone response decrease with age in infancy but the implicit time of the rod response varies little with age (7).

Maturation of Pattern ERG

Maturation studies of pattern ERG in infants are somewhat limited because of required fixation for pattern ERG recording (18–20). Developmental changes are particularly pronounced during the first 8 weeks after birth with the peak latency of the pattern ERG approaching adult values at about age 6 months (19). For children between age 7 and 18 years, an increasing predominance of the macular contribution seems to occur (20).

Maturation of EOG

The maturation of EOG is difficult to study in infants due to required accurate eye movements. However, EOG can be recorded by eliciting passive eye movements related to the oculo-vestibular reflex (21,22). The infant is placed in the supine position held by the mother in a rocking chair, and a distracting visual stimulus encourages fixation from the infant while the infant is being nursed and rocked. EOG studies indicate that EOG light-peak to dark-trough amplitude ratios of infants are comparable to adult values.

Maturation of VEP

Both flash and pattern reversal VEP responses are small and very prolonged with P1 latency of over 200 msec at birth for term newborns as well as for preterm infants as young as 30 weeks after conception (6,23). VEP latencies shorten rapidly in a logarithmic fashion during the first 6 months of life and essentially reach adult values by age 1 year (Fig. 6.2) (24–26). The rates of improvement of pattern reversal VEP responses are similar for large and small check sizes with responses to small check sizes having longer latencies. In addition, monocular pattern reversal VEP responses have slightly longer latencies than binocular responses with this difference being invariant with age but significantly greater

VEP Maturation

Pattern Reversal VEP P100 Latency

LARGE CHECKS   SMALL CHECKS

48-minute Checks   12-Minute Checks

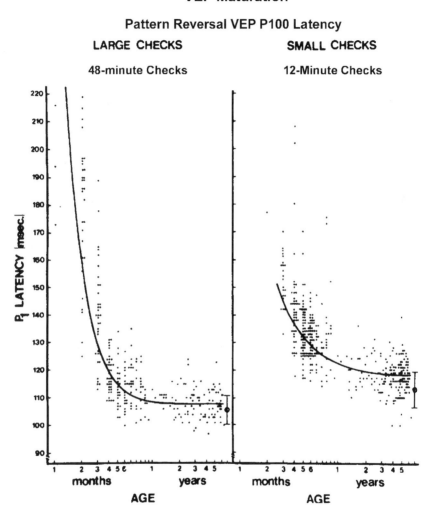

Figure 6.2 Maturation of pattern reversal VEP P100 latency. The P100 latency decreases and reaches near adult values by age 1 year with the most rapid development occurring during the first 4 months of life. The rates of improvement are similar for large and small checks with responses to small checks having longer latencies. (From Ref. 25 with permission from Elsevier.)

with larger check stimuli (24). For preterm infants, the maturation of pattern reversal VEP is related more to their gestational or corrected age rather than their postnatal age (27,28). In addition, for normal infants, some specialized VEP responses such as those to pattern chromatic stimuli may not reach adult waveforms until well into childhood (29).

DELAYED VISUAL MATURATION

Delayed visual maturation refers to an idiopathic disorder characterized by visual inattention during infancy. The diagnosis is made by excluding any recognizable ophthalmic or neurologic conditions that impair visual development (30). Infants with delayed visual maturation may frequently demonstrate other signs of delayed neurological development, but the prognosis is generally excellent if visual impairment is the presenting feature (31). Visual behavior develops usually by age 1 year or less, and normal visual function is obtained later in childhood. Diagnostic tests that are beneficial in establishing the diagnosis of delayed visual maturation include magnetic resonance imaging, full-field ERG, and VEP. Full-field ERG is helpful to exclude conditions such as Leber congenital amaurosis and achromatopsia. VEP responses are variable. Several studies have shown reduced or delayed flash and pattern reversal VEP responses in affected infants, which normalize over time (32–35). However, in a study by Lambert et al. (36), eight of nine infants with delayed visual maturation consistently demonstrated normal VEP responses comparable to age-matched controls. Differences in study results are likely due to differences in methodology and patient population as well as the fact that variability in VEP responses is high among infants during early development, necessitating the use of adequate age-matched control.

ELECTROPHYSIOLOGIC TESTING IN INFANTS

Recording visual electrophysiologic responses from infants and young children present special challenges (37,38). Their attention span is short and they do not want to hold still. Crying is a common reaction to situations that they do not understand. Explaining the purpose and procedure of the test to the parents is critical to assure parents that their child will be handled gently and to alleviate any anxieties. The goal is to create a quiet, calm environment devoid of any unnecessary distractions and to minimize the recording period (39). The mother or the person best in calming the child should accompany the child during testing. Deferring bottle feeding for an infant until test time may calm the infant enough for testing, and the use of soft background music will work in some infants. However, gentle restraints may be required in some cases, and even in the best of hands, sedation with pharmacologic agent may be necessary at times. In general, infants and young children are more likely to tolerate recording of responses from only one eye at a time and may not cooperate long enough for successful recordings from both eyes. The use of a hand-held rather than a desk-top full-field stimulus for full-field ERG and flash VEP recordings may be helpful. Recording artifacts from blink, eye, and head movements are frequent in this age group, which necessitate multiple recordings of the same stimulus until repeatable responses are obtained, or averaging of multiple responses may be used to reduce the effect of artifacts. Cooperation notably improves beyond age 5 years, and testing becomes easier in school-age children.

Recording electrophysiologic responses from infants and young children under pharmacologic sedation reduces recording time by quieting the child and minimizing blink, eye, or head movement artifacts and allows full-field ERG and flash VEP recordings. Because of the small risk of life-threatening complications of sedation, participation of an anesthesiologist and strict adherence to hospital guidelines are essential. Virtually all sedative agents are likely to cause some effect on visual electrophysiologic responses, and to facilitate interpretation, each laboratory should ideally obtain age-related normative electrophysiologic values for the specific sedative agent used. However, realistically, obtaining electrophysiologic values from normal healthy infants or young children by exposing them to risks of a sedative agent is not typically performed. Therefore, information on the specific electrophysiologic effects of a sedative agent may be limited, and the laboratory may have to utilize values from normal-appearing responses from other patients. Nevertheless, distinguishing normal and abnormal responses under sedation and obtaining valid diagnostic information are generally possible.

Numerous sedative agents have been used in infants and young children for visual electrophysiologic recordings (40,41). Short acting barbituates such as methohexital (Brevital) usually provide an adequate level of sedation and may produce transient nystagmus and prolonged full-field ERG responses (Fig. 6.3). Chloral hydrate causes depressed cortical

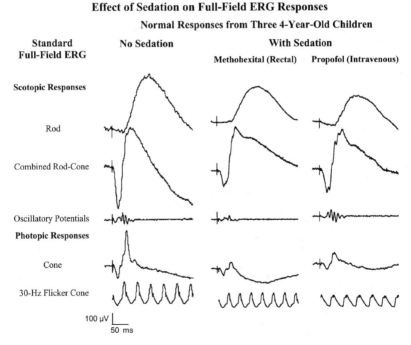

Figure 6.3 Effects of sedative agents on the normal full-field ERG. Note the reduced and prolonged responses under light sedation with methohexital or propofol.

function without altering vital signs, but vomiting and hyperactivity may occur during induction. Recording valid, interpretable pattern reversal VEP responses is possible under chloral hydrate sedation (42). Propofol (Diprivan®) is an intravenous sedative–hypnotic agent that can be titrated to provide different levels of sedation or anesthesia and has the advantage of rapid, predictable awakening (Fig. 6.3). Diazepam and chlordiazepoxide may also be used but are not typically given to young infants. Inhalation anesthetics such as halothane, methoxyflurane, enflurane, diethylether, and chloroform require tracheal intubation and retard retinal dark adaptation (43–46). The deeper anesthesia provided by these anesthetic agents is seldom necessary for visual electrophysiologic recording.

ESTIMATING VISUAL ACUITY IN INFANTS

Preferential-looking behavior and VEP are the two primary methods of estimating visual acuity in infants and preverbal children. The differences between these techniques are outlined in Table 6.1. In the Teller forced-choice preferential-looking technique, pattern stimulus cards, consisting of alternating black-and-white vertical stripes with different strip widths but the same average luminance, are presented to the infant one at the time, either to the right or left of the center in front of a homogenous screen (47). An observer behind the peephole of the background screen determines the location of the grating stimulus and based on the infant's viewing behavior records the percent correct for each strip width. The visual acuity is estimated from the stimulus with the narrowest strip width, that is, the highest spatial frequency, that consistently elicits the preferential-looking behavior. Estimate of monocular visual acuity is obtained with one eye patched.

VEP estimates of visual acuity in preverbal children may be obtained primarily by two methods: transient responses to pattern reversal stimuli or steady-state responses using specialized techniques such as sweep VEP. In both methods,

Table 6.1 Methods for Estimating Visual Acuity in Infants and Preverbal Children

	Teller preferential looking	Pattern reversal VEP	Sweep VEP
Basic principle	Preferential looking behavior	Transient VEP response	Steady-state VEP activity
Primary physiologic area tested	Cortical area 17 and areas of higher behavior processing	Cortical area 17	Cortical area 17
Cooperation level required from subject	Indicate viewing behavior toward stimulus which is presented to the right or left of the infant	Sufficient amount of fixation at the stimulus in front of the infant	Sufficient amount of fixation at the stimulus in front of the infant
Patient exclusion factors	Significant motor dysfunction or neurologic developmental delay	Nystagmus, marked abnormal EEG	Nystagmus, marked abnormal EEG
Stimulus	Cards with stationary alternating black-and-white vertical stripes of different spatial frequency	Dynamic reversing stimulus of alternating black-and-white checks of different spatial frequency	Dynamic reversing stimulus of alternating black-and-white vertical stripes with increasing spatial frequency
Threshold measure for estimating visual acuity	Spatial frequency of the card with the smallest grating that consistently elicits the preferential looking behavior	Spatial frequency of the stimulus at which VEP response can no longer be discriminated from noise	Spatial frequency of the stimulus at which VEP activity can no longer be discriminated from noise
Time and cost of equipment setup	+	++	+++
Time for testing and data analysis	+	+++	++
Estimated visual acuity level	Generally worse than visual acuity estimated by VEP	Generally better than visual acuity estimated by preferential looking	Generally better than visual acuity estimated by preferential looking

recording is made with the child sitting on parent's lap and in a dark room where the only visual stimulus is the monitor displaying the black-and-white stimulus. One recording electrode is placed at the midline occipital position (O_z) and more recording electrodes may be placed at other occipital positions if desired. An observer behind the monitor starts the recording with a hand-held switch when the child looks into the stimulus and stops the recording when fixation is inadequate or when head movement is excessive.

In estimating visual acuity from pattern reversal VEP, responses to a reversing black-and-white checkerboard stimulus of various check sizes are obtained (48,49). The results are analyzed graphically by plotting the stimulus check sizes against the corresponding amplitudes of the P1 component of the responses. Visual acuity is estimated from the smallest check that corresponds to zero or noise level amplitude based on extrapolating the best-fit curve (Fig. 6.4, Table 6.2). Similar to other pattern reversal VEP recordings, averaging of multiple responses is obtained to improve response-to-noise ratio. Binocular testing is usually performed first followed by monocular testing. Children older than age 6 months with normal visual acuity of 20/20 should produce a detectable response to 15 min of arc checks. For infants younger than age 6 months, optimal check sizes for eliciting VEP responses are larger, 120–240 min of arc for age 1 month, 60–120 min of arc for age 2 months, and 30–60 min of arc for age 3–5 months. Initially, the child is tested with these corresponding age-related check sizes, and if no detectable responses are obtained, the check size is doubled until there is a detectable response. If no detectable responses are obtained even with large checks, a flash VEP is performed to see if there is any response. After obtaining a binocular response, monocular testing is performed with the other eye patched, and the procedure is repeated starting with the smallest check size that elicited the binocular response.

In estimating visual acuity from sweep VEP, VEP activity to a varying stimulus lasting several seconds is obtained (50–52). The stimulus usually consists of vertically oriented alternating black-and-white stripes, and the width of the stripes becomes smaller either in linear or logarithmic steps during recording, that is, the spatial frequency of the reversing grating stimulus increases in steps. The recordings obtained are not individual waveforms but reflects the amount of VEP activity at each spatial frequency. The results are displayed graphically by plotting the width of the stripes

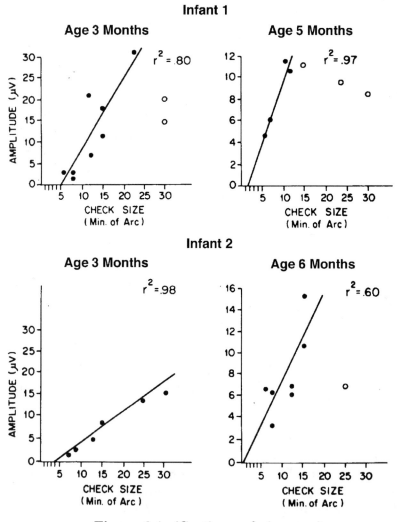

Figure 6.4   (*Caption on facing page*)

in cycles per degree against the corresponding VEP amplitudes (Fig. 6.5, Table 6.2). Visual acuity is estimated from the narrowest stripe, the one with the highest spatial frequency, that produces no or background noise level amplitude based on extrapolating of the graph. The level of estimated visual acuity is similar for a rate of stimulus reversal between 8 and 24 reversals per second, that is, 8–24 Hz of temporal frequency (51).

Reported success rates of preferential-looking testing in infants and young children vary from about 60% to nearly 100% (53–55). Likewise, reported success rates of VEP acuity testing vary from about 60% to 90% (53,54). These rate variations among studies are likely due to differences in patient population and methodology. In addition, patients with significant motor dysfunction or neurologic developmental delay may be unable to reliably perform preferential-looking testing, and patients with nystagmus or marked abnormal EEG may not be able to provide adequate recorded VEP responses.

Visual acuity estimates from forced-choice preferential looking are generally worse than those estimated from VEP (56,57). In normal controls, VEP acuity estimates indicate rapid acuity improvement after birth with a Snellen equivalent acuity of near 20/20 attained by age 6 months. In contrast,

Figure 6.4 (*Facing page*) Estimating visual acuity in infants with pattern reversal VEP. The amplitudes of the pattern reversal VEP responses for stimulus of different check sizes are shown for two infants. Regression lines are fit to the data points shown by the closed circles; data shown by open circles are not included in the regression line analysis but are shown to demonstrate where the peak VEP amplitude occurs. For subject 1, the peak VEP shifts from check size 24′ at age 3 months to check size 12′ at age 5 months. For age 3 months, extrapolation of the regression line to 0 μV reveals a value of 5′, equivalent to visual acuity of 20/100, and for age 5 months, the extrapolated regression line shows a value of 1.5′, equivalent to 20/30. For subject 2, the peak VEP is 30′ for age 3 months and 15′ for age 6 months. Extrapolation of the regression line to 0 μV reveals visual acuity equivalent of 20/80 and 20/20 at age 3 months and age 6 months, respectively. (From Ref. 49 with permission from Elsevier.)

Table 6.2 Visual Acuity and Spatial Frequency Equivalent

Visual acuity Snellen fraction		Decimal notation	Minimal angle of resolution (MAR) (minutes of arc)[a]	Log MAR	Spatial frequency equivalent (cycles/ degree)[a]
Metric (m/m)	English (ft/ft)				
6/3	20/10	2.0	0.5	−0.3	60
6/6	20/20	1.0	1.0	0	30
6/7.5	20/25	0.8	1.25	0.1	24
6/9	20/30	0.67	1.5	0.18[b]	20
6/12	20/40	0.5	2.0	0.3	15
6/15	20/50	0.4	2.5	0.4	12
6/18	20/60	0.33	3.0	0.48[b]	10
6/24	20/80	0.25	4.0	0.6	7.5
6/30	20/100	0.2	5.0	0.7	6
6/60	20/200	0.1	10.0	1.0	3

[a] Applicable to pattern reversal and grating stimuli.

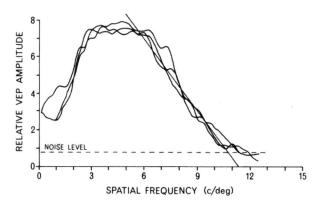

Estimating Visual Acuity with Sweep VEP

Figure 6.5 Estimating visual acuity with steady-state sweep VEP. Three traces of the VEP amplitude vs. spatial frequency plot of a child are superimposed to show the repeatability of the data. The solid line is drawn visually and extrapolated through the noise (dashed line) to the 0 μV level to determine the estimated VEP acuity (12 cycle/degree = 20/50). (From Ref. 52 with permission of *Investigative Ophthalmology and Visual Science*.)

preferential-looking acuity estimates demonstrate a Snellen equivalent of 20/50 by age 1 year followed by improvement to 20/20 by about age 4 years (58). The rate of development is steeper for Teller preferential-looking acuity than sweep VEP acuity with Teller preferential-looking acuity starting at a much lower level (57). Differences in Snellen equivalent acuity between preferential-looking and VEP estimates are due to the fact that each test provides different information about the visual system (Table 6.1). Preferential-looking acuity tests functional or behavioral acuity while VEP acuity reflects potential acuity measured at the visual cortex. In addition, the magnitude of differences between clinical recognition Snellen acuity and preferential-looking acuity or VEP acuity depends on the ocular condition (53). For example, preferential-looking grating acuities are similar to clinical recognition Snellen acuities in normal children, but preferential-looking acuities are better than recognition acuities among patients with an abnormal fovea such as oculocutaneous albinism, macular coloboma, and persistent hyperplastic primary vitreous (55).

AMBLYOPIA

Amblyopia is a developmental anomaly that usually produces impaired visual function in one eye although binocular involvement may also occur. The condition is the result of persistent blurred image from one or both eyes during visual development due to anisometropia, strabismus, or visual deprivation from cataract, corneal opacity, or ptosis. The cellular layers of the visual cortex normally receive binocular projections from corresponding visual field areas, but in amblyopia, the projections are predominantly monocular from the non-amblyopic eye. Amblyopia develops during the first 3 years of life and responds more favorably if treatment is instituted before age 6 years. In young children, treatment of the underlying cause as well as a regimen of part-time or full-time occlusion of the non-amblyopic eye should be initiated as soon as amblyopia is identified.

The most prominent feature of amblyopia is a reduction in visual acuity, but amblyopic deficits are numerous and include impaired contrast sensitivity and stereoacuity. In preverbal children, amblyopia is commonly diagnosed by determining fixation pattern or by estimating visual acuity using either the Teller preferential-looking technique or VEP. In assessing fixation pattern, the inability to maintain fixation with one eye or the other while the opposite eye is covered suggests a fixation preference and is an indication of reduced visual acuity. Other methods of estimating visual acuity such as Teller preferential-looking technique, pattern reversal VEP, and sweep VEP are discussed in detail earlier in this chapter.

Several studies have demonstrated improved pattern reversal VEP P100 amplitude and implicit time in the amblyopic eye with contralateral monocular occlusion treatment (59–61). Although the P100 latencies of the pattern VEP are prolonged in amblyopic eyes, the latencies of the second positive component may be shorter than normal eyes, perhaps as a reflection of selective loss of the contrast-specific evoked potential mechanism (54,62). Multifocal VEP in amblyopic eyes shows greater deficits at the fovea and greater impairment in the temporal field than the nasal field in esotropic amblyopes (63). Some strabismic amblyopes but not anisometropic amblyopes may have supranormal flash VEP response at higher temporal frequencies (64).

The binocularity of the visual cortex may be assessed by a specialized VEP technique called the binocular beat technique (65). In this technique, the stimulus consists of two uniform fields whose luminances are modulating sinusoidally at different temporal frequencies. During testing, one field is seen by one eye while the other field is seen by the other eye. The two luminance modulating fields have different frequencies and come in and out of phase with each other so that the monocular signals summate and cancel each other at the visual cortex. Steady-state VEP of normal subjects shows a modulating waveform response with a frequency (beat frequency) corresponding to the arithmetic difference between the two frequencies of the stimulus fields. In subjects with binocular vision deficits such as those with amblyopia, the VEP beat response is severely reduced (66–68).

Full-field ERG responses are normal in amblyopic eyes, and EOG responses are mildly reduced (69). The amount of EOG amplitude reduction is very modest and its clinical significance is doubtful since the light-peak to dark-trough amplitude ratio is unaffected compared to the contralateral eye. Studies of pattern ERG responses in amblyopia are conflicting. Some studies showed mild decreases of the P50 component (70,71) while other studies found no pattern ERG abnormalities (72,73).

AGING

Gradual decline of visual function and electrophysiologic responses in the absence of any recognizable disease such as cataract or retinal degeneration is a normal part of aging and is the result of age-related physiologic changes of the neuronal visual pathway, ocular media, and pupil size. Therefore, ideally, each laboratory should obtain age-related normative values for each electrophysiologic test to facilitate clinical interpretation.

Aging Effects on Full-Field ERG

The amplitudes and implicit times of virtually all components of the full-field ERG worsen with aging (Fig. 6.1) (74–81). Although a gradual decline begins not long after ERG maturation, age-dependent changes are generally less likely to be clinically significant until after about age 50 years. In a study of standard full-field ERG in 268 normal subjects, Birch and Anderson (12) found the logarithm of the rod and cone amplitudes decreased exponentially with age in adults such that the amplitudes for rod and cone responses declined to one half those in the young adult level by about age 70 (Fig. 6.6). The decline in amplitude was gradual from ages 5 to 54 years and was followed by a rapid decline beyond age 55 years. The amplitudes were converted to logarithm values for analysis, because the distributions of the full-field ERG

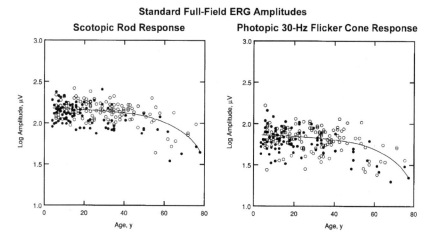

Figure 6.6 Full-field ERG response in aging. The relationship between age in years and log b-wave amplitude is shown. For the rod response, the curve is best-fit exponential with half amplitude at age 69 years. For the 30-Hz flicker cone response, the curve is best-fit exponential with half amplitude at age 70 years. Open circles indicate female; and solid circles indicate male. (From Ref. 12 with permission from the American Medical Association.)

amplitudes and b-wave implicit times in normal subjects do not follow a normal bell-shaped distribution and are skewed. Conversion to logarithm values normalizes the distribution making statistical analyses, which are normal distribution based, more meaningful. Likewise, the maximal b-wave amplitude (V_{max}) of the Naka–Rushton function plot for scotopic intensity response series also declines with age (Fig. 6.7). The V_{max} at age 68 years is half that at age 20 years. However, the semisaturation constant, $\log k$, of the scotopic intensity response Naka–Rushton function plot (the light intensity which elicits half of the maximal response) was only 0.1 log unit higher at age 70 years than at age 20 years, indicating that the loss in retinal sensitivity is modest with aging. This finding is consistent with previous studies showing little decrease in density of photopigment with aging (82,83). Further studies on phototransduction of cone and rod photoreceptors using high-intensity stimuli and analyses of the

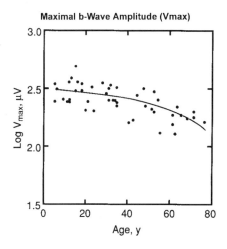

Maximal b-Wave Amplitude (Vmax)

Figure 6.7 Aging and the full-field ERG maximal b-wave amplitude (V_{max}). The V_{max} was obtained from the Naka–Rushton best-fit plot relating b-wave amplitude to retinal illuminance from a series of scotopic responses to increasing stimulus intensity. The relationship between age in years and $\log V_{max}$ is shown for 50 normal subjects. Solid curve is best-fit exponential relating V_{max} to age. The V_{max} declines with age, and at age 68 years, the V_{max} is half that at age 20 years. (From Ref. 12 with permission from the American Medical Association.)

leading edge of the a-wave have shown that the sensitivity variable (S) for cone- and rod-only responses decreases modestly with age while maximum cone and rod photoreceptor responses (Rm_{p3}) remain constant (84,85).

Aging Effects on Focal and Multifocal ERG

Age-related decline of focal and multifocal ERG cone responses is most striking at the fovea and less pronounced in the parafoveal and eccentric regions (86–89). The decline is definitely clinical notable after age 50 years (90–92). Amplitude ratio between macular and paramacular focal ERG responses tends to be more independent of age (93). Both first-order and second-order multifocal ERG responses decrease with age, and a relationship between logarithm of the first-order responses and age has been demonstrated

(92,94). With sophisticated analysis, age-related changes are also found on responses to stimuli presented in isolation as well as in backward and forward interactions between consecutive flash responses (95).

Aging Effects on Pattern ERG

Because pattern ERG is a measure of predominantly retinal ganglion cell function, factors that influence age-related decline of pattern ERG responses involve not only age-related physiologic changes of the ocular media and the retina but also retinal ganglion cells. The age-associated decline of retinal function as shown by full-field, focal, and multifocal ERG responses will cause decreased inputs to retinal ganglion cells. In addition, the number of retinal ganglion cell fibers decreases with age (96). However, a large variability of ganglion cell counts exists among individuals (97). In any case, several studies have demonstrated age-related decline of amplitude and increase in latency of the P50 and N95 components of the transient pattern ERG (98–100). This age relationship appears more prominent for amplitude than for latency. For instance, one study found no age-related increase in latency with analysis being performed after decreasing the latency of older adults by 3.5 msec to compensate for age-related miosis (101). Similarly, steady-state pattern ERG responses decrease with age along with a phase lag (100,102,103). The phase lag is likely to be due to age-related miosis but the reduction in amplitude cannot be attributed to age-related miosis alone (100,104). In general, a pattern ERG amplitude reduction of about 40% occurs from age 20 to 70 over most spatial and temporal frequencies (104).

Aging Effects on EOG

Age-related declines of EOG occur and are due in part to alterations of retinal function as reflected by declines of ERG as well as other physiologic changes that affect the standing potential of the retina (105,106). A notable decrease in both light-peak amplitude and dark-trough amplitude is found after age 40 years, and a mild decline in light-peak to dark-trough amplitude ratio (Arden ratio) occurs with aging (106).

Aging Effects on VEP

Because VEP latency rather than amplitude is the more reliable clinical measure, several studies have shown an age-related increase in latency of the P100 component of the pattern reversal VEP, that generally becomes clinically significant after age 40 years (Fig. 6.8) (107–109). This age-related increase of VEP latency is more pronounced for stimulus of smaller sizes (high spatial frequency) and for slower stimulus pattern alterations (lower temporal frequencies) (104). For instance, age-associated increase in latency is nearly twice as fast for smaller checks (12 min of arc) as compared to larger checks (48 min of arc)

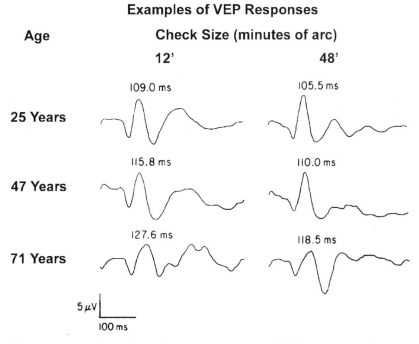

Figure 6.8 Examples of pattern reversal VEP responses demonstrating increasing P100 latency with aging. (From Ref. 107 with permission from Elsevier.)

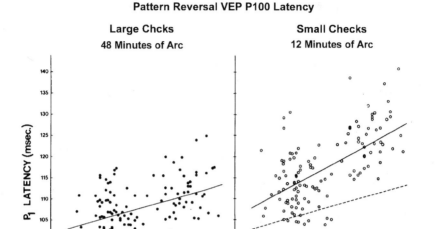

Figure 6.9 Aging and pattern reversal VEP P100 latency. Age-associated increase in latency is nearly twice as fast for small checks (12 min of arc; regression line: $y = 0.26x + 105.6$) as compared to large checks (48 min of arc; regression line: $y = 0.14x + 101.8$). For comparison, the regression line for 48-min checks is repeated as a dashed line on the plot for 12-min checks. (From Ref. 107 with permission from Elsevier.)

(Fig. 6.9) (107). Although some studies have indicated that the increase in VEP latency is at least in part due to age-related miosis, the alteration of the VEP cannot be explained completely by age-related miosis alone (75,101,103). Because of repeat variability, age-related changes in VEP amplitudes are less consistent than those of latency (75,101).

GENDER

Several studies have demonstrated slightly larger full-field ERG responses in women compared to men (12,78,79,110).

This difference may be due in part to the fact that reduction in both scotopic and photopic ERG amplitudes correlates directly with increased axial eye length, and men tend to have longer axial eye lengths than women (111–114). Despite the statistical significance of this gender difference in ERG responses, the difference is quite modest and is not substantiated in all studies (81). Therefore, its clinical significance is unclear. Likewise, light-peak to dark-trough EOG amplitude ratios are slightly higher in women than men (115). Of interest, latency of the P100 component of the pattern reversal VEP response may be shorter in female newborns and young infants as compared to males with no differences in amplitude (116).

REFERENCES

1. Birch DG, Birch EE, Hoffman DR, Uauy RD. Retinal development in very-low-birthweight infants fed diets differing in omega-3 fatty acids. Invest Ophthalmol Vis Sci 1992; 33: 21–32.

2. Birch DG, Birch EE, Petrig B, Uauy RD. Retinal and cortical function of very-low-birth-weight infants at 37 and 57 weeks postconception. Clin Vis Sci 1989; 5:363–373.

3. Horsten GP, Winkelman JE. The electric activity of the eye in the first days of life. Acta Physiol Pharmacol Neerl 1965; 13:196–198.

4. Mactier H, Dexter JD, Hewett JE, Latham CB, Woodruff CW. The electroretinogram in preterm infants. J Pediatr 1988; 113:607–612.

5. Mactier H, Hamilton R, Bradnam MS, Turner TL, Dudgeon J. Contact lens electroretinography in preterm infants from 32 week after conception: a development in current methodology. Arch Dis Child Fetal Neonatal Ed 2000; 82:F233–F23.

6. Leaf AA, Green CR, Esack A, Costeloe KL, Prior PF. Maturation of electroretinograms and visual evoked potentials in preterm infants. Dev Med Child Neurol 1995; 37:814–826.

7. Fulton AB, Hansen RM, Westall CA. Development of ERG responses: the ISCEV rod, maximal and cone responses in normal subjects. Doc Ophthalmol 2003; 107:235–241.

8. Berezovsky A, Moraes NSB, Nusinowitz S, Salomao SR. Standard full-field electroretinography in healthy preterm infants. Doc Ophthalmol 2003; 107:243–249.

9. Barnet AB, Lodge A, Armington JC. Electroretinogram in newborn human infants. Science 1965; 148:651–654.

10. Zetterstrom B. The clinical electroretinogram IV: the electroretinogram in children during the first year of life. Acta Ophthalmol 1951; 29:295–304.

11. Horsten GPM, Winkelman JE. Electrical activity of the retina in relation to histological differentiation in infants born prematurely and at full-term. Vision Res 1962; 2:269–276.

12. Birch DG, Anderson JL. Standardized full-field electroretinography: normal values and their variations with age. Arch Ophthalmol 1992; 110:1571–1576.

13. Fulton AB, Hansen RM. The development of scotopic sensitivity. Invest Ophthalmol Vis Sci 2000; 41:1588–1596.

14. Breton ME, Quinn GE, Schueller AW. Development of electroretinogram and rod phototransduction response in human infants. Invest Ophthalmol Vis Sci 1995; 36: 1588–1602.

15. Fulton AB, Hansen RM. Background adaption in human infants: analysis of b-wave responses. Doc Ophthalmol Proc Ser 1982; 31:191–197.

16. Nusinowitz S, Birch DG, Birch EE. Rod photoresponses in 6-week and 4-month-old human infants. Vision Res 1998; 38:627–635.

17. Hansen RM, Fulton AB. The course of maturation of rod-mediated visual thresholds in infants. Invest Ophthalmol Vis Sci 1999; 40:1883–1886.

18. Odom JV, Maida TM, Dawson WW, Romano PE. Retinal and cortical pattern responses: a comparison of infants and adults. Am J Optom Physiol Opt 1983; 60:369–375.

19. Fiorentini A, Trimarchi C. Development of temporal properties of pattern electroretinogram and visual evoked potentials in infants. Vision Res 1992; 32:1609–1621.

20. Brecelj J, Struel M, Zidar I, Tekavcic-Pompe M. Pattern ERG and VEP maturation in schoolchildren. Clin Neurophysiol 2002; 113:1764–1770.

21. Hansen RM, Fulton AB. Corneoretinal potentials in human infants. Doc Ophthalmol Proc Ser 1983; 37:81–86.

22. Trimble JL, Ernest JT, Newell FW. Electro-oculography in infants. Invest Ophthalmol Vis Sci 1977; 16:668–670.

23. Harding GF, Grose J, Wilton A, Bissenden JG. The pattern reversal VEP in short-gestation infants. Electroencephalogr Clin Neurophysiol 1989; 74:76–80.

24. McCulloch DL, Skarf B. Development of the human visual system: monocular and binocular pattern VEP latency. Invest Ophthalmol Vis Sci 1991; 32:2372–2381.

25. Moskowitz A, Sokol S. Development changes in the human visual system as reflected by the latency of the pattern reversal VEP. Electroencephalogr Clin Neurophysiol 1983; 56:1–15.

26. Porciatti V. Temporal and spatial properties of the pattern-reversal VEP's in infants below 2 months of age. Hum Neurobiol 1984; 3:97–102.

27. Roy MS, Barsoum-Homsy M, Orquin J, Benoit J. Maturation of binocular pattern visual evoked potentials in normal full-term and preterm infants from 1 to 6 months of age. Pediatr Res 1995; 37:140–144.

28. Tsuneishi S, Casaer P. Effects of preterm extrauterine visual experience in the development of the human visual system: a flash VEP study. Dev Med Child Neurol 2000; 42:663–668.

29. Madrid M, Cregnale MA. Long-term maturation of visual pathways. Vis Neurosci 2000; 17:831–817.

30. Scher MS, Richardson GA, Robles N, Geva D, Goldschmidt L, Dahl RE, Sclabassi RJ, Day NL. Effects of prenatal substance exposure: altered maturation of visual evoked potentials. Pediatr Neurol 1998; 18:236–243.

31. Tresidder J, Fielder AR, Nicholson J. Delayed visual maturation: ophthalmic and neurodevelopmental aspects. Dev Med Child Neurol 1990; 32:872–881.

32. Harel S, Holtzman M, Feinsod M. Delayed visual maturation. Arch Dis Child 1983; 58:298–309.

33. Mellor DH, Fielder AR. Dissociated visual development: electrodiagnostic studies in infants who are 'slow to see'. Dev Med Child Neurol 1980; 22:327–335.

34. Fielder AR, Russell-Eggitt IR, Dodd KL, Mellor DH. Delayed visual maturation. Trans Ophthalmol Soc UK 1965; 104: 653–661.

35. Hoyt CS, Jastrzebski G, Merg E. Delayed visual maturation in infancy. Br J Ophthalmol 1983; 67:127–130.

36. Lambert SR, Kriss A, Taylor D. Delayed visual maturation. A longitudinal clinical and electrophysiological assessment. Ophthalmology 1989; 96:524–528.

37. Jones RM, France TD. Recording ERGs and VERs from unsedated children. J Pediatr Ophthalmol 1977; 14:316–319.

38. Marmor MF. Corneal electroretinograms in children without sedation. J Pediatr Ophthalmol 1976; 13:112–116.

39. Fulton AB, Hartmann EE, Hansen RM. Electrophysiological testing techniques in children. Doc Ophthalmol 1989; 71:341–354.

40. Bagolini B, Penne A, Fonda S, Mazzetti A. Pattern reversal visually evoked potentials in general anesthesia. Graefes Arch Clin Exp Ophthalmol 1979; 209:231–238.

41. Wahitacre MM, Ellis PP. Outpatient sedation for ocular examination. Surv Ophthalmol 1984; 28:643–652.

42. Wright KW, Eriksen KJ, Shors TJ, Ary JP. Recording pattern visual evoked potentials under chloral hydrate sedation. Arch Ophthalmol 1986; 104:718–721.

43. van Norren D, Padmos P. Halothane retards dark adaption. Doc Ophthalmol Proc Ser 1974; 4:155–159.

44. van Norren D, Padmos P. The influence of various inhalation anesthetics on dark adaption. Doc Ophthalmol Proc Ser 1975; 11:149–151.

45. van Norren D, Padmos P. Cone dark adaptation: the influence of halothane anesthesia. Invest Ophthalmol 1975; 14:212–227.

46. Wongpichedchai S, Hansen RM, Koda B, Gudas VM, Fulton AB. Effects of halothane on children's electroretinogram. Ophthalmology 1992; 99:1309–1312.

47. Teller DY, Morse R, Borton R, Regal D. Visual acuity for vertical and diagonal gratings in human infants. Vision Res 1974; 14:1433–1439.

48. Sokol S, Hansen VC, Moskowitz A, Greenfield P, Towle VL. Evoked potential and preferential looking estimates of visual acuity in pediatric patients. Ophthalmology 1983; 90:552–562.

49. Sokol S. Measurement of infant visual acuity from pattern reversal evoked potentials. Vision Res 1978; 18:33–39.

50. McCulloch DL, Taylor LJ, Whyte HE. Visual evoked potentials and visual prognosis following perinatal asphyxia. Arch Ophthalmol 1991; 109:229–233.

51. Gottlob I, Fendick MG, Guo S, Zubcov AA, Odom JV, Reinecke RD. Visual acuity measurements by swept spatial frequency visual-evoked-cortical potentials (VECPs): clinical application in children with various visual disorders. J Pediatr Ophthalmol Strabismus 1990; 27:40–47.

52. Tyler CW, Apkarian P, Levi DM, Nakayama K. Rapid assessment of visual function: and electronic sweep technique for the pattern visual evoked potential. Invest Ophthalmol Vis Sci 1979; 18:703–713.

53. Bane MC, Birch EE. VEP acuity, FPL acuity and visual behavior of visually impaired children. J Pediatr Ophthalmol Strabismus 1992; 29:202–209.

54. Sokol S. Abnormal evoked potential latencies in amblyopia. Br J Ophthalmol 1983; 67:310–314.

55. Mayer DL, Fulton AB, Hansen RM. Preferential looking acuity obtained with a staircase procedure in pediatric patients. Invest Ophthalmol Vis Sci 1982; 23:538–543.

56. Dobson V, Teller DY. Visual acuity in human infants: a review and comparison of behavioural and electrophysiologic studies. Vision Res 1978; 18:1233–1238.

57. Riddell PM, Ladenheim B, Mast J, Catalano T, Rita N, Hainline L. Comparison of measures of visual acuity in infants: Teller acuity cards and sweep visual evoked potentials. Optom Vis Sci 1997; 74:702–707.

58. Mayer DL, Dobson V. Visual acuity development in infants and young children as assessed by operant preferential looking. Vision Res 1982; 22:1141–1151.

59. Arden GB, Bernard WM. Effect of occlusion of the visual evoked response in amblyopia. Trans Ophthalmol Soc UK 1979; 99:419–426.

60. Henc-Petrinovic L, Deban N, Gabric N, Petrinovic J. Prognostic value of visual evoked responses in childhood amblyopia. Eur J Ophthalmol 1993; 3:114–120.

61. Odom JV, Hoyt CS, Marg E. Effect of natural deprivation and unilateral eye patching on visual acuity of infants and children: evoked potential measurements. Arch Ophthalmol 1981; 99:1412–1416.

62. Sokol S, Bloom B. Visually evoked cortical responses of amblyopes to a spatially alternating stimulus. Invest Ophthalmol 1973; 12:936–939.

63. Yu M, Brown B, Edwards MH. Investigation of multifocal visual evoked potential in anisometropic and esotropic amblyopes. Invest Ophthalmol Vis Sci 1998; 39:2033–2040.

64. Davis ET, Bass SJ, Sherman J. Flash visual evoked potential (VEP) in amblyopia and optic nerve disease. Optom Vis Sci 1995; 72:612–618.

65. Baitch LW, Levi DM. Binocular beats: psychophysical studies of binocular interaction in normal and stereoblind humans. Vision Res 1989; 29:27–35.

66. Sloper JJ, Garnham C, Gous P, Dyason R, Plunkett D. Reduced binocular beat visual evoked responses and stereoacuity in patients with Duane syndrome. Invest Ophthalmol Vis Sci 2001; 42:2826–2830.

67. Stevens JL, Berman JL, Schmeisser ET, Baker RS. Dichoptic luminance beat visual evoked potentials in the assessment of binovularity in children. J Pediatr Ophthalmol Strabismus 1994; 31:368–373.

68. Struck MC, Ver Hoeve JN, France TD. Binocular cortical interactions in the monofixation syndrome. J Pediatr Ophthalmol Strabismus 1996; 33:291–297.

69. Williams C, Papakostopoulos D. Electro-oculographic abnormalities in amblyopia. Br J Ophthalmol 1995; 79: 218–224.

70. Arden GB, Wooding SL. Pattern ERG in amblyopia. Invest Ophthalmol Vis Sci 1985; 26:88–96.

71. Persson HE, Wanger P. Pattern-reversal electroretinograms in squint amblyopia, artificial anisometropia and simulated eccentric fixation. Acta Ophthalmol (Copenh) 1982; 60: 123–132.

72. Gottlob I, Welge-Lussen L. Normal pattern electroretinograms in amblyopia. Invest Ophthalmol Vis Sci 1987; 28:187–191.

73. Hess RF, Baker C Jr, Verhoeve JN, Keesey UT, France TD. The pattern evoked electroretinogram: its variability in normals and its relationship to amblyopia. Invest Ophthalmol Vis Sci 1985; 26:1610–1623.

74. Weleber RG. The effect of age on human cone and rod ganzfeld electroretinograms. Invest Ophthalmol Vis Sci 1981; 20:392–399.

75. Wright CE, Williams DE, Drasdo N, Harding GF. The influence of age on the electroretinogram and visual evoked potential. Doc Ophthalmol 1985; 59:365–384.

76. Lehnert W, Wunsche H. [The electroretinogram at different ages of life]. Graefes Arch Clin Exp Ophthalmol 1966; 170:147–155.

77. Peterson H. The normal B-potential in the single flash clinical electroretinogram: a computer technique study of the influence of sex and age. Acta Ophthalmol 1968; 99 (suppl):7–77.

78. Zeidler I. The clinical electroretinogram, IX: the normal electroretinogram-value of the b-potential in different age groups and its differences in men and women. Acta Ophthalmol 1959; 37:294–301.

79. Karpe G, Rickenbach K, Thomasson S. The clinical electroretinogram, I: the normal electroretinogram above fifty years of age. Acta Ophthalmol 1950; 28:301–305.

80. Martin DA, Heckenlively JR. The normal electroretinogram. Doc Ophthalmol Proc Ser 1982; 31:135–144.

81. Iijima H. Distribution of ERG amplitudes, latencies, and implicit times. In: Heckenlively J, Arden G, eds. Principles and Practice of Clinical Electrophysiology of Vision. St Louis: Mosby Year Book, 1991:289–290.

82. Elsner AE, Berk L, Burns SA, Rosenberg PR. Aging and human cone pigments. J Opt Soc Am 1988; 5:2106–2112.

83. Keunen JEE, van Norren D, van Meel GJ. Density of foveal cone pigments at older age. Invest Ophthalmol Vis Sci 1979; 28:985–991.

84. Birch DG, Hood DC, Locke KG, Hoffman DR, Tzekov RT. Quantitative electroretinogram measures of phototransduction in cone and rod photoreceptors: normal aging, pregression with disease, and test–retest variability. Arch Ophthalmol 2002; 120:1045–1051.

85. Cideciyan AV, Jacobson SG. An alternative phototransduction model for human rod and cone ERG a-waves: normal parameters and variation with age. Vision Res 1996; 36:2609–2621.

86. Anzai K, Mori K, Ota M, Murayama K, Yoneya S. Aging of macular function as seen in multifocal electroretinogram. Nippon Ganka Gakkai Zasshi 1998; 102:49–53.

87. Birch DG, Fish GE. Focal cone electroretinograms: aging and macular disease. Doc Ophthalmol 1988; 69:211–220.

88. Fortune B, Johnson CA. Decline of photopic multifocal electroretinogram responses with age is due primarily to preretinal optical factors. J Opt Soc Am A Opt Image Sci Vis 2002; 19:173–184.

89. Jackson GR, Ortega J, Girkin CA, Rosenstiel CE, Owsley C. Aging-related changes in the multifocal electroretinogram. J Opt Soc Am A Opt Image Sci Vis 2002; 19:185–189.

90. Hayashi H, Miyake Y, Horiguchi M, Tanikawa A, Kondo M, Suzuki S. [Aging the focal macular electroretinogram]. Nippon Ganka Gakkai Zasshi 1997; 101:417–422.

91. Mohidin N, Yap MK, Jacobs RJ. Influence of age on the multifocal electroretinography. Ophthalmic Physiol Opt 1999; 19:481–488.

92. Nabeshima T, Tazawa Y, Mita M, Sano M. Effects of aging on the first and second-order kernels of multifocal electroretinogram. Jpn J Ophthalmol 2002; 46:261–269.

93. Bagolini B, Porciatti V, Falsini B, Scalia G, Neroni M, Moretti G. Macular electroretinogram as a function of age of subjects. Doc Ophthalmol 1988; 70:37–43.

94. Gerth C, Garcia SM, Ma L, Keltner JL, Werner JS. Multifocal electroretinogram: age-related changes for different luminance levels. Graefes Arch Clin Exp Ophthalmol 2002; 240:202–208.

95. Gerth C, Sutter EE, Werner JS. mfERG response dynamics of the aging retina. Invest Ophthalmol Vis Sci 2003; 44:4443–4450.

96. Balazsi AG, Rootman J, Drance SM, Schulzer M, Douglas GR. The effect of age on the nerve fiber population of the human optic nerve. Am J Ophthalmol 1984; 97:760–766.

97. Repka MX, Quigley HA. The effect of age on normal human optic nerve fiber number and diameter. Ophthalmology 1989; 96:26–32.

98. Celesia GG, Kaufman D, Cone S. Effect of age and sex on pattern electroretinograms and visual evoked patients. Electroencephalogr Clin Neurophysiol 1987; 68:161–171.

99. Hull RM, Drasdo N. The influence of age on the pattern-reversal electroretinogram. Ophthalmic Physiol Opt 1990; 10:49–53.

100. Trick GL, Nesher R, Cooper DG, Shields SM. The human pattern ERG: alterations of response properties with aging. Optom Vis Sci 1992; 69:122–128.

101. Trick LR. Age-related alterations in retinal function. Doc Ophthalmol 1987; 65:35–43.

102. Porciatti V, Falsini B, Scalia G, Fadda A, Fontanesi G. The pattern electroretinogram by skin electrodes: effect of spatial frequency and age. Doc Ophthalmol 1988; 70:117–122.

103. Tomoda H, Celesia GG, Brigell MG, Toleikis S. The effects of age on steady-state pattern electroretinograms and visual evoked potentials. Doc Ophthalmol 1991; 77:201–211.

104. Porciatti V, Burr DC, Morrone MC, Fiorentini A. The effect of aging on the pattern electroretinogram and visual evoked potential in humans. Vision Res 1992; 32:1199–1209.

105. Wakana K. [Effects of aging on electrooculography in normal eyes]. Nippon Ganka Gakkai Zasshi 1982; 86:613–622.

106. Alexandridis E, Bittighofer U. [Age-dependent changes in the electrooculogram]. Ber Zusammenkunft Dtsch Ophthalmol Ges 1974; 72:461–646.

107. Sokol S, Moskowitz A, Towle VL. Age-related changes in the latency of the visual evoked potential: influence of check size. Electroencephalogr Clin Neurophysiol 1981; 51:559–562.

108. Kooi KA, Bagchi BK. Visual evoked responses in man: normative data. Ann NY Acad Sci 1964; 112:254–269.

109. Straumanis JJ, Shagass C, Schwartz M. Visually evoked cerebral response changes associated with chronic brain syndromes and aging. J Gerontol 1965; 20:498–506.

110. Vianio-Mattila B. The clinical electroretinogram, II: the difference between the electroretinogram in men and in women. Acta Ophthalmol 1951; 29:25–32.

111. Pallin O. The influence of the axial length of the eye on the size of the recorded b-potential in the clinical single-flash electroretinogram. Acta Ophthalmol 1969; 101 (suppl):1–57.

112. Perlman I, Meyer E, Haim T, Zonis S. Retinal function in high refractive error assessed electroretinographically. Br J Ophthalmol 1984; 68:79–84.

113. Westall CA, Dhaliwal HS, Panton CM, Sigesmon D, Levin AV, Nischal KK, Heon E. Values of electroretinogram responses according to axial length. Doc Ophthalmol 2001; 102:115–130.

114. Chen JF, Eisner AE, Burns SA, Hansen RM, Lou PL, Kwong KK, Fulton AB. The effect of eye shape on retinal responses. Clin Vision Sci 1992; 7:521–530.

115. Jones RM, Stevens TS, Gould S. Normal EOG values of young subjects. Doc Ophthalmol Proc Ser 1977; 13:93–97.

116. Malcolm CA, McCulloch DL, Shepherd AJ. Pattern-reversal visual evoked potentials in infants: gender differences during early visual maturation. Dev Med Child Neurol 2002; 44: 345–351.

7

Overview: Clinical Indications and Disease Classification

Clinical indications of visual electrophysiologic testing are evolving with the development of new electrophysiologic techniques. For instance, the rapid development of multifocal ERG has allowed assessment of local retinal function. The visual electrophysiologic tests are described in detail in Chapters 1–5, and the commonly available tests are summarized in Table 7.1. In addition, disease classification is also evolving with advances in the understanding of pathophysiologic mechanisms of established and newly discovered conditions. This chapter discusses issues pertinent to clinical use of ERG, EOG, and VEP and to disease classification.

CLINICAL INDICATIONS OF VISUAL ELECTROPHYSIOLOGIC TESTS

Ultimately, the key determinant of ordering a diagnostic test is whether the test results will alter the management of the patient. Medical management is viewed in the broad context

Table 7.1 Overview of Clinical Visual Electrophysiologic Tests

	Stimulus	Activities measured	Localization	Pupil dilation	Steady fixation required
Electroretinography					
Full-field	Panretinal flash from a full-field bowl	Rod and cone associated retinal responses	Panretinal, non-localizing response	Yes	No
Multifocal	Pattern of black and white hexagons, each hexagon reversing at a predetermined pseudo-random sequence	Cone associated retinal responses	Topographical, local responses	Yes	Yes
Pattern	Reversing black and white checkerboard	Retinal ganglion cells (optic nerve), inner retina	Non-localizing, macular dominated response	No	Yes
Electro-oculography	Light phase with background light	Retinal pigment epithelium	Non-localizing standing potential	Yes or No[a]	Yes[b]
Visual evoked potential					
Pattern	Reversing black and white checkerboard	Occipital visual cortex	Non-localizing macular dominated cortical response	No	Yes
Flash	Flash subtending ≤20° visual angle	Occipital visual cortex	Non-localizing macular dominated cortical response	No	No

[a] Depending on available luminance for light phase.
[b] Adequate fixation for accurate saccades.

of providing not only treatment but also diagnostic and prognostic information. For instance, counseling a patient with an untreatable condition is an essential and appropriate part of medical management.

Modern medical practice demands that decisions be made on the basis of scientific evidence rather than anecdotal conjecture or hypothetical thinking. The concept of evidence-based medicine is rooted in the principle of incorporating the highest quality of available scientific information into the context of clinical care. In addition, current practice environment dictates efficiency as well as cost-effectiveness. Therefore, the usefulness of visual electrophysiologic tests such as ERG, EOG, and VEP is not simply judged by whether the probability of a disease is increased or decreased given the test results. Rather, the sensitivity and specificity of these procedures in diagnosing and detecting visual function change of a given disease must be critically compared to other available diagnostic tests. For instance, ERG is essential in the early diagnosis of cancer-associated retinopathy where the ERG responses are impaired even when the retina appears normal. In contrast, even though ERG impairment is associated with retinal detachment, ERG is rarely performed in retinal detachment because ophthalmoscopic retinal examination is by far the most helpful diagnostic procedure.

The indications of performing a diagnostic test must also take into account the fact that there are sometimes substantial differences among clinicians in the management of medical conditions. These differences may stem from many factors. First, there may be a relative lack of general medical consensus or a lack of evidence-based information or both. Many medical organizations such as the American Academy of Ophthalmology have published preferred practice patterns for specific medical conditions but this is not available for all disease categories. Second, the standard of care may vary somewhat among local communities due, in part, to differences in the number and quality of available diagnostic tests. Like other tests, accessibility to quality ERG, EOG, and VEP support is crucial to its effective clinical use, and productive communication between the clinician and the electrophysiologist is helpful so that useful recordings are obtained. For example, in fundus albipunctatus, rod ERG responses increase with prolonged dark adaptation, and if this diagnosis is suspected, prolonged dark-adapted ERG responses are required.

Because the clinical indications of when to perform a diagnostic test are determined by numerous factors, a list of conditions for which visual electrophysiologic tests would be of clinical value is difficult to generate. Nevertheless, consensus regarding the key diagnostic value of electrophysiologic testing exists in many conditions including achromatopsia, Leber congenital amaurosis, cone dystrophy, X-linked retinoschisis, enhanced S cone syndrome, and thioridazine toxicity.

DISEASE CLASSIFICATION

Traditionally, many disorders are defined by clinical features. For instance, numerous retinal conditions are defined or grouped mostly on the basis of retinal appearance. However, recent advances in the understanding of basic disease mechanisms have caused disease classification to evolve.

A case in point is the retinal dystrophies. Rapid advances in molecular genetics have identified alterations of specific genes that are responsible for many of the hereditary retinal conditions. These advances have led to accurate molecular diagnosis, even during the early stages of the disease and have improved understanding of the underlying disease mechanism. The genotypes for the hereditary retinal degenerations are numerous and diverse, and the fundamental biochemical aberrations which produce these disorders are correspondingly complex. In addition, the expressivity or manifestation of a particular hereditary disorder is often variable even for affected persons with identical disease-causing genotype in the same family. Because these disorders have been classified traditionally on basis of clinical findings, that is, expressivity, a great deal of disparity between traditional disease classification and genetic categorization has emerged.

For example, genetic mutations associated with a clinical diagnosis of retinitis pigmentosa are found on numerous genes including genes encoding rhodopsin, peripherin, cGMP phosphodiesterase, and retinal pigment epithelium protein RPE65. Conversely, a specific disease-causing peripherin gene mutation within a single family may produce different phenotypes compatible with clinical diagnoses of not only retinitis pigmentosa but also macular pattern dystrophy and adult-onset vitelliform macular dystrophy.

No doubt, with further advances in the future, the classification of diseases will become more rooted in physiologic mechanisms. Nevertheless, both clinical classification and physiologic classification have a role in the management of patients. Clinical classification helps to categorize patients on the basis of clinical features, and physiologic classification, such as genotypic classification as in the case of retinal dystrophies, identifies the pathophysiologic origin of the condition.

8

Retinitis Pigmentosa and Pigmentary Retinopathies

Diffuse retinal pigmentary alteration is a feature in a number of distinct disorders ranging from retinal dystrophies to systemic metabolic disorders. In addition, congenital infections such as rubella and syphilis may also produce pigmentary retinopathy. The clinical applications and findings of electrophysiologic tests in pigmentary retinopathies are covered in this chapter with the following outline:

- Retinitis pigmentosa (rod–cone dystrophy)
- Leber congenital amaurosis
- Usher syndrome
- Bardet–Biedl syndrome
- Refsum syndrome
- Abetalipoproteinemia
    (Bassen–Kornzweig syndrome)
- Neuronal ceroid lipofuscinosis
- Kearns–Sayre syndrome—mitochondrial retinopathy
- Rubella retinopathy
- Syphilitic retinopathy

- Enhanced S cone syndrome
- Goldmann–Favre syndrome
- Dominant late-onset retinal degeneration
- Cone–rod dystrophy
- Alström syndrome

RETINITIS PIGMENTOSA
(ROD–CONE DYSTROPHY)

Retinitis pigmentosa (RP) refers to a large group of genetically heterogeneous disorders characterized by early rod photoreceptor dysfunction and progressive rod and cone dysfunction. The prominent retinal pigmentary changes, which occurs in most but not all patients with RP led Donders to use the term "retinita pigmentosa" in 1857. Pigmentary retinal degenerations associated with systemic findings such as Refsum syndrome, Bardet–Biedl syndrome, Bassen–Kornsweig syndrome, and neuronal ceroid lipofuscinosis (Batten disease) have occasionally been clumped under the broad category of RP or secondary RP. However, to avoid confusion, "retinitis pigmentosa" is recommended to be reserved only for primary rod–cone photoreceptor dystrophies and not as a synonym for pigmentary retinal degeneration (1).

Retinitis pigmentosa affects approximately 1 in 3000–4500 persons of the general population (2). Symptoms and clinical findings in RP patients are variable, even among patients with the same genotype and within the same family. Night vision impairment, peripheral vision loss, and light sensitivity generally begin insidiously between the second and fifth decades of life (3). Visual acuity and macular function are usually relatively spared until late in the disease. Diffuse or patchy areas of retinal atrophy with vascular attenuation and pigmentary clumping (bone spicules) are typically evident initially in the mid-periphery regions of the retina producing a ring-shaped scotoma surrounding fixation on visual field testing (Fig. 8.1). In some cases, the inferior mid-peripheral regions of the retina may be preferentially involved in early disease. With time, progressive diffuse

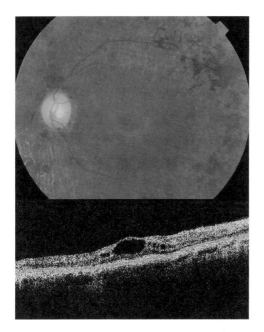

Figure 8.1 *Top*: Diffuse retinal atrophy, vascular attenuation, and pigmentary clumping in a patient with advanced RP. *Bottom*: Cystoid macular edema may occur in RP and was present in this patient as demonstrated by optic coherence tomography. (Refer to the color insert.)

retinal degeneration occurs. Other ocular findings of RP include optic nerve atrophy, atrophic macular lesions, cystoid macular edema, vitreous syneresis with vitreous cells, and posterior subcapsular cataracts (3,4).

Autosomal recessive, autosomal dominant, and X-linked recessive forms of RP are all found. Approximately 50% of RP patients have no family history of RP and have sporadic or isolated RP. The hereditary pattern in sporadic RP patients is presumably mostly autosomal recessive implying that this mode of inheritance is the most common (2). X-linked recessive forms of RP are the least common and are generally more severe. Advances in molecular genetics have helped to determine the specific hereditary pattern as well as the fundamental biochemical defect in RP patients.

The genotypes of RP are extremely numerous and complex. Mutations on at least 40 genes are associated with the RP phenotype. Identification of RP genotypes suggests that several biochemical mechanisms may produce the RP phenotype including defects involving the renewal and shedding of photoreceptor outer segments, the visual transduction cascade, and retinol (vitamin A) metabolism (5). For example, mutations of the rhodopsin gene account for less than 25% of all autosomal dominant RP, but at least 90 different point mutations of the rhodopsin gene are associated with RP. On the other hand, mutations of the peripherin/RDS gene are associated not only with autosomal dominant RP but also with pattern dystrophy and fundus flavimaculatus (6). Examples of autosomal recessive RP genotypes include mutations of the cGMP phosphodiesterase genes, α-subunit cGMP-gated channel gene, the retinal pigment epithelium protein RPE65 gene, and the arrestin gene. Further, defects in the RP GTPase regulator (RPGR) gene account for 20–30% of X-linked recessive RP.

Full-Field ERG Findings in RP

Full-field ERG responses are reduced in early stages of RP even when symptoms and clinical findings are mild; therefore, ERG testing is helpful in diagnosing or confirming RP (7,8). For those patients with detectable ERG responses, ERG testing serves as an objective measure of retinal function, which may be used to follow the degree of progression. Among RP patients ERG responses are variable, and this variability may occur among affected persons of the same family. In general, patients with early stages of RP have reduced and prolonged rod ERG responses and near normal or slightly reduced cone responses which may or may not be prolonged (Fig. 8.2) (9). With further progression of the disease, the rod and cone ERG responses diminish, prolong, and become non-detectable (Fig. 8.2). In RP patients with moderate to severe disease, the full-field ERG responses are likely to be very small or non-detectable. In some patients with mild disease, referred to as "delimited" or "self-limited"

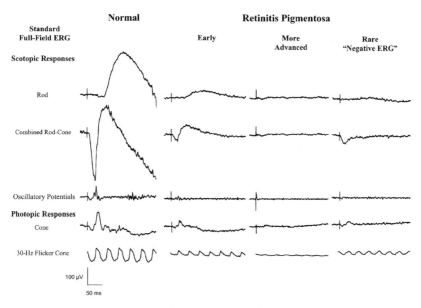

Figure 8.2 Examples of full-field ERG responses in RP. Both rod and cone responses are impaired early in RP with a preferential impairment of rod responses. In more advanced cases, the responses are non-detectable except for residual cone flicker responses. Very rarely, a "negative ERG" may occur where a selective reduction of the b-wave produces a b-wave to a-wave amplitude ratio of less than 1 in the scotopic bright-flash combined rod–cone response.

disease, the ERG responses are substantial and the prognosis more favorable (8,10,11). Patients with normal or mildly delayed photopic cone response implicit times are also more likely to have better prognosis (12).

For RP patients with detectable full-field ERG responses, the average yearly loss of 30-Hz cone flicker response amplitude ranges from 10% to 17%. However, because of considerable individual variation, these population ERG results should be applied with caution in predicting ERG declines in individual patients. Further, fluctuation in ERG responses due to normal re-test variations need to be considered in determining progression. Impaired 30-Hz cone flicker response in RP is likely due to a sensitivity change at the photoreceptor and a delay in the response of the inner retina (13,14). In a 4-year study of 67 RP patients with detectable rod and cone full-field ERG responses by Birch et al. (15), the percentages of RP patients with a decline in ERG amplitudes were 64% and 60% for rod and cone responses, respectively, and the mean annual increase in rod ERG threshold was 28% per year (0.14 log unit) compared to 13% per year (0.06 log unit) for cone ERG threshold. In the same study, RP patients, on the average, lost 13.3% of the remaining 30-Hz cone flicker ERG response amplitude per year. These results are comparable to those of a previous 3-year study by Berson et al. (16), where 94 RP patients with detectable cone but not necessarily detectable rod full-field ERG demonstrated an average annual of decline of 17.1% of 30-Hz cone response amplitude. In a subsequent randomized clinical trial by Berson et al. (17), the average annual decline of 30-Hz cone flicker ERG response amplitude was 10% for untreated RP patients.

Prior to genetic advances in RP, the classification of RP was based on hereditary pattern as well as clinical and ERG findings. Discrimination among dominant, autosomal recessive, and X-linked RP is not possible based on ERG responses (11,18). Massof and Finkelstein (19) identified two types of autosomal dominant RP based on measures of rod sensitivity relative to cone sensitivity. One category of patients was characterized by an early diffuse loss of rod sensitivity and later loss of cone sensitivity while the other category had regional and combined loss of rod and cone sensitivity. Subsequently, other subgroups of dominant RP patients were also identified who did not fit into this classification scheme (20). Fishman et al. (10) classified dominant RP patients based on clinical and ERG criteria: type 1—diffuse retinopathy with non-detectable ERG; type 2—preferential inferior retinal involvement with marked loss in ERG rod response with prolonged cone implicit times; type 3—same as type 2 but with normal cone implicit times; and type 4—"delimited" form with mild disease with substantial cone and rod ERG amplitudes and normal implicit times.

Narrow-Band Filtering of Low-Amplitude Cone ERG in RP

In patients with advanced RP and full-field ERG responses that are very small, computer averaging alone or in combination with a narrow-band electronic filter may allow the measurement of 30-Hz cone responses of less than $1\,\mu V$ (21). Averaging hundreds of 30-Hz cone responses smooths out and reduces the effect of random background electrical noise. Further, a narrow-band electronic filter with bandpass of 29–31 Hz and a center frequency of 30 Hz alters the recorded signal so that only the 30-Hz recorded signals are preserved. This technique increases the signal-to-noise ratio for responses that are predominantly sinusoidal at the 30-Hz frequency, but those signals that are outside the range of the narrow-band filter will be lost, potentially altering the amplitude of the response. Andréasson et al. (21) found that narrow-band filtering reduces the computer-averaged amplitude by an average of 7%, but this reduction in amplitude was independent of the size of the unbandpassed response. Critics of narrow-band filtering point out that because of the nature of the narrow-band filter, the small processed signals ($<0.5\,\mu V$) obtained in patients with advanced disease will resemble 30-Hz sinusoidal waves regardless of whether the signals are generated by retinal activity or by background noise.

Correlation of ERG and Visual Fields in RP

Correlations between full-field ERG amplitudes and visual field areas in RP patients have been demonstrated by several studies (22–28). Because of individual variations, correlations between ERG and visual field in individual patients are not always precise (29). Fahle et al. (23) showed significant relationships between all parameters of the full-field ERG and visual field diameters obtained by the Goldmann and Tübinger perimeters with regression coefficients ranging from 0.4 to 0.67. Iannaccone et al. (25) noted significant correlations between the scotopic bright-flash b-wave amplitude and Goldmann areas obtained by the I4e, III4e, V4e isopters. Further, in a study of 601 RP patients, Sandberg et al. (27) noted that significant correlations between Gold-mann V4e isopter equivalent diameter and full-field ERG amplitude were generally higher for the photopic 30-Hz cone flicker response than the photopic cone flash response. The correlations were also higher for patients with dominant or recessive RP than for patients with X-linked RP, most likely because X-linked RP patients generally have smaller ERG amplitudes.

ERG Response and Functional Disability in RP

Studies indicate that visual acuity and visual field measures are better correlates of difficulty with daily activities than ERG parameters. Szlyk et al. (30) administered question-naires to 160 patients with RP and seven patients with Usher syndrome type 2 and found that perceived difficulty in per-forming common tasks such as mobility, driving, negotiating steps, eating meals, and activities involving central vision is strongly related to level of visual acuity and visual fields. Although some ERG amplitude measures did correlate with difficulty with some self-reported activities, overall, the ERG amplitude measures showed the least relationship with patients' self reports. In another study, the same research group evaluated driving performance in RP patients by self-reported accident frequency and by performance on an inter-active driving simulator (31). Visual field loss was found to be a primary correlate of automotive accidents in individuals with RP.

Use of ERG in Clinical Treatment Trial of RP

Favorable ERG outcomes in clinical treatment trials of RP have not necessarily been associated with better visual func-tion outcomes. Using narrow-band filtering of the 30-Hz cone response in a randomized trial, Berson et al. (17) found that, compared to the placebo group, RP patients treated with oral 15,000 I.U. vitamin A palmitate daily had a slower rate of decline in 30-Hz cone response and those treated with oral vitamin E of 400 I.U. daily had a faster rate of decline. How-ever, no significant differences in change of visual acuity or visual field were noted among the patient groups. In a randomized clinical trial of patients with X-linked RP receiving either supplemental docosahexaenoic acid (DHA) or placebo, Hoffman et al. (32) noted that DHA supplementation significantly reduced rod ERG function loss in patients aged <12 years and preserved cone ERG function in patients ≥12 years, but neither visual acuity nor visual fields showed any significant change compared to the placebo group.

Unilateral RP

Although RP is usually a bilateral condition, patients with unilateral RP are occasionally encountered. The criteria for the diagnosis of unilateral RP are: (1) retinal, functional, and ERG changes consistent with RP in the affected eye; (2) normal function and normal ERG and EOG in the fellow eye; (3) exclusion of inflammatory, infectious, vascular, and traumatic causes of the retinopathy in the affected eye; (4) a sufficient period of observation to exclude a delayed onset of RP in the unaffected eye (33). Acquired disorders that may produce unilateral retinal pigmentary degeneration include ophthalmic artery occlusion, inflammatory retinopathies from syphilis, rubeola, onchocerciasis, and diffuse unilateral subacute neuroretinitis, and traumatic retinal injuries (34–37). Serial ERG and EOG testing of both eyes over time is helpful to determine that the "good" eye is normal and to exclude the possibility of subsequent development of bilateral asymmetric RP (37–39). Based on these criteria, true unilateral RP is rare, and most RP patients with unilateral symptoms have asymmetric disease (Fig. 8.3). Further, the lack of positive family history in virtually all unilateral RP patients implies that this disorder is acquired or recessively inherited.

Sector RP

Sector RP occurs when retinal atrophy, attenuated retinal vessels, and bone-spicule-like pigmentary clumping are localized to one or two quadrants of the retina. This rare disorder is typically bilateral, often autosomal dominant, and generally mildly progressive (40–44). However, some

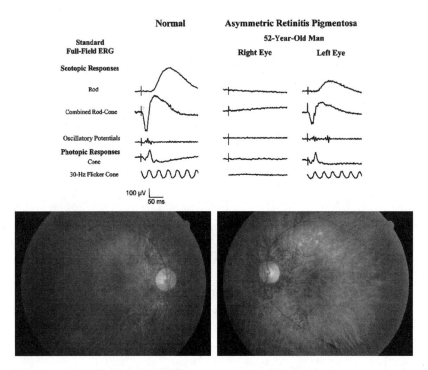

Figure 8.3 Full-field ERG responses and retinal appearance of a 52-year-old man with asymmetric RP. Visual acuity was 20/20 in each eye. Goldmann visual fields showed marked constriction in the right eye and mild constriction in the left eye. *Top*: The ERG responses were asymmetric with non-detectable responses in the right eye and impaired responses in the left eye. *Bottom*: Retinal atrophy and pigmentary clumping were present in both eyes with the left eye having less vascular attenuation.

cases of presumptive "sector" RP may represent early stages of widespread RP. In sector RP, rod and cone full-field ERG responses are reduced, but the implicit times are normal (43,44). Although the ERG responses are somewhat proportional to the extent of visible retinal involvement, perimetric visual thresholds, dark adaptometry, ERG, and EOG studies have also revealed dysfunction of the normal-appearing areas of the retina (41,42,44). This has led Krill and Archer to suggest that "asymmetrical" rather than "sector" RP better describes this condition.

ERG in X-Linked RP Carriers

Heterozygous female carriers of X-linked RP show a broad spectrum of clinical features ranging from normal retinal appearance to widespread retinal degeneration, presumably due to lyonization, the degree of whether the normal or the abnormal X chromosome is inactivated (45–48). Full-field ERG responses in X-linked RP carriers correlate with the extent of retinal findings, and ERG responses and prognosis are more favorable for those carriers with normal retinal appearance or tapetal-like retinal reflex only (49,50). Impaired full-field ERG responses may be demonstrated in 50–96% of X-linked RP carriers (47,51,52). In general, both the cone and rod responses are reduced in carriers, and the a-wave is reduced but not prolonged and the b-wave is both reduced and prolonged (53). The most consistent full-field ERG abnormality in X-linked RP carriers is likely delay in cone b-wave implicit times (54,55). Retinal examination combined with full-field ERG can lead to the identification of virtually all X-linked RP carriers (47). Multifocal ERG demonstrates patchy areas of retinal dyfunction in most X-linked RP carriers, and this mosaic pattern of dysfunction may be observed even in the absence of any visible retinal and full-field ERG abnormalities (56,57).

Negative ERG in RP

A negative ERG where a selective reduction of the b-wave produces a b-wave to a-wave amplitude ratio of less than 1 in the scotopic bright-flash combined rod–cone full-field ERG response is rarely found in RP (Fig. 8.2). Cideciyan and Jacobson (58) examined seven patients who had typical clinical features of RP with negative ERG pattern and found that the derived PII component of the rod ERG was abnormally reduced relative to the PIII component. Many of the patients also had a disproportionate reduction of the ON ERG component as compared to the OFF component. Photopic oscillatory potentials were also reduced and delayed or not detectable. Taken together, these findings indicate that in this rare subset of RP patients, dysfunction occurs not only at the level of the photoreceptor outer segment but also at or proximal to the photoreceptor terminal region.

Low Frequency Damped ERG Wavelets in RP

Low frequency damped wavelet is a very rare full-field ERG finding noted in patients with early stages of RP (59). A series of 3–5 wavelets with reducing frequency and a period of 25–37 ms are observed in the scotopic bright-flash combined rod–cone response and the photopic cone flash response. Other ERG features in these patients include a non-detectable rod response and an increased b-wave to a-wave ratio for the photopic cone flash response presumably due to contribution of the first wavelet of the low frequency wavelets to the b-wave. Because the rod ERG responses are non-detectable, the low frequency damped wavelets are presumably cone-driven and may be due to a reverberating of the OFF-pathway. The wavelets diminish over time as the disease progresses.

Multifocal ERG in RP

In general, multifocal ERG assesses cone function, because recording of multifocal rod ERG is difficult due to poor signal-to-noise ratio produced by the need for blank frames and the slower recovery of the rods to successive stimulation (60). Multifocal ERG studies indicate decreased amplitudes and increase implicit times especially eccentric to the fovea in RP patients (61,62). Loss of amplitude of a multifocal ERG test area is not a good predictor of visual sensitivity obtained with Humphrey visual field, but delayed timing of the test area appears to be an early indicator of local retinal damage to the cone system (61).

VEP in RP

In general, VEP responses in RP are impaired due to retinal dysfunction. However, several studies have noted detectable VEP responses in RP patients (63–66). For instance, Jacobson et al. (63) performed flash VEP in the dark-adapted and light-adapted states in 50 RP patients and found all but one of the patients had a detectable VEP responses. Detectable VEP was present in some patients with non-detectable ERG responses, and the authors concluded VEP may be a useful objective measure in assessing patients with residual central visual fields only.

LEBER CONGENITAL AMAUROSIS

Leber congenital amaurosis (LCA), described by Leber (67) in 1869, refers to a group of genetically heterogeneous autosomal recessive retinal dystrophies characterized by severe visual impairment noted within a few months after birth, infantile nystagmus, and the subsequent development of pigmentary retinal degeneration. However, at the time of diagnosis in infancy, the retinal appearance may be normal or demonstrate macular dysplasia or coloboma. Other associated features of LCA include hyperopia, keratoconus, cataracts, mental retardation, cystic renal disease, skeletal disorders, and hydrocephalus (68,69).

Leber congenital amaurosis is associated with several genetic loci (70). LCA1 is caused by mutations of the gene encoding retinal guanylate cyclase (GUCY2D) on chromosome 17p (71). LCA2 is due to mutations of the RPE65 (retinal pigment epithelium-specific 65-kD protein) gene on chromosome 1 (72). LCA3 is mapped to chromosome 14q. LCA4 is produced by mutations of the AIPL1 (arylhydrocarbon interacting protein-like 1) gene on chromosome 17p (73). LCA5 is mapped to chromosome 6q. LCA6 is associated with mutations of the RPGR-interacting (RPGRIP1) protein. Genetic loci of other forms of LCA include the photoreceptor-specific homeo box gene CRX on chromosome 19 and the Crumbs homolog 1 gene (74).

In infants with congenital blindness, full-field ERG is the key test for determining retinal dysfunction and the diagnosis of LCA. Several studies have demonstrated nondetectable rod and cone full-field ERG responses in most patients with LCA with a few having detectable but severely reduced and attenuated responses (69,75–79). Patients with

LCA associated with heterozygous compound RPE 65 mutations (LCA2) have non-detectable rod ERG response and residual cone ERG response and may retain some useful visual function at age 10 (77). Full-field cone ERG impairment with mild cone–rod dysfunction is found in some carrier parents of patients with LCA associated with GUCY2D mutation consistent with the higher expression of GUCY2D in cone as compared to rod photoreceptors (80).

A non-detectable ERG in blind children with pigmentary retinopathy is not specific for LCA, and systemic diseases such as infantile Refsum disease, Zellweger syndrome, neuronal ceroid lipofuscinosis should be considered (76). Further, rare patients with autosomal recessive congenital stationary night blindness may have nystagmus, notable visual impairment in infancy, and reduced ERG and may be misdiagnosed as having LCA (81).

Despite mostly non-detectable full-field ERG responses, flash VEP responses are detectable in many infants and children with LCA (76,82). One hypothesis of this phenomenon is that the sensitivity of the VEP is higher in lower stimulus luminance due to the magnification of the foveal contribution (83).

USHER SYNDROME

Usher syndrome refers to a genetically heterogeneous group of autosomal recessive disorders characterized by sensorineural hearing loss and progressive retinal pigmentary degeneration. Usher syndrome, described in the 1800s, is named after Charles Usher, a British ophthalmologist of the early 1900s. Usher syndrome is classified into three main types, all of which are associated with early onset of progressive pigmentary retinopathy and marked reduction of full-field ERG responses. Patients with type I Usher syndrome have severe congenital deafness and vestibular dysfunction, patients with type II Usher syndrome have less profound congenital hearing loss and normal vestibular function, and patients with type III Usher syndrome have congenital near normal hearing with progressive hearing loss. Therefore, hearing testing with audiometry is valuable in differentiating types of Usher syndrome (84).

Usher syndrome is extremely heterogeneous with numerous genetic subtypes. Type I Usher syndrome is associated with at least five genetic loci located on chromosomes 14 q (type 1A), 11q (type 1B), 11p (type 1C), 10q (type 1D), and 21q (type 1E). Type 1B accounts for about 75% of patients with type 1 Usher syndrome and is caused by mutations of the gene encoding myosin VIIA, a cytoskeletal protein (85). Abnormal myosin VIIA results in abnormal organization of microtubules of photoreceptor cells and degeneration of organ of Corti. Type II Usher syndrome is associated with at least three genetic located on chromosomes 1q (type IIA), 3p (type IIB), and 5q (type IIC). Type IIA accounts to about 90% patients with type 1I Usher syndrome and is caused by mutations of the gene designated as usherin (86). Type III Usher syndrome is the least common type but more common in Finnish families and is associated with mutations of the USH3A gene on chromosome 3q.

Ocular findings and degree of visual impairment are variable in Usher syndrome even patients with similar genetypes (87). Ocular symptoms and signs of Usher syndrome are similar to severe, early-onset RP. Night vision impairment, peripheral vision loss, and light sensitivity generally begin insidiously by the second decade of life. Visual acuity and macular function are relatively more preserved early in the disease. Retinal atrophy with vascular attenuation and pigmentary clumping (bone spicules) develop, and with progression, optic nerve atrophy, atrophic macular lesions, cystoid macular edema, vitreous syneresis with mild vitritis, and posterior subcapsular cataracts ccour.

Full-field ERG responses in Usher syndrome are severely reduced even in early disease with greater impairment of rod response than cone response. With disease progression, full-field ERG responses become non-detectable. Patients with type I Usher syndrome generally have earlier onset and more severe progressive retinopathy compared with type II patients. At any given age, visual acuity, visual field area, and ERG responses are likely to be more impaired in type I patients than type II patients (88,89). Likewise, the prevalence of atrophic or cystic foveal lesions is greater in type I patients (90). However, considerable overlap of the degree of impairment of these clinical parameters occurs between type I and type II; this makes typing Usher patients difficult on ophthalmologic grounds (89). Further, Bharadwaj et al. (91) have shown that visual acuity, visual field area, and ERG responses are not significantly different between type IB and other type I patients. Of interest, Seeliger et al. (92) found similar first-order multifocal ERG amplitude reduction among patients with RP, type I Usher syndrome, and type II Usher syndrome, but patients with type I Usher syndrome had only slightly delayed implicit times in the periphery of the 30° tested area compared to more delayed implicit times for patients with RP and type II Usher syndrome.

Full-field ERG is an important diagnostic test in combination with an ophthalmologic examination to screen for Usher syndrome in children with profound, preverbal sensorineural hearing loss (93). Although the prevalence of Usher syndrome in the United States has been estimated at 4.4 per 100,000, up to 6% of hearing-impaired children have Usher syndrome (94).

Heterozygous carriers of Usher syndrome have mild hearing loss and tend to have mildly reduced light-peak to dark-trough EOG amplitude ratios, but these findings are not sensitive or specific enough for reliable detection of carriers (95–97).

BARDET–BIEDL SYNDROME

Bardet–Biedl syndrome (BBS), described by Bardet in 1920 and Biedl in 1922, is a rare autosomal recessive disorder characterized by obesity, mild mental retardation, severe progressive pigmentary retinopathy, polydactyly, and hypogonadism (98,99). Other common clinical features of BBS include renal abnormalities and diabetes mellitus (100). Bardet–Biedl syndrome (BBS) is a genetically heterogeneous disorder associated with several genetic loci including chromosomes 11q (BBS1), 16q (BBS2), 3p (BBS3), 15q (BBS4),

2q (BBS5), and 20p (BBS6). BBS2 is due to mutations of the BBS2 gene, and BBS6 is related to mutations of the MKKS (Mckusick–Kaufman syndrome) gene (101–103).

Visual impairment in patients with Bardet–Biedl syndrome is usually apparent in the first two decades of life. Ocular findings include optic nerve atrophy and progressive pigmentary retinal degeneration with vascular attenuation and macular atrophy (Fig. 8.4) (104–106). Full-field ERG responses are severely impaired early in the disease and are severely prolonged and reduced to less than 10% of normal values for age (104,107). In those patients with detectable full-field ERG responses, cone responses are more likely to be greater than rod responses (104,106–108). Pattern VEP responses are likely to be more preserved in patients with better macular function (109). Obligatory carriers of BBS generally have normal or near normal clinical full-field ERG but have diminished PII sensitivity demonstrable with specialized ERG analysis; PII is a positive inner retinal potential related mostly to bipolar cell activity (110).

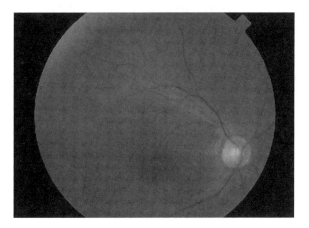

Figure 8.4 Retinal atrophy in a 14-year-old boy with Bardet–Biedl syndrome. The patient had obesity, short stature, and polydactyly. Visual acuity was 20/20 in each eye with constricted and depressed visual fields. Although the retinal atrophy appeared mild, the full-field ERG responses were non-detectable. (Refer to the color insert.)

Bardet–Biedl syndrome and Alström syndrome   share similar clinical features such as obesity, pigmentary retinopathy, and diabetes mellitus. However, Alström syndrome is not associated with mental retardation and polydactyly, and in contrast to BBS, Alström syndrome is associated with nystagmus, early loss of central vision, and generalized cone–rod rather than rod–cone dysfunction.

REFSUM SYNDROME

Refsum disease, described by Refsum in the mid 1900s, is a rare autosomal recessive disorder associated with abnormal metabolism resulting in the accumulation of phytanic acid, a branched-chain fatty acid (111,112). Refsum disease is due to dysfunction of the peroxisome, an organelle found in cells of most tissues, and is genetically heterogeneous (113). Infantile form of Refsum disease is due to defective assembly or biogenesis of peroxisome. Clinical features of infantile Refsum disease include mental retardation, failure to thrive, pigmentary retinopathy, sensorineural hearing loss, minor facial dysmorphism, hepatomegaly, neuromuscular hypotony, and peripheral neuropathy. Infantile Refsum disease can be caused by mutations of the PEX1 and PEX2 genes. Examples of other peroxisomal biogenesis disorders include neonatal adrenoleukodystrophy and Zellweger syndrome, both of which have overlapping features with infantile Refsum disease. In contrast, classic form of Refsum disease is associated with point mutations and deletions of the PAHX gene which encodes phytanonyl-CoA hydroxylase, an enzyme which activates phytanic acid to phytanoyl-CoA before it is oxidized. Clinical features of classic Refsum disease include pigmentary retinopathy, polyneuropathy, and cerebellar dysfunction.

Early diagnosis of Refsum disease is critical because the condition is treatable with dietary restriction of phytanic acid and plasma exchange. Serum phytanic acid is typically consistently elevated. Visual symptoms such as night visual impairment and decreased vision may be the only early presenting symptoms. Progressive pigmentary retinal degeneration with vascular attenuation and macular atrophy is the primary ocular finding. Nystagmus may be present. Full-field ERG is usually markedly impaired early in the disease and is a helpful diagnostic tool especially in infantile Refsum disease (7). Both rod and cone responses are reduced and prolonged, and the b-wave may be more affected than the a-wave suggesting greater inner retinal dysfunction; a negative pattern of the scotopic combined rod–cone response with a b-wave to a-wave amplitude of less than 1 may occur (114–116). With treatment, neurologic symptoms improve and visual function stabilizes (114). Rarely, older adults with pigmentary retinopathy, mildly impaired ERG, and elevated serum phytanic acid are found and are considered as having a variant of Refsum disease (117).

ABETALIPOPROTEINEMIA
(BASSEN–KORNZWEIG SYNDROME)

In 1950, Bassen and Kornzweig reported an 18-year-old girl with generalized retinal degeneration, Friedreich ataxia, and abnormal red blood cells, and in 1960, an absence of apolipoprotein B in plasma was found to be associated with this rare autosomal recessive disorder which was subsequently called abetalipoproteinemia (118,119). Apolipoprotein B is the only apoprotein of low density lipoprotein (LDL) and accounts for about 35% of apoprotein composition of very low density lipoprotein (VLDL). Apolipoprotein B is also a component of chylomicrons, and patients with abetalipoproteinemia have reduced absorption of fat as well as fat-soluble vitamins such as A and E. Serum levels of cholesterol and triglycerides in abetalipoproteinemia are extremely low. Abetalipoproteinemia is caused by point mutations of the gene encoding microsomal triglyceride transfer protein (MTP) which catalyzes the transport of triglyceride, cholesteryl ester, and phospholipid from phospholipid surfaces (120,121). Clinical features of abetalipoproteinemia start in childhood and include celiac syndrome with steatorrhea, progressive ataxic neuropathy, abnormal red blood cells (acanthocytosis), and pigmentary retinal degeneration. Treatment of abetalipoproteinemia consists of low-fat diet and oral supplementation of vitamins A and E.

Ocular manifestations include pigmentary retinopathy, ophthalmoplegia, ptosis, nystagmus, and angioid streaks. The pigmentary retinopathy occurs in all patients with abetalipoproteinemia and is similar to RP (rod–cone dystrophy) with progressive diffuse retinal atrophy accompanied by vascular attenuation and pigmentary clumping (bone spicules) (122). Visual acuity and macular function are usually relatively spared in early disease. Full-field ERG responses in abetalipoproteinemia are similar to those found in RP with greater impairment of rod response than cone response in early disease although b-wave implicit times tend to be less delayed in abetalipoproteinemia (7). The EOG and VEP responses are correspondingly reduced (123–125). As the disease progresses, full-field ERG responses become non-detectable. With initiation of large doses of oral vitamin A or vitamin A and E in previously untreated patients, partial recovery of visual function and full-field ERG responses may occur in less advance cases even if the ERG responses are non-detectable (126–128). Further, chronic combined vitamin A and E therapy initiated prior to the age of 2 years can markedly lessen but not prevent the development of pigmentary retinopathy and impaired ERG responses (123,129–131). Taken together, investigators have concluded that full-field ERG is useful in monitoring visual function in response to therapy in abetalipoproteinemia. Of interest, patients with hypobetalipoproteinemia, which is associated with mutations in the apolipoprotein B gene, also have reduced apolipoprotein B and demonstrate clinical features and ERG findings similar to abetalipoproteinemia (129).

NEURONAL CEROID LIPOFUSCINOSIS

Neuronal ceroid lipofuscinosis is a group of genetic heterogeneous autosomal recessive disorders with numerous phenotypic variations, characterized by the accumulation of lipopigments in lysosomes (132,133). Primary clinical features include progressive pigmentary retinopathy, regression of intellect, and seizures. The infantile form of the disease [also known as infantile neuronal ceroid lipofuscinosis (INCL), ceroid lipofuscinosis 1 (CLN1), Haltia-Santavuori disease, or Finnish form] with onset before age two is caused by mutations of the gene encoding palmitoyl-protein thioesterase on chromosome 1p32. Patients with CLN1 have blindness and severe psychomotor retardation. The late infantile form (LINCL, CLN2, or Jansky–Bielchoesky disease) with onset between age 2.5 and 4.0 is associated with mutations of the CLN2 gene on chromosome 11p15. Patients with CLN2 have regression of developmental milestones, seizures, and later loss of vision. The late infantile form is also associated with several other genetic loci including 13p22 (CLN5) and 15q22 (CLN6). The juvenile form (JNCL, CLN3, Batten disease, or Vogt–Spielmeyer disease) with onset between age 4.5 and 8.0 is due to mutations of the CLN3 gene on chromosome 16. Patients with CLN3 have rapid progressive loss of vision with slower intellectual regression. The juvenile form is also associated with other genetic loci such as 8p23 (CLN8). The adult form (ANCL, CLN4, or Kufs disease) is associated with psychomotor regression and mild visual symptoms or findings. Of interest, one of the early descriptions of the disorder was by Batten, and the term "Batten disease" has been used occasionally to encompass all neuronal ceroid lipofuscinoses (134).

Visual impairment from progressive pigmentary retinal degeneration with vascular attenuation and macular atrophy is often the presenting symptom especially in patients with the juvenile form of the disease (Fig. 8.5). The diagnosis is confirmed by electron microscopic identification of lipopigments in peripheral blood lymphocytes. Full-field ERG is a helpful ancillary test to detect retinal dysfunction and is severely impaired in the early stages of the disease even when visible retinal changes are still mild (135). With progression, the ERG responses become non-detectable. In INCL, Weleber (136) reported that the earliest full-field ERG manifestation

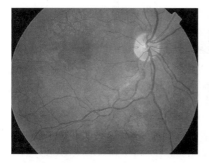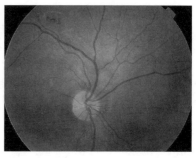

Figure 8.5 Retinal atrophy and pigment clumping in a 9-year-old girl with neuronal ceroid lipofuscinosis, juvenile form (Batten disease). Visual acuity was 20/100 in each eye, and full-field ERG responses were moderately reduced. The patient had insidious progressive visual loss and night vision impairment. She also exhibited periods of inattention, inappropriate behavior, and verbal confusion. The diagnosis was confirmed by electron microscopic identification of cytoplasmic granules in peripheral blood lymphocytes. (Refer to the color insert.)

is a marked loss of the scotopic and photopic b-wave with relative preservation of the a-wave (negative pattern, b-wave to a-wave amplitude ratio <1) suggesting a greater dysfunction of the inner retina. For late infantile form of the disorder, the same author noted severely reduced and prolonged cone responses with impaired but less affected rod response, and in the juvenile form, the rod response was non-detectable with severely reduced, negative pattern photopic cone and bright-flash scotopic responses. Likewise, Horiguchi and Miyake noted similar ERG findings in patients with juvenile neuronal ceroid lipofuscinosis, and Eksandh et al. found non-detectable rod responses and marked diminished cone responses in patients with CLN3 mutations (137,138). In the adult form of the disease, Dawson et al. (139) found severely diminished photopic cone responses. Heterozygous carriers of neuronal ceroid lipofuscinosis generally have mild impairment of rod full-field ERG, pattern ERG, and EOG compared to normals but carriers cannot be accurately determined on an individual basis based on these findings (140).

KEARNS–SAYRE SYNDROME: MITOCHONDRIAL RETINOPATHY

Kearns–Sayre syndrome, Pearson syndrome, and chronic progressive external ophthalmoplegia (CPEO) are associated with identical deletions of the mitochondrial DNA. The variability in clinical manifestations among these disorders is related to the difference in tissue distributions of the mutant mitochondrial DNA. In Kearns–Sayre syndrome, mutant DNAs are more localized to muscles and central nervous system while in Pearson syndrome, mutant DNAs are found in high levels in all tissues. In contrast, in CPEO mutant DNA are likely to be very localized to involve mostly muscles. Initially described in 1958, the clinical features of Kearns–Sayre syndrome include progressive external ophthalmoplegia with ptosis, pigmentary retinopathy, cardiomyopathy, heart block, muscle weakness, cerebellar dysfunction, deafness, short stature, and electroencephalographic changes (141). Aside from mitochondrial DNA analysis, the diagnosis may be supported by the finding of ragged red fibers on muscle biopsy.

When present, the pigmentary retinopathy in Kearns–Sayer syndrome is variable in severity and frequently asymptomatic. Full-field ERG responses are generally mildly to moderately impaired in patients with mild retinopathy but may be markedly diminished in severe cases. EOG impairment also occurs but EOG cannot be obtained in patients with ophthalmoplegia that is severe enough to prevent adequate eye movements for EOG testing. In a study of 61 patients with mitochondrial myopathy, Mullie et al. (142) found 22 (36%) with pigmentary retinopathy. Of these 22 patients, 18 had "salt and pepper" retinal appearance consisting of diffuse stippled areas of hypopigmentation and hyperpigmentation and visual acuity of mostly 20/40 or better. Of the remaining 4 patients, two had RP-like changes with hand-movement and light perception vision, but unlike classic RP, pigment clumping was present at the maculas. The other two patients had severe generalized atrophy of the retinal pigment epithelium and choriocapillaris with severe visual loss. Ten of the 18 patients with "salt and pepper" retinopathy were studied with

EOG and full-field ERG; both the rod and cone ERG responses as well as the EOG light-peak to dark-trough amplitude ratios demonstrated mild to moderate reductions with diminished cone flicker response being the most consistent finding. However, other studies have shown that normal EOG and ERG may occur in Kearns–Sayre retinopathy, and conversely, in some cases the ERG is diminished before the retinal pigmentary changes are visible (143–145). In addition, reduced scotopic with normal photopic ERG responses in a patient with Kearns–Sayre syndrome has also been reported (146), and abnormal scotopic ERG responses are common in children with mitochondrial disorders (147).

Impaired VEP in Kearns–Sayre syndrome is common (148–150). This is likely due in part to retinal dysfunction from the retinopathy as well as from the electroencephalographic alterations associated with central nervous system involvement.

RUBELLA RETINOPATHY

Pigmentary retinopathy may be a manifestation of the post-rubella syndrome. The retinopathy is usually bilateral but may be asymmetric. Although post-rubella retinopathy may mimic RP in appearance, retinal vascular attenuation is generally not present. Electroretinogram is a key diagnostic test in distinguishing the two conditions. Full-field ERG is normal in almost all cases of post-rubella retinopathy but may occasionally be mildly below the normal range (151,152). Of interest, in patients with asymmetric retinal pigmentary changes, ERG amplitudes may be relatively more reduced in the more affected eye (153).

SYPHILITIC RETINOPATHY

Chorioretinitis and pigmentary retinopathy may be a feature of syphilitic or post-syphilitic syndrome. Not surprisingly, impaired ERG responses and impaired EOG are found patients with syphilitic chorioretinitis (154). However, in contrast to RP, the full-field ERG response is generally only mildly or moderately impaired and is more likely to have reduced amplitude than prolonged implicit time (155).

ENHANCED S-CONE SYNDROME

In 1990, Marmor et al. (156) reported eight patients with night blindness, maculopathy, and unusual but characteristic full-field ERG responses which represent increased responses of blue or short-wavelength sensitive cones (S cones), and this rare but distinct autosomal recessive retinal degeneration was named "enhanced S-cone syndrome."

Symptoms of night blindness, reduced visual acuity, and visual field disturbance usually occur within the first two decades of life, but symptoms and signs of this disorder show variable expressivity even within the same family (157). Visual acuity ranges from 20/20 to 20/200, and visual field ranges from full to central and mid-pheripheral ring scotomas. Retinal findings include cystoid maculopathy, yellow fleck-like lesions peripherally or near the vascular arcades, and gray or pigmentary degeneration (Fig. 8.6). Despite the early onset of this disorder, progression is usually slow (156,157).

Full-field ERG is a key test for diagnosing enhanced S-cone syndrome. The dark-adapted ERG shows no response to low-intensity stimuli that normally activate rods. With high-intensity stimuli that normally activate both rods and cones, the dark-adapted ERG demonstrates large, slow responses. The light-adapted ERG flash cone response also shows similar large, slow waveforms that are nearly identical to those elicited by scotopic high-intensity stimuli (Figs. 8.6 and 8.7). Under standardized clinical ERG conditions, the specific findings include: (1) a severely reduced or non-detectable rod response to the scotopic dim flash, (2) a subnormal slow a-wave and a much reduced slow b-wave for both the scotopic bright-flash response and for the photopic flash cone response, (3) reduced oscillatory potentials, and (4) reduced photopic flicker responses. The ERG pattern of

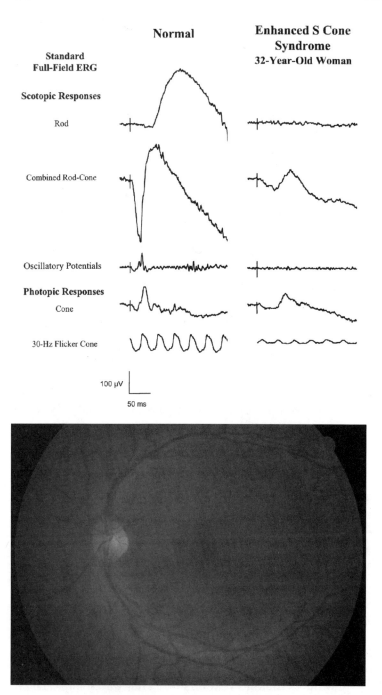

Figure 8.6 (*Caption on facing page*)

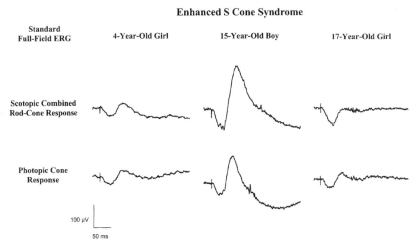

Figure 8.7 Similar standard full-field ERG morphology of the scotopic combined rod–cone response and the photopic cone response in three patients with enhanced S cone syndrome demonstrating inter-individual variation.

increased S-cone sensitivity is not unique to enhanced S-cone syndrome but is also found in Goldmann–Favre syndrome (158). In the enhanced S-cone syndrome, EOG light-peak-to-dark-trough amplitude ratios are reduced (156).

The number of S-cone photoreceptors is increased in patients with enhanced S-cone syndrome. Hood et al. (159) using high intensity flashes and a cone photorecptor activation model (see Chapter 6) found large a-waves in response to blue and white flashes, which were driven almost entirely by photoreceptors containing S-cone pigment. These findings

Figure 8.6 (*Facing page*) Full-field ERG responses and retinal appearance in a 32-year-old woman with enhanced S-cone syndrome. Note the non-detectable rod response and the similar morphology of the tracings of the scotopic combined rod–cone response and the photopic cone response. Gray retinal atrophy with rare pigment clumping is evident particularly near the vascular arcades and in the mid-peripheral region. (Refer to the color insert.)

indicate not only that the number of S cones is increased in affected patients but also that these S cones have replaced some of the normal red, long-wavelength sensitive cones (L cones), green, medium-wavelength sensitive cones (M-cones), and many of the rods. This hypothesis was subsequently supported by further testing with measurements of cone system sensitivities, S-cone acuity, and other psychophysical measurements of the S-cone system (160).

Subsequently, Haider et al. (161) found mutations of a nuclear receptor gene, NR2E3, in 94% of patients with enhanced S-cone syndrome. The NR2E3 protein is a part of a large family of nuclear receptor transcription factors. Nuclear receptors are involved in the regulation of embryonic development, and expression of NR2E3 is thought to be limited to the outer nuclear layer of the human retina. This finding of NR2E3 mutations in affected patients suggests that enhanced S-cone syndrome is a disorder of differentiation of the photoreceptors and that NR2E3 plays a role in determining photoreceptor phenotype during human retinal development. Subsequently, NR2E3 mutations are found also to produce Goldmann–Favre syndrome and clumped pigmentary retinal degeneration (162).

GOLDMANN–FAVRE SYNDROME

Goldmann–Favre syndrome described in 1958 is an autosomal recessive disorder characterized by progressive pigmentary retinal degeneration, peripheral retinoschisis, vitreous strands, macular cystoid changes, and posterior subcapsular cataract (163). Affected persons have night blindness and variably decreased visual acuity and peripheral vision.

In patients with Goldmann–Favre syndrome, both rod and cone ERGs are markedly diminished and may be nondetectable (164). When standard full-field ERG is detectable, the entire light-adapted ERG flash cone response is reduced and prolonged and quite similar to the dark-adapted bright-flash rod–cone maximal response. By using dark-adapted perimetry and spectral ERG, Jacobson et al. (158) showed that the predominant ERG signal was from the short-wave-length sensitive cones. This relative hypersensitivity of the short-wavelength sensitive cones (S-cone, blue-sensitive cones) is similar to ERG features of the enhanced S-cone syndrome which is associated with mutations of the NR2E3 gene. At least some cases of Goldmann–Favre syndrome are also associated with NR2E3 mutations (162).

DOMINANT LATE-ONSET RETINAL DEGENERATION

In 1996, Kuntz et al. (165) reported an autosomal dominant late-onset retinal degeneration characterized by night vision impairment developing in the sixth decade of life with subsequent progressive pigmentary retinopathy. Patchy puncatate yellow–white lesions may be visible in the early stages, and with time, islands of pigmentary disturbance and chorio-retinal atrophy develop in the midperipheral regions of the retina with sparing of the macula and the far peripheral retina (165,166). With further progression, diffuse pigmentary retinal atrophy occurs. The most consistent early manifestation of the condition is abnormal dark adaptation which occurs even in affected but asymptomatic persons. Full-field ERG responses are usually normal early in the disease or may demonstrate mild impairment of the rod response (165,166). As the disease progresses, the ERG responses becomes non-detectable.

CONE–ROD DYSTROPHY

Cone–rod dystrophy refers to a large group of genetically heterogeneous disorders characterized by early cone photoreceptor dysfunction and progressive cone and rod dysfunction. In contrast to RP (rod–cone dystrophy), patients with cone–rod dystrophy generally have decreased central vision rather than night vision impairment, macular pigmentary changes usually with some peripheral retinopathy, and full-field ERG cone responses that are more or equally reduced than rod responses (Fig. 8.8) (24). Aside from reduced visual acuity and impaired color vision, other ocular symptoms and signs of cone–rod dystrophy include photoaversion, reduced visual field, and optic nerve atrophy.

Autosomal recessive, autosomal dominant, and X-linked recessive forms of cone–rod dystrophy are all found. As a group, cone–rod dystrophy is genetically heterogeneous. Genotypes associated with the cone–rod dystrophy phenotype include mutations involving the peripherin/RDS gene (dominant), the guanylate cyclase activator 1A gene (GUCA1A) (dominant), the retinal guanylate cyclase gene (GUCY2D) (dominant), the photoreceptor-specific homeobox gene CRX (dominant), and the ATP-binding

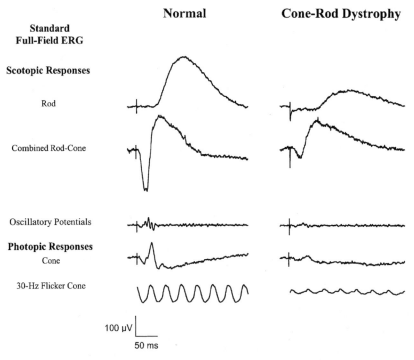

Figure 8.8 Standard full-field ERG responses of a 47-year-old man with sporadic cone–rod dystrophy showing greater impairment of the cone responses compared to rod and combined rod–cone responses.

cassette transporter protein ABCA4 (recessive). Mutations of some of these genes are also associated with other phenotypes such as RP, Leber congenital amaurosis, and Stargardt macular dystrophy.

The clinical features of cone–rod dystrophy are diverse, and the degree of cone as well as rod dysfunction may be variable even among family members with the same genotype (167). Several studies have classified cone–rod dystrophy into subtypes based on clinical and ERG findings. In a study of 14 patients with recessive or sporadic cone–rod dystrophy using full-field ERG and dark-adapted static threshold perimetry, Yagasaki and Jacobson (168) described three patterns of visual dysfunction. The first pattern shows slowly progressive central scotoma with mild peripheral retinal dysfunction equally affecting rod and cone systems. The second pattern is more progressive and characterized by central scotoma, greater cone than rod retinal dysfunction, and earlier peripheral than midperipheral visual field loss. The third pattern is the most progressive with marked central scotoma, no measurable cone function, and patches of rod function retained in the central and inferotemporal regions of the visual field. In another study, Szlyk et al. (169) prospectively examined 33 patients and reviewed clinical records of 150 patients with isolated, autosomal dominant, and autosomal recessive cone–rod dystrophy. Based on the full-field ERG results, two major types of cone–rod dystrophy were differentiated. In type 1, cone amplitudes were reduced more than rod amplitudes, and in type 2, cone and rod amplitudes were decreased to the same extent. These two types were further subdivided based on visual field loss and threshold elevation. In types 1a and 2a, central scotomas were accompanied by more elevated cone thresholds centrally than peripherally, and in types 1b and 2b, central scotoma is absent (1b) or a ring scotoma is present (2b) accompanied by more elevated cone thresholds peripherally than centrally.

In general, the likelihood of progressive ERG amplitude loss is similar among cone–rod dystrophy patients and RP patients. In a 4-year study of 29 cone–rod dystrophy patients and 67 RP patients with detectable rod and cone full-field

ERG responses by Birch and Fish (170), the percentage of patients with RP showing rod amplitude progression (64%) was not significantly different from the percentage of patients with cone–rod dystrophy (45%) ($p = 0.14$). Likewise, the percentage of patients demonstrating cone amplitude progression was similar between RP patients (60%) and cone–rod dystrophy patients (62%) ($p = 0.97$). However, when rod sensitivity as measured by retinal illumination necessary to elicit half of the maximal response ($\log k$, Naka–Rushton function) during the scotopic intensity response series, the rod sensitivity is normal or near normal in cone–rod dystrophy and significantly elevated in RP. Further, patients with advanced cone–rod dystrophy with diffuse pigmentary retinopathy and non-detectable full-field ERG are clinically virtually indistinguishable from patients with advanced RP. On the other end of the spectrum, it may be difficult to distinguish cone dystrophy from cone–rod dystrophy in patients with maculopathy, minimal peripheral retinopathy, and reduced cone but borderline rod ERG responses.

Several reports have studied the clinical features of cone–rod dystrophy associated with specific disease-causing genotypes (167,171–178). The degree of intrafamilial and interfamilial variability associated with a specific genotype ranges from differences only in severity to wide differences in clinical features among affected persons.

Female carriers of X-linked cone–rod dystrophy may appear clinically normal (179). However, some carriers may demonstrate subtle color vision defects, various degree of retinal degeneration, and prolonged 30-Hz cone flicker full-field ERG responses with interocular asymmetry (180).

Rarely in cone–rod dystrophy, one finds a negative ERG pattern where a selective reduction of the b-wave produces a b-wave to a-wave amplitude ratio of less than 1 in the scotopic bright-flash combined rod–cone full-field ERG response (174,181). A negative ERG pattern may be a prominent feature in a kindred or occur in an isolated affected family member.

In 1974, Deutman (182) reported four affected members of a family with a bull's-eye-like maculopathy consisting a ring of depigmentation surrounding a normal central macular area and called this autosomal dominant condition "benign concentric annular macular dystrophy" (182). In a follow-up examination of this kindred 10 years later, van den Biesen et al. (183) noted deterioration of vision and progression of the macular lesions. Some family members were also found to have peripheral pigmentary retinopathy with bone-spicule-like pigmentation. Full-field ERG responses showed equally impaired rod and cone responses. Subsequently, Miyake et al. (184) described four unrelated patients with bull's eye maculopathy and full-field ERG with maculopathy similar to patients with benign concentric annular macular dystrophy. However, the full-field ERG responses demonstrated a negative pattern of the scotopic bright-flash combined rod–cone full-field ERG response as well as markedly reduced oscillatory potentials and elevated dark adaptation rod thresholds. The cone responses were normal or mildly reduced. Whether the patients reported by Deutman and Miyake represent a variant of cone–rod dystrophy or RP is unclear.

ALSTRÖM SYNDROME

Alström syndrome, first described in 1959, is a rare autosomal recessive disorder characterized by obesity, pigmentary retinopathy, sensorineural hearing loss, cardiomyopathy, and diabetes mellitus (185,186). Alström syndrome is associated with mutations of the ALMS1 gene on chromosome 2p13 (187,188). Although the disorder shares some similar features to Bardet–Biedl syndrome, Alström syndrome is not associated with mental retardation and polydactyly and in contrast to Bardet–Biedl syndrome, Alström syndrome is associated with nystagmus, early loss of central vision, and generalized cone–rod rather than rod–cone dysfunction. The predominant ocular feature is the early development of retinal vascular attenuation with progressive diffuse pigmentary retinopathy involving the macula and optic nerve atrophy (185,189). Both cone and rod full-field ERG responses are severely reduced early in the disease and in many patients, the responses are nondetectable on presentation even in infancy (185,186,190). In

those with detectable ERG responses, severe early cone dysfunction occurs with the cone response diminishing rapidly to
become non-detectable (190). The ERG rod response is affected
to a less lesser degree initially but deteriorates rapidly as well.

REFERENCES

1. Marmor MF, Aguirre G, Arden G, Berson E, Birch D,
    Boughman JA, Carr R, Chatrian GE, del Monte M, Dowling
    J, Fishman GA, Fulton A, Garcia CA, Gouras P, Heckenlively
    J, Hu D, Lewis RA, Niemeyer G, Parker JA, Perlman I, Ripps
    H, Sandberg MA, Siegel I, Weleber RG, Wolf ML, Wu L, Young
    RS. Retinitis pigmentosa, a symposium on terminology and
    methods of examination. Ophthalmology 1983; 90:126–131.

2. Pagon RA. Retinitis pigmentosa. Surv Ophthalmol 1988;
    33:137–177.

3. Heckenlively JR, Yoser SL, Friedman LH, Oversier JJ. Clin-
    ical findings and common symptoms in retinitis pigmentosa.
    Am J Ophthalmol 1988; 105:504–511.

4. Fishman GA, Lam BL, Anderson RJ. Racial difference in the
    prevalence of atrophic-appearing macular lesions between
    black and white patients with retinitis pigmentosa. Am J
    Ophthalmol 1994; 118:33–38.

5. van Soest S, Westerveld A, de Dejong PTV, Bleeker-
    Wagemakers EM, Bergen AB. Retinitis pigmentosa: defined
    from a molecular point of view. Surv Ophthalmol 1999;
    43:321–334.

6. Weleber RG, Carr RE, Murphey WH, Sheffield VC, Stone EM.
    Phenotypic variations including retinitis pigmentosa, pattern
    dystrophy, and fundus flavimaculatus in a single family with
    a deletion of codon 153 or 154 of the peripherin/RDS gene.
    Arch Ophthalmol 1993; 111:1531–1542.

7. Berson EL. Retinitis pigmentosa and allied diseases: applica-
    tions of electroretinographic testing. Int Ophthalmol 1981;
    4:7–22.

8. Berson EL. Retinitis pigmentosa. The Friedenwald Lecture.
    Invest Ophthalmol Vis Sci 1993; 34:1659–1676.

9. Gouras P, Carr RE. Electrophysiological studies in early retinitis pigmentosa. Arch Ophthalmol 1964; 72:104–110.

10. Fishman GA, Alexander KR, Anderson RJ. Autosomal dominant retinitis pigmentosa. A method of classification. Arch Ophthalmol 1985; 103:366–374.

11. Marmor MF. The electroretinogram in retinitis pigmentosa. Arch Ophthalmol 1979; 97:1300–1304.

12. Iijima H, Yamaguchi S, Hosaka O. Photopic electroretinogram implicit time in retinitis pigmentosa. Jpn J Ophthalmol 1993; 37:130–135.

13. Birch DG, Sandberg MA. Dependence of cone b-wave implitit time on rod amplitude in retinitis pigmentosa. Vision Res 1987; 27:1105–1112.

14. Hood DC, Birch DG. Abnormalities of the retinal cone system in retinitis pigmentosa. Vision Res 1996; 36:1699–709.

15. Birch DG, Anderson JL, Fish GE. Yearly rates of rod and cone functional loss in retinitis pigmentosa and cone-rod dystrophy. Ophthalmology 1999; 106:258–268.

16. Berson EL, Sandberg MA, Rosner B, Birch DG, Hanson AH. Natural course of retinis pigmentosa over a three-year interval. Am J Ophthalmol 1985; 99:240–251.

17. Berson EL, Rosner B, Sandberg MA, Hayes KC, Nicholson BW, Weigel-DiFranco C, Willett W. A randomized trial of vitamin A and vitamin E supplementation for retinitis pigmentosa. Arch Ophthalmol 1993; 111:761–772.

18. Rothberg DS, Weinstein GW, Hobson RR, Nork TM. Electroretinography and retinitis pigmentosa: no discrimination between genetic subtypes. Arch Ophthalmol 1982; 100:1422–1426.

19. Massof RW, Finkelstein D. Two forms of autosomal dominant primary retinitis pigmentosa. Doc Ophthalmol 1981; 51: 289–346.

20. Arden GB, Carter RM, Hogg CR, Powell DJ, Ernest WJ, Clover GM, Lyness AL, Quinlan MP. Rod and cone activity in patients with dominantly inherited retinitis pigmentosa: comparisons between psychophysical and electroretingrographic measurements. Br J Ophthalmol 1983; 67:405–418.

21. Andréasson SOL, Sandberg MA, Berson EL. Narrow-band filtering for monitoring low-amplitude cone electroretinograms in retinitis pigmentosa. Am J Ophthalmol 1988; 105:500–503.

22. Birch DG, Wesley KH, deFaller JM, Disbrow DT, Birch EE. The relationship between rod perimetric thresholds and full-field rod ERGs in retinitis pigmentosa. Invest Ophthalmol Vis Sci 1987; 28:954–965.

23. Fahle M, Steuhl KP, Aulhorn E. Correlation between electroretinography, morphology and function in retinitis pigmentosa. Graefes Arch Clin Exp Ophthalmol 1991; 229:37–49.

24. Heckenlively JR. RP cone–rod degeneration. Trans Am Ophthalmol Soc 1987; 85:438–470.

25. Iannaccone A, Rispoli E, Vingolo EM, Onori P, Steindl K, Rispoli D, Pannarale MR. Correlation between Goldmann perimetry and maximal electroretinogram response in retinitis pigmentosa. Doc Ophthalmol 1995; 90:129–142.

26. Massof RW, Finkelstein D, Perry C, Starr SJ, Johnson MA. Properties of electroretinographic intensity–response functions in retinitis pigmentosa. Doc Ophthalmol 1984; 57: 279–296.

27. Sandberg MA, Weigel-DiFranco C, Rosner B, Berson EL. The relationship between visual field size and electroretinogram amplitude in retinitis pigmentosa. Invest Ophthalmol Vis Sci 1996; 37:1693–1698.

28. Yagasaki K, Jacobson SG, Apathy PP, Knighton RW. Rod and cone psychophysics and electroretinography: methods for comparison in retinal degenerations. Doc Ophthalmol 1988; 69:119–130.

29. Holopigian K, Greenstein V, Seiple W, Carr RE. Rates of change differ among measures of visual function in patients with retinitis pigmentosa. Ophthalmology 1996; 103: 398–405.

30. Szlyk JP, Fishman GA, Alexander KR, Revelins BI, Derlacki DJ, Anderson RJ. Relationship between difficulty in performing daily activities and clinical measures of visual function in patients with retinitis pigmentosa. Arch Ophthalmol 1997; 115:53–59.

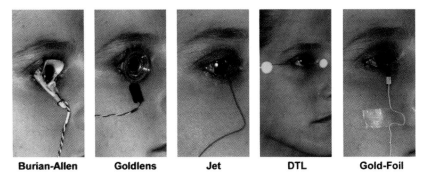

Burian-Allen   **Goldlens**   **Jet**   **DTL**   **Gold-Foil**

Figure 1.2 ERG recording electrodes. The characteristics of the electrodes are summarized in Table 1.2 (pp. 10–11). Proper placement of the electrodes, as described on pp. 8–9 and Table 1.2, is critical to obtain accurate, consistent recordings.

Multifocal ERG - Three-Dimensional (3D) Response Density Plot

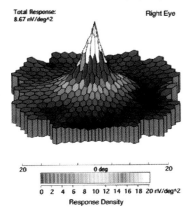

Total Response:
8.67 nV/deg^2   Right Eye

20   0 deg   20

0 2 4 6 8 10 12 14 16 18 20 nV/deg^2
Response Density

Figure 2.7 Normal 3D response density plots of the multifocal ERG: The multifocal ERG trace array of this normal subject is shown in Fig. 2.4. The 3D plot is based on response density (nV/deg^2) obtained by dividing the response amplitude by the area of the hexagon. The fovea has the highest response density consistent with its high cone photoreceptor density.

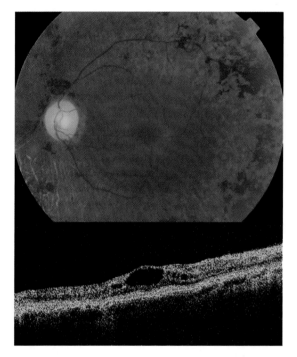

Figure 8.1 *Top*: Diffuse retinal atrophy, vascular attenuation, and pigmentary clumping in advanced RP. *Bottom*: Cystoid macular edema in RP, as demonstrated by optic coherence tomography.

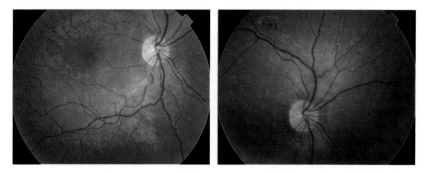

Figure 8.5 Retinal atrophy and pigment clumping in 9-year-old girl with neuronal ceroid lipofuscinosis, juvenile form (Batten disease). Visual acuity: 20/100 in each eye; full-field ERG responses, moderately reduced. Patient had insidious progressive visual loss and night vision impairment, with periods of inattention, inappropriate behavior, and verbal confusion. Diagnosis was confirmed by electron microscopic identification of cytoplasmic granules in peripheral blood lymphocytes.

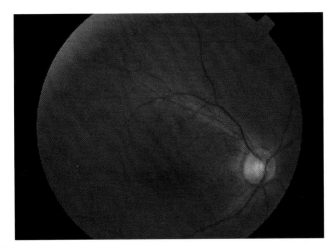

Figure 8.4 Retinal atrophy in 14-year-old boy with Bardet–Biedl syndrome (obesity, short stature, and polydactyly). Visual acuity: 20/20 in each eye; constricted, depressed visual fields. Although the atrophy appeared mild, full-field ERG responses were non-detectable.

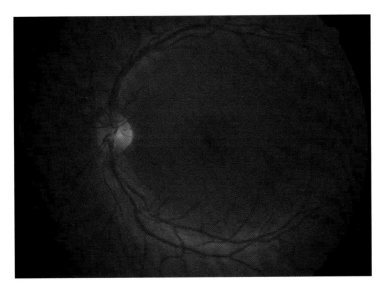

Figure 8.6 Full-field ERG responses and retinal appearance in 32-year-old woman with enhanced S-cone syndrome. Note non-detectable rod response and similar morphology of the tracings of the scotopic combined rod–cone and photopic cone response. Gray retinal atrophy with rare pigment clumping is evident near the vascular arcades and mid-peripheral region.

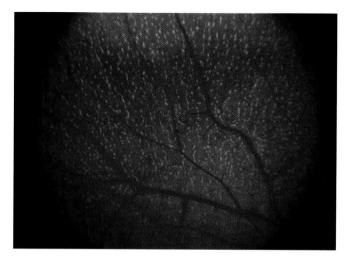

Figure 9.4 Small discrete white-yellow retinal lesions in fundus albipunctatus. The lesions spares the fovea and are scattered throughout the retina. (From Ref. 96.)

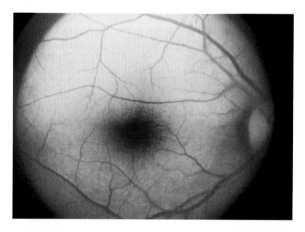

Figure 9.6 Yellowish appearance of the retina in Oguchi disease. The color of the retina and the dark-adapted rod thresholds are restored after very prolonged dark adaptation. (From Ref. 96.)

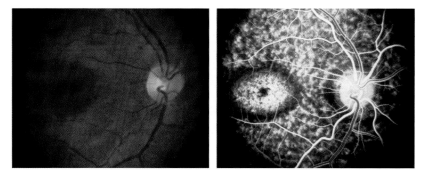

Figure 10.3 *Left*: Fundus appearance with Stargardt macular dystrophy. Note fleck-like lesions. *Right*: Fluorescein angiography shows numerous fleck-like lesions and diffuse blockage of choroidal filling ("choroidal silence") due to accumulation of lipofuscin-like material in retinal pigment epithelium. (From Ref. 202.)

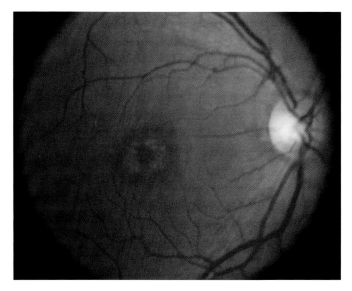

Figure 10.7 "Bull's-eye" macular atrophic lesion with cone dystrophy. This pattern of macular atrophy is not specific for cone dystrophy and may occur in rod–cone dystrophy, chloroquine or hydroxychloroquine retinal toxicity, and Stargardt macular dystrophy. (From Ref. 202.)

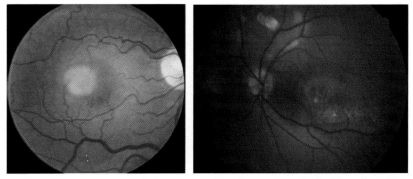

Figure 10.5 Best vitelliform macular dystrophy. *Left*: Foveal yellow egg-yolk-like lesion. *Right*: Multiple lesions. (From Ref. 202.)

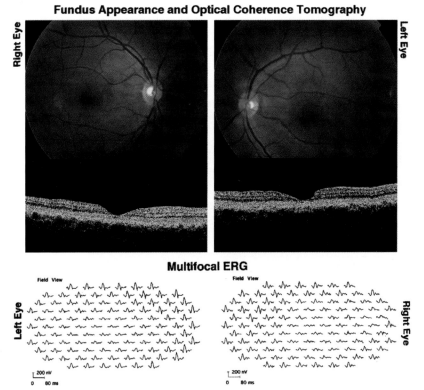

Figure 10.9 31-year-old man with central cone dystrophy (occult macular dystrophy). Photo show normal fundus in each eye. Optical coherence tomography demonstrates thinned foveal thickness to 104 and 97 μm (normal ≈ 200 μm) for right eye and left eye, respectively. The first-order trace arrays reveal impaired responses centrally in each eye.

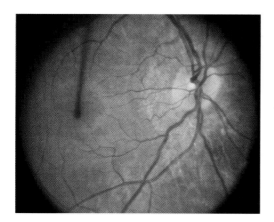

Figure 11.1 Chorioretinal degeneration with choroideremia. (From Ref. 29.)

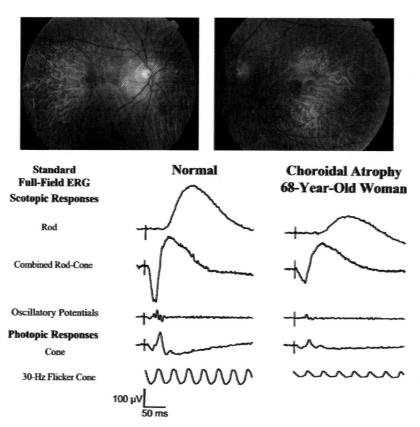

Figure 11.4 *Top (left and right)*: Diffuse choroidal atrophy in 68-year-old woman progressive worsening of vision for 1 year. In contrast to pigmentary retinal degeneration, the retinal arterioles are not significantly attenuated. *Bottom*: Note the reduced, mildly prolonged full-field ERG responses.

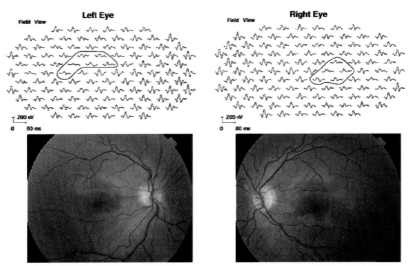

Figure 13.4 Multifocal ERG responses and retinal appearance of 20-year-old woman with acute macular neuroretinopathy. Impaired focal responses (*circled*) correlate with gray-reddish petal-shaped macular abnormality in each eye (*bottom left*: right eye; *bottom right*: left eye). Visual acuity was 20/20 in each eye.

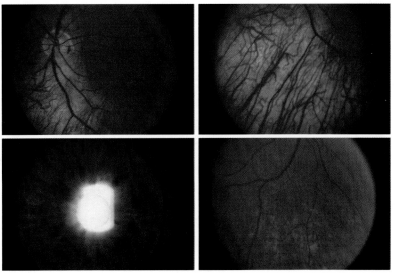

Figure 16.2 X-linked ocular albinism. *Top left*: Fundus of left eye of 25-year-old man with 20/60 vision, indistinct fovea, and retinal depigmentation. *Bottom left*: Iris illumination defects in 76-year-old affected maternal cousin. *Bottom right*: "Mud-splattered" retinal appearance of the 55-year-old mother who is an obligatory carrier. The full-field ERG responses of affected males family were normal.

31. Szlyk JP, Alexander KR, Severing K, Fishman GA. Assessment of driving performance in patients with retinitis pigmentosa. Arch Ophthalmol 1992; 110:1709–1713.

32. Hoffman DR, Locke KG, Wheaton DH, Fish GE, Spencer R, Birch DG. A randomized, placebo-controlled clinical trial of docosahexaenoic acid supplementation for x-linked retinitis pigmentosa. Am J Ophthalmol 2004; 137:704–718.

33. François J, Verriest G. Retinopathie pigmentaire unilaterale. Ophthalmologica 1952; 124:65–87.

34. Carr RE, Siegel IM. Unilateral retinitis pigmentosa. Arch Ophthalmol 1973; 90:21–26.

35. Spadea L, Magni R, Rinaldi G, Dragani T, Bianco G. Unilateral retinitis pigmentosa: clinical and electrophysiological report of four cases. Ophthalmologica 1998; 212:350–354.

36. Kandori F, Tamai A, Watanabe T, Kurimoto S. Unilateral pigmentary degeneration of the retina. Report of two cases. Am J Ophthalmol 1968; 66:1091–1101.

37. Henkes HE. Does unilateral retinitis pigmentosa really exist? In: Burian H, Jacobson J, eds. Clinical Electroretinography. Proceedings of the Third International Symposium 1964. Elmsford, NY: Pergamon Press, 1966:327–350.

38. Auerbach E, Rowe H. The 'good' eye in unilateral retinitis pigmentosa. Ophthalmologica 1968; 155:98–116.

39. Kolb H, Galloway NR. Three cases of unilateral pigmentary degeneration. Br J Ophthalmol 1964; 48:471–479.

40. Fulton AB, Hansen RM. The relation of rhodopsin and scotopic retinal sensitivity in sector retinitis pigmentosa. Am J Ophthalmol 1988; 105:132–140.

41. Massof RW, Finkelstein D. Vision threshold profiles in sector retinitis pigmentosa. Arch Ophthalmol 1979; 97:1899–1904.

42. Krill AE, Archer D, Martin D. Sector retinitis pigmentosa. Am J Ophthalmol 1970; 69:977–987.

43. Berson EL, Howard J. Temporal aspects of the electroretinogram in sector retinitis pigmentosa. Arch Ophthalmol 1971; 86:653–665.

44. Abraham FA. Sector retinitis pigmentosa. Electrophysiological and psychophysical study of the visual system. Doc Ophthalmol 1975; 39:13–28.

45. Andréasson S, Ponjavic V, Abrahamson M, Ehinger B, Wu W, Fujita R, Buraczynska M, Swaroop A. Phenotypes in three Swedish families with X-linked retinitis pigmentosa caused by different mutations in the RPGR gene. Am J Ophthalmol 1997; 124:95–102.

46. Fishman GA, Grover S, Buraczynska M, Wu W, Swaroop A. A new 2-base pair deletion in the RPGR gene in ablack family with X-linked retinitis pigmentosa. Arch Ophthalmol 1998; 116:213–218.

47. Fishman GA, Weinberg AR, MacMahon TT. X-linked recessive retinitis pigmentosa: clinical characteristics of carriers. Arch Ophthalmol 1986; 104:1329–1335.

48. Weleber RG, Butler NS, Murphey WH, Sheffield VC, Stone EM. X-linked retinitis pigmentosa associated with a 2-based pair insertion in codon 99 of the RP3 gene RPGR. Arch Ophthalmol 1997; 115:1429–1435.

49. Grover S, Fishman GA, Anderson RJ, Lindeman M. A longitudinal study of visual function in carriers of X-linked recessive retinitis pigmentosa. Ophthalmology 2000; 107:386–396.

50. Jacobson SG, Roman AJ, Cideciyan AV, Robey MG, Iwata T, Inana G. X-linked retinitis pigmentosa: functional phenotype of an RP2 genotype. Invest Ophthalmol Vis Sci 1992; 33:3481–3492.

51. Arden GB, Carter RM, Hogg CR, Powell DJ, Ernst WJ, Clover GM, Lyness AL, Quinlan MP. A modified ERG technique and the results obtained in X-linked retinitis pigmentosa. Br J Ophthalmol 1983; 67:419–430.

52. Berson EL, Gouras P, Gunkel RD, Myrianthopoulos NC. Rod and cone responses in sex-linked retinitis pigmentosa. Arch Ophthalmol 1969; 81:215–225.

53. Peachey NS, Fishman GA, Derlacki DJ, Alexander KR. Rod and cone dysfunction in carriers of X-linked recessive retinitis pigmentosa. Ophthalmology 1988; 95:677–685.

54. Andréasson SOL, Ehinger B. Electroretinographic diagnosis in families with X-linked retinitis pigmentosa. Acta Ophthalmol 1990; 68:139–144.

55. Berson EL, Rosen JB, Simonoff EA. Electroretinographic testing as an aid in detection of carriers of X-choromosome-linked retinitis pigmentosa. Am J Ophthalmol 1979; 87: 460–468.

56. Vajaranant TS, Seiple W, Szlyk JP, Fishman GA. Detection using the multifocal electroretinogram of mosaic retinal dysfunction in carriers of X-linked retinitis pigmentosa. Ophthalmology 2002; 109:560–568.

57. Jacobson SG, Buraczynka M, Milam AH, Chen C, Jarvalainen M, Fujita R, Wu W, Huang Y, Cideciyan AV, Swaroop A. Disease expression in X-linked retinitis pigmentosa caused by putative null mutation in the RPGR gene. Invest Ophthalmol Vis Sci 1997; 38:1983–1997.

58. Cideciyan AV, Jacobson SG. Negative electroretinograms in retinitis pigmentosa. Invest Ophthalmol Vis Sci 1993; 34: 3253–3263.

59. Lam BL, M L, I HD. Low-frequency damped electroretinographic wavelets in young asymptomatic patients with dominant retinitis pigmentosa: a new electroretinographic finding. Ophthalmology 1999; 106:1109–1113.

60. Hood DC, Wladis EJ, Shady S, Holopigian K, Li J, Seiple W. Multifocal rod electroretinograms. Invest Ophthalmol Vis Sci 1998; 39:1152–1162.

61. Hood DC, Holopigian K, Greenstein V, Seiple W, Li J, Sutter EE, Carr RE. Assessment of local retinal function in patients with retinitis pigmentosa using the multi-focal ERG technique. Vis Res 1998; 38:163–179.

62. Seeliger M, Kretschmann U, Apfelstedt-Sylla E, Ruther K, Zrenner E. Multifocal electroretinography in retinitis pigmentosa. Am J Ophthalmol 1998; 125:214–226.

63. Jacobson SG, Knighton RW, Levene RM. Dark- and light-adapted visual evoked cortical potentials in retinitis pigmentosa. Doc Ophthalmol 1985; 60:189–196.

64. Jacobson JH, Hirose T, Suzuki T. Simultaneous ERG and VER in lesions of the optic pathway. Invest Ophthalmol 1968; 7:279–292.

65. Lennerstrand G. Delayed visual evoked cortical potentials in retinal disease. Acta Ophthalmol 1982; 60:497–504.

66. Nakamura Z, Ohzeki T. Electroretinograms and visual evoked potentials in the primary retinal dystrophies. Doc Ophthalmol Proc Ser 1982; 31:155–164.

67. Leber T. Ueber Retinitis pigmentosa und augeborene Amaurose. Albrecht von Graefes Arch Ophthalmol 1869; 15:1–25.

68. Nickel B, Hoyt CS. Leber's congenital amaurosis: is mental retardation a frequent associated defect? Arch Ophthalmol 1982; 100:1089–1092.

69. Schroeder R, Mets MB, Maumenee IH. Leber's congenital amaurosis: retrospective review of 43 cases and a new fundus finding in two cases. Arch Ophthalmol 1987; 105: 356–359.

70. Lotery AJ, Namperumalsamy P, Jacobson SG, Weleber RG, Fishman GA, Musarella MA, Hoyt CS, Heon E, Levin A, Jan J, Lam BL, Carr RE, Franklin A, Radha S, Andorf JL, Sheffield VC, Stone EM. Mutation analysis of 3 genes in patients affected with Leber's congenital amaurosis. Arch Ophthalmol 2000; 118:538–543.

71. Perrault I, Rozer JM, Calvos P, Gerber S, Camuzat A, Dolfus H, Chatelin S, Souied E, Ghazi I, Leowski C, Bonnermaison M, Le Paslier D, Frézal J, Dufer J-L, Pittler S, Munnich A, Kalpan J. Retinal-specific guanylate cyclase gene mutations in Leber's congenital amaurosis. Nat Genet 1996; 14: 461–464.

72. Marlhens F, Bareil C, Griffoin JM, Zrenner E, Amalric P, Eliaou C, Liu S-Y, Harris E, Redmond TM, Arnaud B, Claustres M, Hamel CP. Mutations in RPE65 cause Leber's congenital amaurosis. Nat Genet 1997; 17:139–141.

73. Sohocki MM, Bowne SJ, Sullivan LS, Blackshaw S, Cepko CL, Payne AM, Bhattacharya SS, Khaliq S, Mehdi Q, Birch DG, Harrison WR, Elder FFB, Heckenlively JR, Daiger SP.

Mutations in a new photoreceptor-pineal gene on 17q cause Leber congenital amaurosis. Nat Genet 2000; 24:79–83.

74. Swaroop A, Wang QL, Wu W, Cook J, Coats C, Xu S, Chen S, Zack DJ, Sieving PA. Leber congenital amaurosis caused by a homozygous mutation (R90W) in the homeodomain of the retinal transcription factor CRX: direct evidence for the involvement of CRX in the development of photoreceptor function. Hum Mol Genet 1999; 8:299–305.

75. Good PA, Searle AET, Campbell S, Crewa SJ. Value of the ERG in congenital nystagmus. Br J Ophthalmol 1989; 73:512–515.

76. Lambert SR, Kriss A, Taylor D, Coffey R, Pembrey M. Follow-up and diagnostic reappraisal of 75 patients with Leber's congenital amaurosis. Am J Ophthalmol 1989; 107:624–631.

77. Lorenz B, Gyurus P, Presiing M, Bremser D, Gu S, Andrassi M, Gerth C, Gal A. Early-onset severe rod–cone dystrophy in young children with RPE 65 mutations. Invest Ophthalmol Vis Sci 2000; 41:2735–2742.

78. Vaizy MJ, Sanders MD, Wybar KC, J W. Neurological abnormalities in congenital amaurosis of Leber. Review of 30 cases. Arch Dis Child 1977; 52:399–402.

79. Weiss AH, Biersdorf WR. Visual sensory disorders in congenital nystagmus. Ophthalmology 1989; 96:517–523.

80. Koenekoop RK, Fishman GA, Iannaccone A, Ezzeldin H, Ciccarelli ML, Baldi A, Suness JS, Lotery AJ, Jablonski MM, Pittler SJ, Manumenee I. Electroretinographic abnormalities in parents of patients with Leber congenital amaurosis who have heterozygous GUCY2D mutations. Arch Ophthalmol 2002; 120:1325–1330.

81. Weleber RG, Tongue AC. Congenital stationary night blindness presenting as Leber's congenital amaurosis. Arch Ophthalmol 1987; 105:360–365.

82. Brecelj J, Stirn-Kranic B. ERG and VEP follow-up study in children with Leber's congenital amaurosis. Eye 1999; 13:47–54.

83. Brigell M, Marchese AL. The luminance-amplitude function of simultaneously recorded flash visual evoked potential and electroretinogram. Clin Vis Sci 1993; 8:41–46.

84. Smith RJ, Berlin CI, Hejtmancik JF, Keats BJ, Kimberling WJ, Lewis RA, Moller CG, Pelias MJ, Tranebjaerg L. Clinical diagnosis of the Usher syndromes. Usher syndrome consortium. Am J Med Genet 1994; 50:32–38.

85. Weil D, Blanchard S, Kaplan J, Guilford P, Gibson F, Walsh J, Mburu P, Varela A, Levilliers J, Weston MD, Kelley PM, Kimberling WJ, Wagenaar M, Levi-Acobas F, Larget-Piet D, Munninich A, Steel KP, Brown SDM, Pelit C. Defective myosin VIIA gene responsible for Usher syndrome 1B. Nature 1995; 374:60–61.

86. Weston MD, Eudy JD, Fujita S, Yao-S-F, Usami S, Cremers C, Greenberg J, Ramesar R, Martini A, Moller CG, Smith RJ, Sumegi J, Kimberling WJ. Genomic structure and identification of novel mutations in usherin, the gene responsible for Usher syndrome type IIa. Am J Hum Genet 2000; 66:2020.

87. Van Aarem A, Wagenaar M, Pinckers AJ, Huygen PL, Bleeker-Wagemakers EM, Kimberling BJ, Cremers CW. Ophthalmologic findings in Usher syndrome type 2A. Ophthalmic Genet 1995; 16:151–158.

88. Pazza L, Fishman GA, Farber M, Derlacki D, Anderson RJ. Visual acuity loss in patients with Usher's syndrome. Arch Ophthalmol 1988; 104:1336–1339.

89. Tsilou ET, Rubin BI, Caruso RC, Reed GF, Pikus A, Hejimancik JF, Iwata F, Redman JB, Kaiser-Kupfer MI. Usher syndrome clinical types I and II: could ocular symptoms and signs differentiate between the two types? Acta Ophthalmol Scand 2002; 80:196–201.

90. Fishman GA, Anderson RJ, Lam BL, Derlacki DJ. Prevalence of foveal lesions in type 1 and type 2 Usher's syndrome. Arch Ophthalmol 1995; 113:770–773.

91. Bharadwaj AK, Kasztejna JP, Huq S, Berson EL, Dryja TP. Evaluation of the myosin VIIA gene and visual function in patients with Usher syndrome type I. Exp Eye Res 2000; 71:173–181.

92. Seeliger MW, Zrenner E, Apfelstedt-Sylla E, Jaissle GB. Identification of Usher syndrome subtypes by ERG implicit time. Invest Ophthalmol Vis Sci 2001; 42:3066–3071.

93. Mets MB, Young NM, Pass A, Lasky JB. Early diagnosis of Usher syndrome in children. Trans Am Ophthalmol Soc 2000; 98:237–242.

94. Boughman J, Vernon M, Shaver K. Usher's syndrome: definition and estimate of prevalence from 2 high risk population. J Chronic Dis 1983; 36:595–603.

95. Pinckers A, van Aarem A, Brink H. The electrooculogram in heterozygote carriers of Usher syndrome, retinitis pigmentosa, neuronal ceroid lipofuscinosis, Senior syndrome and choroideremia. Ophthalmic Genet 1994; 15:25–30.

96. van Aarem A, Cremers CW, Pinckers AJ, Huygen PL, Hombergen GC, Kimberling BJ. The Usher syndrome type 2A: clinical findings in obligate carriers. Int J Pediatr Otorhinolaryngol 1995; 31:159–174.

97. Wagenaar M, ter Rahe B, van Aarem A, Huygen P, Admiraal R, Bleeker-Wagemakers E, Pinckers A, Kimberling W, Cremers C. Clinical findings in Obligate carriers of type I Usher syndrome. Am J Med Genet 1995; 59:375–379.

98. Bardet G. Sur un syndrome d'obesite infantile avec polydactlie et retinite pigmentaire (contribution a l'etude des formes cliniques de l'obesite hypophysaire). Vol. Ph.D. thesis, Paris, France, 1920.

99. Biedl A. Ein Geschwisterpaar mit adiposo-genitaler Dystrophie. Disch Med Woschenschr 1922; 48:1630.

100. Green JS, Parfrey PS, Harnett JD, Farid NR, Cremer BC, Johnson G, Heath O, McManamon PJ, O'Leary E, Pryse-Phillips W. The cardinal manifestations of Bardet-Biedl syndrome. a form of Laurence–Moon–Biedl syndrome. New Eng J Med 1989; 321:1002–1009.

101. Nishimura DY, Searby CC, Carmi R, Elbedour K, van Maldergem L, Fulton AB, Lam BL, Powell BR, Swiderski RE, Bugge KE, Halder NB, Kwitek-Black AE, Ying L, Duhi DM, Gorman SM, Heon E, Iannacconne A, Jacobson SG, Stone EM, Sheffield VC. Positional cloning of novel gene on

chromosome 16q causing Bardet–Biedl syndrome (BBS2). Hum Mol Genet 2001; 10:865–874.

102. Katsanis N, Beales PL, Woods ML, Lewis RA, Green JS, Parfrey PS, Anslay SJ, Davidson WS, Lupuki JR. Mutations in MKKS cause obesity, retinal dystrophy and renal malformations associated with Bardet–Biedl syndrome. Nat genet 2000; 26:67–70.

103. Slavotinek AM, Stone EM, Mykytyn K, Heckenlively JR, Green JS, Heon E, Mussarella MA, Parfrey PS, Sheffleid VC, Biesecker LG. Mutations in MKKS cause Bardet–Biedl syndrome. Nat genet 2000; 26:15–16.

104. Fulton AB, Hansen RM, Glynn RJ. Natural course of visual functions in the Bardet–Biedl syndrome. Arch Ophthalmol 1993; 111:1500–1506.

105. Iannaccone A, De Propris G, Roncati S, Rispoli E, Del Porto G, Pannarale MR. The ocular phenotype of the Bardet–Biedl syndrome. Comparison to non-syndromic retinitis pigmentosa. Ophthalmic Genet 1997; 18:13–26.

106. Spaggiari E, Salati R, Nicolini P, Borgatti R, Pozzoli U, Polenghi F. Evolution of ocular clinical and electrophysiological findings in pediatric Bardet–Biedl syndrome. Int Ophthalmol 1999; 23:61–67.

107. Jacobson SG, Borruat FX, Apáthy PP. Patterns of rod and cone dysfunction in Bardet–Biedl syndrome. Am J Ophthalmol 1990; 109:676–688.

108. Iannaccone A, Vingolo EM, Rispoli E, De Propris G, Tanzilli P, Pannarale MR. Electroretinographic alterations in the Laurence–Moon–Bardet–Biedl phenotype. Acta Ophthalmol Scand 1996; 74:8–13.

109. Lavy T, Harris CM, Shawkat F, Thompson D, Taylor D, Kriss A. Electrophysiological and eye-movement abnormalities in children with the Bardet–Biedl syndrome. J Pediatr Ophthalmol Strabismus 1995; 32:364–367.

110. Cox GF, Hansen RM, Quinn N, Fulton AB. Retinal function in carriers of Bardet–Biedl syndrome. Arch Ophthalmol 2003; 121:804–810.

111. Refsum S. [Heredopathia atactica polyneuritiformis, Hexade-canoic acid storage disease (Refsum's disease) definition treatment and pathogenesis. A short review]. Psychiatr Neurol Med Psychol Beih 1977; 22-23:11–18.

112. Refsum S, Salomonsen L, Skatvedt M. Heredopathia atactica polyneuritiformis in children. J Pediatr 1949; 35: 335–343.

113. Wills AJ, Manning NJ, Reilly MM. Refsum's disease. QJM 2001; 94:403–406.

114. Hansen E, Bachen NI, Flage T. Refsum's disease. Eye manifestations in a patient treated with low phytol low phytanic acid diet. Acta Ophthalmol (Copenh) 1979; 57:899–913.

115. Rinaldi E, Cotticelli L, Di Meo A, Romano A. Ocular findings in Refsum's disease. Metab Pediatr Ophthalmol 1981; 5: 149–154.

116. Weleber RG, Tongue AC, Kennaway NG, Budden SS, Buist NR. Ophthalmic manifestations of infantile phytanic acid storage disease. Arch Ophthalmol 1984; 102:1317–1721.

117. Yamamoto S, Onozu H, Yamada N, Hayasaka S, Watanabe A. Mild retinal changes in a 47-year-old patient with phytanic acid storage disease. Ophthalmologica 1995; 209:251–255.

118. Bassen FA, Kornzweig AL. Malformation of the erythrocytes in a case of atypical retinitis pigmentosa. Blood 1950; 5: 381–387.

119. Salt HB, Wolff OH, Lloyd JK, Fosbrooke AS, Cameron AH, Hubble DV. On having no beta-lipoprotein: a syndrome comprising abetalipoproteineaemia, acanthocytosis, and steatorrhoea. Lancet 1960; 11:325–329.

120. Wetterau JR, Aggerbeck LP, Bouma M-E, Eisenberg C, Munck A, Hermier M, Schmitz J, Gay G, Rader DJ, Gregg RE. Absence of microsomal triglyceride transfer protein in individuals with abetalipoproteinemia. Science 1992; 258: 999–1001.

121. Sharp D, Blinderman L, Combs KA, Kienzle B, Ricci B, Wager-Smith K, Gil CM, Turck CW, Bouma M-E, Rader DJ, Aggerneck LP, Gregg RE, Gordon DA, Wetterau JR.

Cloning and gene defects in microsomal triglyceride transfer protein associated with abetalipoproteinemia. Nature 1993; 365:65–69.

122. Carr RE. Abetalipoproteinemia and the eye. Birth Defects Orig Artic Ser 1976; 12:385–408.

123. Bishara S, Merin S, Cooper M, Azizi E, Delpre G, Deckelbaum RJ. Combined vitamin A and E therapy prevents retinal electrophysiological deterioration in abe talipoproteinaemia. Br J Ophthalmol 1982; 66:767–770.

124. Brin MF, Pedley TA, Lovelace RE, et al. Electrophysiologic features of abetalipoproteinemia: functional consequences of vitamin E deficiency. Neurology 1986; 36:669–673.

125. Fagan ER, Taylor MJ. Longitudinal multimodal evoked potential studies in abetalipoproteinaemia. Can J Neurol Sci 1987; 14:617–621.

126. Gouras P, Carr RE, Gunkel RD. Retinitis pigmentosa in abetalipoproteinemia: effects of vitamin A. Invest Ophthalmol 1971; 10:784–793.

127. Judisch GF, Rhead WJ, Miller DK. Abetalipoproteinemia. Report of an unusual patient. Ophthalmologica 1984; 189:73–79.

128. Sperling MA, Hiles DA, Kennerdell JS. Electroretinographic responses following vitamin A therapy in abetalipoproteinemia. Am J Ophthalmol 1972; 73:342–351.

129. Chowers I, Banin E, Merin S, Cooper M, Granot E. Long-term assessment of combined vitamin A and E treatment for the prevention of retinal degeneration in abetalipoproteinaemia and hypobetalipoproteinaemia patients. Eye 2001; 15: 525–530.

130. Muller DP, Lloyd JK, Bird AC. Long-term management of abetalipoproteinemia: possible role for vitamin E. Arch Dis Child 1977; 52:209–214.

131. Runge P, Muller DP, McAllister J, Calver D, Lloyd JK, Taylor D. Oral vitamin E supplements can prevent the retinopathy of abetalipoproteinaemia. Br J Ophthalmol 1986; 70:166–173.

132. Goebel HH. The neuronal ceroid-lipofuscinoses. J Child Neurol 1995; 10:424–437.

133. Mole SE. Batten's disease: eight genes and still counting? Lancet 1999; 354:443–445.

134. Batten PE. Cerebral degeneration with symmetrical changes in the maculas in two members of a family. Trans Ophthalmol Soc UK 1903; 23:386–390.

135. Copenhaver RM, Goodman G. The electroretinogram in infantile, late infantile, and juvenile amaurotic family idocy. Arch Ophthalmol 1960; 63:559–566.

136. Weleber RG. The dystrophic retina in multisystem disorders: the electroretinogram in neuronal ceroid lipofuscinosis. Eye 1998; 12:580–590.

137. Eksandh LB, Ponjavic VB, Munroe PB, Eiberg HE, Uvebrant PE, Ehinger BE, Mole SE, Andreasson S. Full-field ERG in patients with Batten/Speilmeyer-Vogt disease caused by mutations in the CLN3 gene. Ophthalmic Genet 2000; 21:69–77.

138. Horiguchi M, Miyake Y. Batten disease-deteriorating course of ocular findings. Jpn J Ophthalmol 1992; 36:91–96.

139. Dawson WW, Armstrong D, Greer M, Maida TM, Samuelson DA. Disease-specific electrophysiological findings in adult ceroid-lipofuscinosis (Kufs disease). Doc Ophthalmol 1985; 60:163–171.

140. Gottlob I, Leipert KP, Kohlschutter A, Goebel HH. Electrophysiological findings of neuronal ceroid lipofuscinosis in heterozygotes. Graefes Arch Clin Exp Ophthalmol 1988; 226:516–521.

141. Kearns TP, Sayre GP. Retinitis pigmentosa, external ophthalmoplegia, and complete heart block: unusual syndrome with histologic study in one of two cases. Arch Ophthalmol 1958; 60:280–289.

142. Mullie MA, Harding AE, Petty RK, Ikeda H, Morgan-Hughes JA, Sanders MD. The retinal manifestations of mitochondrial myopathy. A study of 22 cases. Arch Ophthalmol 1985; 103:1825–1830.

143. Berdjis H, Heider W, Demisch K. ERG and VECP in chronic
      progressive external ophthalmoplegia (CPEO). Doc Ophthal-
      mol 1985; 60:427–4334.

144. Ota I, Miyake Y, Awaya S. [Studies of ocular fundus and
      visual functions in Kearns–Sayre syndrome—with special
      reference to the new stage classification]. Nippon Ganka
      Gakkai Zasshi 1989; 93:329–338.

145. Ota Y, Miyake Y, Awaya S, Kumagai T, Tanaka M, Ozawa T.
      Early retinal involvement in mitochondrial myopathy with
      mitochondrial DNA deletion. Retina 1994; 14:270–276.

146. Bastiaensen LA, Notermans SL, Ramaeckers CH, van Dijke
      BJ, Joosten EM, Jaspar HH, Standhouders AM, Beljaars
      CT. Kearns syndrome or Kearns disease: further evidence
      of a genuine entity in a case with uncommon features.
      Ophthalmologica 1982; 184:40–50.

147. Cooper LL, Hansen RM, Darras BT, Korson M, Dougherty
      FE, Shoffner JM, Fulton AB. Rod photoreceptor function in
      children with mitochondrial disorders. Arch Ophthalmol
      2002; 120:1055–1062.

148. Ambrosio G, De Marco R, Loffredo L, Magli A. Visual
      dysfunction in patients with mitochondrial myopathies. I.
      Electrophysiologic impairments. Doc Ophthalmol 1995;
      89:211–218.

149. Rigaudiere F, Manderieux N, Le Gargasson JF, Guez JE,
      Grall Y. Electrophysiological exploration of visual function
      in mitochondrial diseases. Electroencephalogr Clin Neuro-
      physiol 1995; 96:495–501.

150. Sartucci F, Rossi B, Tognoni G, Siciliano G, Guerrini V,
      Murri L. Evoked potentials in the evaluation of patients with
      mitochondrial myopathy. Eur Neurol 1993; 33:428–435.

151. Isaeff WB, Niswonger J. Survey of 336 deaf students for reti-
      nitis pigmentosa. Ann Ophthalmol 1981; 13:1131–1132.

152. Obenour LC. The electroretinogram in rubella retinopathy.
      Int Ophthalmol Clin 1972; 12:105–110.

153. Fishman GA, Birch DG, Holder GE, Brigell MG. Choroidere-
      mia. Electrophysiologic Testing in Disorders of the Retina,

Optic Nerve, and Visual Pathway. San Francisco: The Foundation of the American Academy of Ophthalmology, 2001:66–68.

154. Rice NSC, Jones BR, Wilkinson AE. Study of late ocular syphilis. Demonstration of treponemes in aqueous humour and cerebrospinal fluid. Trans Ophthalmol Soc UK 1968; 88:257–273.

155. Berson EL, Gouras P, Hoff M. Temporal aspects of the electroretinogram. Arch Ophthalmol 1969; 81:207–214.

156. Marmor M, Jacobson S, Foerster M, Kellner U, Weleber R. Diagnostic clinical findings of a new syndrome with night blindness, maculopathy, and enhanced S cone sensitivity. Am J Ophthalmol 1990; 110:124–134.

157. Kellner U, Zrenner E, Sadowski B, Foerster MH. Enhanced S cone sensitivity syndrome: long-term follow-up: electrophysiological and psychophysical findings. Clin Vis Sci 1993; 8:425–434.

158. Jacobson SG, Roman AJ, Roman MI, Gass JDM, Parker JA. Relatively enhanced S cone function in the Goldmann–Favre syndrome. Am J Ophthalmol 1991; 111:446–453.

159. Hood DC, Cideciyan AV, Roman AJ, Jacobson SG. Enhanced S cone syndrome: evidence for an abnormally large number of S cones. Vis Res 1995; 10:1473–1481.

160. Greenstein VC, Zaidi Q, Hood DC, Spehar B, Cideciyan AV, Jacobson SG. The enhanced S cone syndrome: an analysis of receptoral and post-receptoral changes. Vis Res 1996; 36:3711–3722.

161. Haider NB, Jacobson SG, Cideciyan AV, Swiderski R, Streb LM, Searby C, Beck G, Hockey R, Hanna DB, Gorman S, Duhl D, Carmi R, Bennett J, Weleber RG, Fishman GA, Wright AF, Stone EM, Sheffield VC. Mutation of a nuclear receptor gener, NR2E3, causes enhanced S cone syndrome, a disorder of retinal cell fate. Nat Genet 2000; 24:127–131.

162. Sharon D, Sandberg MA, Caruso RC, Berson EL, Dryja TP. Shared mutations in NR2E3 in enhanced S-cone syndrome, Goldmann–Favre syndrome, and many cases of clumped pigmentary retinal degeneration. Arch Ophthalmol 2003; 121:1316–1623.

163. Favre M. A propos de deux cas de degenerescence hyaloideor-
      etinienne. Ophthalmologica 1958; 135:604–609.

164. Fishman GA, Jampol LM, Goldberg MR. Diagnostic features
      of the Favre–Goldmann syndrome. Br J Ophthalmol 1976;
      60:345–353.

165. Kuntz CA, Jacobson SG, Cideciyan AV, Li Z-Y, Stone EM,
      Possin D, Milam AH. Sub-retinal pigment epithelial deposits
      in a dominant late-onset retinal degneration. Invest Ophthal-
      mol Vis Sci 1996; 37:1772–1782.

166. Milam AH, Curcio CA, Cideciyan AV, Saxena S, John SK,
      Kruth HS, Malek G, Heckenlively JR, Weleber RG, Jacobson
      SG. Dominantlate-onset retinal degeneration with regional
      variation of sub-retinal pigment epithelium deposits, retinal
      function, and photoreceptor degeneration. Ophthalmology
      2000; 107:2256–2266.

167. Downes SM, Holder GE, Fitzke FW, Payne AM, Warren MJ,
      Battacharya SS, Bird AC. Autosomal dominant cone and
      cone–rod dystrophy with mutations in the guanylate cyclase
      activator 1A gene-encoding guanylate cyclase activating pro-
      tein-1. Arch Ophthalmol 2001; 119:96–105.

168. Yagasaki K, Jacobson SG. Cone–rod dystrophy. Phenotypic
      diversity by retinal function testing. Arch Ophthalmol 1989;
      107:701–708.

169. Szlyk JP, Fishman GA, Alexander KR, Peachey NS, Derlacki
      DJ. Clinical subtypes of cone–rod dystrophy. Arch Ophthal-
      mol 1993; 111:781–788.

170. Birch DG, Fish GE. Rod ERGs in retinitis pigmentosa and
      cone–rod degeneration. Invest Ophthalmol Vis Sci 1987;
      28:140–150.

171. Birch DG, Peters AY, Locke KL, Spencer R, Megarity CF,
      Travis GH. Visual function in patients with cone–rod dystro-
      phy (CRD) associated with mutations in the ABCA4 (ABCR)
      gene. Exp Eye Res 2001; 73:877–886.

172. Downes SM, Payne AM, Kelsell RE, Fitzke FW, Holder GE,
      Hunt DM, Moore AT, Bird AC. Autosomal dominant cone–
      rod dystrophy with mutations in the guanylate cyclase 2D

gene encoding retinal guanylate cyclase-1. Arch Ophthalmol 2002; 119:1667–1673.

173. Evans K, Duvall-Young J, Fitzke FW, Arden GB, Bhatta-charya SS, Bird AC. Chromosome 19q cone–rod dystrophy: ocular phenotype. Arch Ophthalmol 1995; 113:195–201.

174. Gregory-Evans K, Kelsell RE, Gregory-Evans CY, Downes SM, Fitzke FW, Holder GE, Stimunovic M, Mollon JD, Taylor R, Hunt DM, Bird AC, Moore AT. Autosomal dominant cone–rod retinal dystrophy (CORD6) from heterozygous mutation of GUCY2D, which encodes retinal guanylate cyclase. Ophthalmology 2000; 107:55–61.

175. Jacabson SG, Cidenciyan AV, Huang Y, Hanna DB, Freund CL, Affatigato LM, Carr RE, Zack DJ, Stone EM, Melness RR. Retinal degenerations with truncation mutations in the cone–rod hoemobox (CRX) gene. Invest Ophthalmol Vis Sci 1998; 39:2417–2426.

176. Klevering BJ, Blankenagel A, Maugeri A, Cremers FP, Hoyng CB, Rohrschneider K. Phenotypic spectrum of autoso-mal recessive cone–rod dystrophies caused by mutations in the ABCA4 (ABCR) gene. Invest Ophthalmol Vis Sci 2002; 43:1980–1985.

177. Nakazawa M, Maoi N, Wada Y, Nakazaki S, Maruiwa F, Sawada A, Tamai M. Autosomal dominant cone–rod dystro-phy associated with Val200Glu mutation of the peripher-in/RDS gene. Retina 1996; 16:405–410.

178. Nakazawa M, Kikawa E, Chida Y, Wada Y, Shiono T, Tamai M. Autosomal dominant cone–rod dystrophy asso-ciated with mutations in codon 244 (Asn244His) and codon 184 (Tyr184Ser) of the perihperin/RDS gene. Arch Ophthal-mol 1996; 114:72–78.

179. Mantyjarvi M, Nurmenniemi P, Partanen J, Myohanen T, Peippo M, Alitalo T. Clinical features and a follow-up study in a family with X-linked progressive cone–rod dystrophy. Acta Ophthalmol Scand 2001; 79:359–365.

180. Brown JJ, Kimura AE, Gorin MB. Clinical and electroretino-graphic findings of female carriers and affected males in a progressive X-linked cone–rod dystrophy (COD-1) pedigree. Ophthalmology 2000; 107:1104–1110.

181. Fujii N, Shiono T, Wada Y, Nakazawa M, Tamai M, Yamada N. Autosomal dominant cone–rod dystrophy with negative electroretinogram. Br J Ophthalmol 1995; 79:916–921.

182. Deutman AF. Benign concentric annular macular dystrophy. Am J Ophthalmol 1974; 78:384–396.

183. van den Biesen PR, Deutman AF, Pinckers AJ. Evolution of benign concentric annular macular dystrophy. Am J Ophthalmol 1985; 100:73–78.

184. Miyake Y, Shiroyama N, Horiguchi M, Saito A, Yagasaki K. Bull's-eye maculopathy and negative electroretinogram. Retina 1989; 9:210–215.

185. Russell-Eggitt IM, Clayton PT, Coffey R, Kriss A, Taylor DS, Taylor JF. Alström syndrome. Report of 22 cases and literature review. Ophthalmology 1998; 105:1274–1280.

186. Alström CH, Hallgren B, Nilsson LB, Asander H. Retinal degeneration combined with obesity, diabetes mellitus and neurogenous deafness: a specific syndrome (not hitherto described) distinct from the Laurence–Moon–Biedl syndrome. A clinical endocrinological and genetic examinaton based on a large pedigree. Acta Psychiat Neurol Scand 1959; 34:129 (suppl):1–35.

187. Collin GB, Marshall JD, Ikeda A, So WV, Russel-Eggitt I, Maffei P, Beck S, Boerkoel CF, Sicolo N, Martin M, Nishina PM, Naggert JK. Mutations in ALMS1 cause obesity, type 2 diabetes and neurosensory degeneration in Alstrom syndrome. Nat Genet 2002; 31:74–78.

188. Hearn T, Renforth GL, Spalluto C, Hanley NA, Piper K, Brickwood S, White C, Connolly V, Taylor JFN, Russel-Eggitt I, Bonneau D, Walker M, Wilson DI. Mutation of ALMS1, a large gene with tandem repeat encoding 47 amino acids, causes Alstrom syndrome. Nat Genet 2002; 31:79–83.

189. Millay RH, Weleber RG, Heckenlively JR. Ophthalmologic and systemic manifestations of Alström's disease. Am J Ophthalmol 1986; 102:482–490.

190. Tremblay F, LaRoche RG, Shea SE, Ludman MD. Longitudinal study of the early electroretinographic changes in Alström's syndrome. Am J Ophthalmol 1993; 115:657–665.

9

Stationary Night Blindness and Stationary Cone Dysfunction Disorders

Hereditary retinal conditions may be stationary or relatively mildly progressive rather than dystrophies with progressive degeneration. Among the stationary disorders, the full-field ERG is an important diagnostic test particularly for congenital stationary night blindness and rod monochromatism. This chapter focuses on the electrophysiologic findings of this group of relatively non-progressive congenital hereditary retinal conditions with the following outline:

Stationary night blindness disorders:

- Congenital stationary night blindness (CSNB)
- Fundus albipunctatus
- Oguchi disease
- Fleck retina of Kandori

Stationary cone dysfunction disorders:

- Hereditary congenital color vision deficiencies

- Rod monochromatism (autosomal recessive achromatopsia)
- Blue cone monochromatism (x-linked incomplete achromatopsia)

STATIONARY NIGHT BLINDNESS DISORDERS

Congenital Stationary Night Blindness

Congenital stationary night blindness (CSNB) refers to a group of genotypically diverse and phenotypically diverse disorders characterized by non-progressive dysfunction of the rod system. The prevalence of CSNB is approximately 1 in 10,000 (1). Night vision impairment is the predominant symptom of CSNB but because this is congenital rather than acquired, some affected persons may not recognize the significance of the symptom and may not complain of impaired night vision if the disease is mild and visual acuity is preserved.

The subtyping of CSNB is complex and is summarized in Fig. 9.1. Autosomal recessive, X-linked recessive, and autosomal dominant forms of CSNB are all found. CSNB subtyping is based on ERG findings and hereditary pattern. Full-field ERG is the key diagnostic test in CSNB because the ERG has distinct findings and retinal appearance is normal except for non-specific myopic changes if present.

Aside from impaired night vision, other clinical findings of CSNB such as reduced visual acuity, myopia, strabismus, and congenital nystagmus may occur and are most consistently found in the X-linked Schubert–Bornschein type. Visual fields in CSNB are normal, and the retinal appearance is unremarkable except for accompanying myopic changes. Tilted, misshapen, or pale optic nerve heads in CSNB have been described (2). However, clinical findings in CSNB are variable even within the same family, and some patients may have normal examination with 20/20 vision so that the diagnosis is not evident unless a full-field ERG is performed. On the other end of spectrum, some autosomal recessive CSNB patients with notable visual impairment in infancy

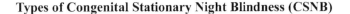

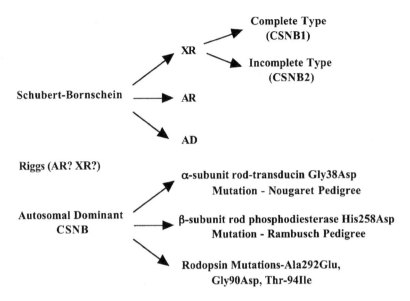

AR = Autosomal Recessive, AD = Autosomal Dominant, XR = X-Linked Recessive

Figure 9.1 Types of congenital stationary night blindness (CSNB). The classification of CSNB is complex and evolving. The diagram presents subtypes of CSNB based on historical subtyping, hereditary pattern, ERG characteristics, and genetic findings.

with decreased vision and nystagmus may be misdiagnosed as having Leber congenital amaurosis (3).

Schubert–Bornschein Type

Described in 1952, Schubert–Bornschein type (4) is the most common type of CSNB and is characterized by a negative full-field ERG. This means that an impairment of the b-wave occurs such that the b-wave to a-wave amplitude ratio is less than 1 so that the peak of the b-wave does not rise above baseline. This distinct pattern is most apparent on the scotopic bright-flash combined rod–cone response although it may also be noted on the photopic cone flash response.

The Schubert–Bornschein type occurs most commonly in X-linked recessive or autosomal recessive pedigrees. However, rare autosomal dominant CSNB pedigrees with negative ERG pattern have also been reported (5,6).

In 1986, Miyake et al. (7) studied mostly X-linked recessive Schubert–Bornschein CSNB patients and proposed a new classification of complete and incomplete types based on ERG responses. The complete type, designated as CSNB1, was later discovered to be due to mutations of the NYX gene located in the p11.4 region of the X-chromosome (8,9). The NYX gene encodes nyctalopin, a glycosylphosphatidyl (GPI) -anchored extracellular protein which is expressed in tissues including retina, brain, testis, and muscles. Nyctalopin regulates cell growth, adhesion, and migration, and mutant nyctalopin disrupts synapse between neurons and circuitry of the retina. ERG responses of CSNB1 patients are similar to those of monkeys after intravitreal injection of 2-amino-4-phosphonobutyric acid, a glutamate analog, which selectively blocks signal transmission from photoreceptors to ON-bipolar cells (10). Other ERG studies have also supported that CSNB1 is due to abnormality of the ON-depolarizing bipolar cell pathway (11–13). The incomplete type, designated as CSNB2, was later found to be due to mutations of a retinal specific calcium-channel α_{1F}-subunit gene, CACNA1F, located in the p11.23 region of the X chromosome (14–16). Mutations of CACNA1F impairs the influx of Ca^{2+} required for neurotransmitter release from photoreceptors and limits the activity of the bipolar cells. Impairment of OFF-bipolar cell activities in CSNB2 has been proposed (10).

Reduced visual acuity, myopia, strabismus, and congenital nystagmus are common features of X-linked Schubert–Bornschein CSNB. Ruether et al. (17) compared clinical features between 13 CSNB1 patients and 10 CSNB2 patients and found no significant differences between the two subgroups. Nearly all patients were myopic with a mean refractive error of about −6.00 diopters, mean visual acuity was close to 20/60, 57% had nystagmus, and 53% had strabismus. However, clinical findings in X-linked Schubert–Bornschein CSNB are highly variable (18,19). Pearce et al. (19) in a study of 42 patients found that at least one of main clinical features of Schubert–Bornschein CSNB, such as impaired night vision, nystagmus, and myopia, was absent in 75% of the patients. Further, considerable variability in clinical expression exists even for a specific genotype. Boycott et al. (20) studied 66 males with CSNB2 from 15 families with a common mutation of CACNA1F (L1056insC) and noted widely variable features both between and within families. Only 60% of the patients reported night vision problem, visual acuity varied widely and ranged from 20/25 to 20/400, 85% had myopia, 43% had nystagmus, and 22% had strabismus.

Examples of standard full-field ERG responses for complete (CSNB1) and incomplete (CSNB2) forms of Schubert–Bornschein CSNB are shown in Fig. 9.2 and the differences in ERG findings are summarized in Table 9.1 (7,21). The most

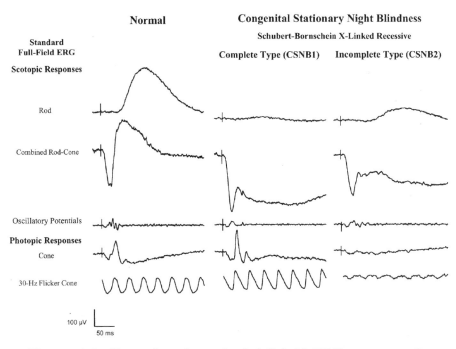

Figure 9.2 Examples of standard full-field ERG responses for complete (CSNB1) and incomplete (CSNB2) forms of X-linked recessive Schubert–Bornschein congenital stationary night blindness (CSNB). The ERG characteristics of CSNB are summarized in Table 9.1.

Table 9.1 ERG Characteristics of Complete and Incomplete Types of X-Linked Recessive Schubert–Bornschein Congenital Stationary Night Blindness

	Complete type (CSNB1)	Incomplete type (CSNB2)
Standard full-field ERG		
Scotopic		
Rod flash response	Not detectable	Reduced
Rod-cone bright flash response	Normal a-wave, marked reduced negative b-wave	Normal a-wave, marked reduced negative b-wave
Oscillatory potentials	Not detectable	Present but delayed
Photopic		
Cone flash response	Normal or mildly reduced, Square-shaped a-wave	Reduced
Cone 30-Hz flicker	Normal or mildly reduced	Reduced
Other full-field ERG findings		
Photopic long-duration flash response	Normal a-wave, reduced b-wave (ON-response), large d-wave (OFF-response)	Small a-wave, relatively large b-wave with elevated plateau (ON-response), small d-wave (OFF-response)
Scotopic threshold response (STR)	Not detectable	Present but delayed
Short-wavelength sensitive cone (S-cone) response	Not detectable	Present

striking ERG finding in both CSNB1 and CSNB2 is a negative full-field ERG for the scotopic bright-flash combined rod–cone response where the a-wave is preserved and the b-wave is marked reduced but not prolonged. However, in CSNB1, the scotopic rod response is non-detectable, the scotopic oscillatory potentials are absent, and the photopic cone flash and 30-Hz responses are normal or mildly reduced. In contrast, in CSNB2, the scotopic rod response is reduced but detectable, the scotopic oscillatory potentials are present but delayed, and the photopic cone flash and 30-Hz responses are reduced. Of interest, in CSNB patients with moderate to severe myopia, generalized reduction in ERG components associated with myopia may also occur and are superimposed on the CSNB ERG.

In addition to findings on standard full-field ERG, there are several other notable differences in specialized full-field ERG responses between CSNB1 and CSNB2. In CSNB1, the photopic long-duration flash response is characterized by a normal a-wave, a reduced b-wave (ON-response) and a large d-wave (OFF-response) (Fig. 9.3) (22,23). This is similar to ERG responses of monkeys after intravitreal injection of 2-amino-4-phosphonobutyric acid, a glutamate analog, which selectively blocks signal transmission from photoreceptors to ON-bipolar cells supporting the hypothesis that dysfunction of the ON-pathway is the primary defect in CSNB1 (10). In contrast, in CSNB2, the photopic long-duration flash response is characterized by a small a-wave, a relatively large b-wave with elevated plateau (ON-response) and a small d-wave (OFF-response) (Fig. 9.3). This has some similarity to ERG responses of monkeys after intravitreal injection of kynurenic acid, a glutamate analog, which selectively blocks signal transmission from cone photoreceptors to OFF-bipolar cells supporting the hypothesis that dysfunction of the OFF-pathway may be the primary defect in CSNB2 (10). Further, in CSNB1, the scotopic threshold response (STR) is not detectable, but in CSNB2 the STR is delayed and detectable at an elevated threshold than normal (24). STR is a negative scotopic wave recorded with very dim flashes and represents the initial threshold ERG response. Scotopic threshold response

Congenital Stationary Night Blindness (CSNB)
Photopic Long-Duration Flash Responses

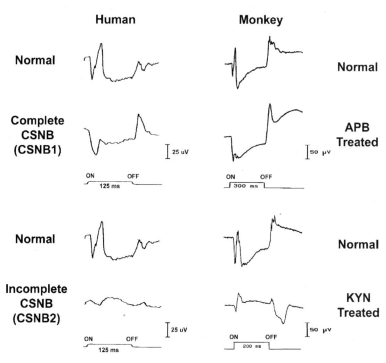

Rod and Cone Visual Pathways

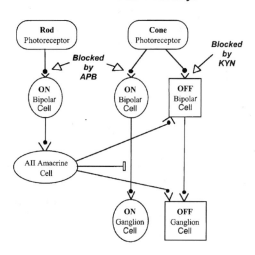

Figure 9.3   *(Caption on facing page)*

originates postsynaptic to the photoreceptors and is maximal in the region of the inner plexiform layer, and impaired STR suggests proximal retinal dysfunction especially of the rod pathway. Moreover, in CSNB1, the short wavelength sensitive cone (S-cone) full-field ERG is not detectable, but in CSNB2, the S-cone ERG response is present (25). The function of the three types of cones can be tested with ERG by using wavelength-specific (i.e., spectral) stimuli. The difference in S-cone ERG response between CSNB1 and CSNB2 has been postulated to be due to the defect of the ON-pathway in CSNB1 and its effect on the predominantly ON-nature of the S-cone pathway. However, despite a non-detectable S-cone ERG, color vision is normal in CSNB1 patients, and using blue-on-yellow perimetry, Terasaki et al. (26) showed that S-cone function CSNB1 is preserved in the foveal region but is abnormal toward the peripheral retina.

Figure 9.3 (*Facing page*) Photopic long-duration flash responses for complete (CSNB1) and incomplete (CSNB2) forms of X-linked recessive Schubert–Bornschein congenital stationary night blindness (CSNB). The responses suggest dysfunction of the ON-pathway is the primary defect in CSNB1 and dysfunction of the OFF-pathway is the primary defect in CSNB2. The response of CSNB1 has a normal a-wave, a reduced b-wave (ON-response) and a large d-wave (OFF-response) and is similar to that of monkeys after intravitreal injection of 2-amino-4-phosphonobutyric acid (APB), a glutamate analog, which selectively blocks the synapse between photoreceptors and depolarizing ON-bipolar cells. The response of CSNB2 has a small a-wave, a relatively large b-wave with elevated plateau (ON-response) and a small d-wave (OFF-response) and is similar to that of monkeys after intravitreal injection of kynurenic acid (KYN), a glutamate analog, which selectively blocks the synapse between photoreceptors and hyperpolarizing OFF-bipolar cells. Note the rod photoreceptors contact only ON-rod bipolar cells which synapse with AII-amacrine cells. The AII-amacrine cells make large gap junction with ON-cone bipolar cells and have synapses with OFF-cone bipolar cells and OFF-ganglion cells. (From Refs. 22 and 95, with permission from the Japanese Ophthalmological Society and the American Ophthalmological Society.)

In terms of multifocal ERG, in a study of four patients with CSNB1 and without nystagmus, Kondo et al. (27) found normal amplitude but delayed first-order kernels for nearly the entire field tested. The authors postulated that the delay of first-order kernels may be related to the severe amplitude reduction of the second-order kernel.

In general, heterozygous female carriers of X-linked CSNB are asymptomatic and have normal dark-adaptation retinal thresholds (28). Miyake and Kawase (28) found normal full-field ERG responses except for reduced oscillatory potentials with normal implicit times in X-linked CSNB female carriers. These findings were confirmed by Young et al. (13) who demonstrated that reduced oscillatory potentials were most apparent with a blue flash stimulus under scotopic condition. Reduced photopic 30-Hz flicker cone responses are also occasionally found in obligatory female CSNB carriers (29). Rarely, female CSNB carriers may manifest the disease and demonstrated typical CSNB ERG responses, presumably due to uneven X-chromosomal lyonization where disproportionate inactivation of the normal allele of the X chromosome occurs so that the abnormal allele is expressed in the retina (30). Affected homozygous females of X-linked CSNB have been reported (31).

Riggs Type

In 1956, Riggs (32) described three CSNB patients, two of whom were sisters, with detectable but markedly impaired dark-adaptation and full-field ERG responses consisting of reduced b-waves, which, in contrast to the Schubert–Bornschein type, remained positive with b-wave to a-wave amplitude ratios of greater than one. In 1969, Auerbach et al. (33) reported findings on 95 CSNB patients, 82 of whom were males, and classified 59 patients into the Schubert–Bornschein type and 36 patients into the Riggs type. Of the 36 CSNB patients with Riggs type, details of mode of inheritance were not available but most were males, and 12 of the patients were offsprings of consanguineous marriages. Taken together, this suggests that the Riggs type is likely inherited as X-linked recessive or autosomal recessive. In the same study, the authors found that myopia and nystagmus were less common in Riggs type patients than Schubert–Bornschein type patients.

Although often mentioned as a distinct type of CSNB, the Riggs type is rare as no large series of Riggs type patients have been reported since Auerbach et al. (33) in 1969. Miyake and Kawase (28) have suggested that the scotopic b-wave ERG responses of incomplete type Schubert–Bornschein CSNB patients do not become negative until stronger stimulus intensity, and under lower stimulus intensities, incomplete type Schubert–Bornschein CSNB patients have reduced but positive b-wave ERG responses which resembles those responses described by Riggs. Therefore, at least some of the incomplete type Schubert–Bornschein CSNB patients are likely to have the same clinical entity as the Riggs type.

Autosomal Dominant CSNB

In addition to the rare autosomal dominant Schubert–Bornschein type, several other pedigrees of autosomal dominant CSNB have been described. The Nougaret type derives its name from the first recognized affected individual, Jean Nougaret (1637–1719), a butcher who lived in Vendemian in Southern France (34). Dryja et al. (35) found that affected descendants have a heterozygous missense mutation (Gly38Asp) in the gene encoding the α-subunit of rod-specific transducin, the G-protein that couples rhodopsin to cGMP-phosphodiesterase in the phototransduction cascade. Sandberg et al. (36) noted non-detectable scotopic full-field ERG responses to dim blue flash in a father and son with Nougaret CSNB, implying that the standard scotopic dim white-flash rod response may also be non-detectable. The scotopic white bright-flash combined rod–cone responses demonstrated decreased biphasic a-wave with a b-wave amplitude that was positive and at least 50% of normal indicating that the loss of rod function was not complete. The cone responses were only slightly impaired. These Nougaret CSNB ERG findings are similar to the ERGs described for the Riggs CSNB type. The EOG light-peak to dark-tough amplitude ratios were only mildly decreased and ranged from 1.4 to 2.0 (normal $\geq$1.8). Taken together, the results suggest that these abnormalities can be simulated by light-adapting the normal retina and are compatible with the proposal that the defective rod transducin is constitutively active in darkness but produces partial desensitization of rods.

Another type of autosomal dominant CSNB was described by Rambusch in 1909 in a Danish family (37). The ancestor of the Rambusch pedigree is Niels Sorensen, a farmer who was born about 1660. Gal et al. (38) found that affected descendants have a heterozygous missense mutation (His258Asp) in the gene encoding the β-subunit of the rod cGMP phosphodiesterase. Full-field ERG responses of affected individuals of the Rambusch pedigree are similar to those of Nougaret CSNB type and resembles the ERG responses of the Riggs CSNB type. Rosenberg and colleagues (37) noted non-detectable scotopic full-field ERG responses to dim blue flash in six affected descendents indicating that the standard scotopic dim white-flash rod response may also be non-detectable. The scotopic white bright-flash combined rod–cone responses demonstrated moderately decreased a-waves and more pronounced b-wave depressions but the b-waves were usually positive or nearly equal to the amplitudes of the a-waves. Cone responses were normal or only slightly impaired. The authors also reported one descendent who seemed to be affected in one eye only with reduced rod and cone full-field ERG responses and a normal ERG in the other eye.

Several types of autosomal dominant CSNB associated with rhodopsin mutations have been described. Dryja et al. (39) noted a heterozygous missense mutation (Ala292Glu) of the rhodopsin gene in a 34-year-old man with CSNB. The patient showed no scotopic full-field ERG rod response to dim blue flash and reduced a-wave and b-waves with shortened implicit times for the scotopic white bright-flash combined rod–cone response. The cone 30-Hz white-flash flicker response was at the low end of normal.

Sieving et al. (40) reported a rhodopsin mutation (Gly90Asp) in a 22 member kindred with autosomal dominant

CSNB. All seven affected individuals had no scotopic full-field ERG rod response to dim blue flash. The cone flash and 30-Hz flicker responses were normal in all but one person. The results of the scotopic white bright-flash combined rod–cone response were not reported.

Another rhodopsin mutation (Thr94Ile) associated with autosomal dominant CSNB was described by al-Jandal et al. (41) in an Irish family. All affected persons had no scotopic full-field ERG rod responses. The scotopic white bright-flash combined rod–cone responses showed moderately reduced a-waves and markedly reduced b-waves that were severe enough to produce a negative b-wave but the b-wave implicit time was shorter than normal. However, the negative ERG in this case differs from Schubert–Bornschein CSNB types in that the a-wave in the latter is near normal rather than reduced. Other ERG features of this rhodopsin phenotype include well-preserved oscillatory potentials and normal photopic flash and 30-Hz flicker cone responses. The authors hypothesized that constitutive activation of transducin by the altered rhodopsin may be the mechanism of this type of autosomal dominant CSNB.

Other CSNB Types

Affected patients with Åland Island eye disease may have similar ERG findings as incomplete CSNB. Åland Island eye disease is X-linked recessive and was described by Forsius and Eriksson in 1964 (42). Clinical features include ocular albinism, myopia, and nystagmus. Genetic changes associated with both Åland Island eye disease and incomplete CSNB are located in the same region of the X chromosome, and the question of whether the two disorders are one and the same has been raised (43).

Barnes et al. (44) described a distinctive form of CSNB with cone ON-pathway dysfunction in a 30-year-old man whose mother had retinitis pigmentosa. In this case, the scotopic rod full-field response was non-detectable and the scotopic combined rod–cone response had markedly reduced a-wave with a severely diminished negative b-wave.

EOG and VEP in CSNB

While the full-field ERG is a key diagnostic test in CSNB, EOG and VEP have no proven diagnostic value in CSNB. Of interest, the EOG light-peak to dark-trough amplitude ratio in CSNB may be normal or reduced (45–47). In terms of VEP, Tremblay et al. (48) found crossed visual evoked potential asymmetry in patients with CSNB2 indicating excessive decussation of retinal ganglion cell fibers at the optic chiasm. This finding not only implies impaired binocularity in CSNB2 but also demonstrates that this finding which is also found in albinism is not to be considered as pathognomonic for albinism.

Fundus Albipunctatus

Fundus albipunctatus is a rare autosomal recessive disorder characterized by impaired night vision and numerous small discrete white-yellow retinal lesions scattered throughout the retina except the fovea. This disorder is caused by mutations in the RDH5 gene (chromosome 12q13–14) which encodes the enzyme 11-*cis* retinol dehydrogenase (49). The enzyme expressed in the retinal pigment epithelium has an important role in the synthesis of rhodopsin by catalyzing the conversion of 11-*cis* retinol to 11-*cis* retinal with cofactor NAD+. Missense mutations (e.g., homozygous Gly238Trp, compound heterozygous Gly238Trp and Ser73Phe) of the RDH5 gene are associated with fundus albipunctatus. In addition, a homozygous one base deletion with four base insertion (1085delC/insGAAG) in the RDH5 gene may be the cause of fundus albipunctatus in most Japanese patients (50). The resulting defect in the enzyme 11-*cis* retinol dehydrogenase produces a prolonged regenerative cycle of visual pigment (51).

Because impaired night vision is congenital, affected persons may or may not be symptomatic. However, the numerous small discrete white-yellow retinal lesions are easily recognized on routine ophthalmic examination (Fig. 9.4). Visual acuity and fields are normal but are reduced if tested with dim stimulus. The retinal lesions evolve in appearance from

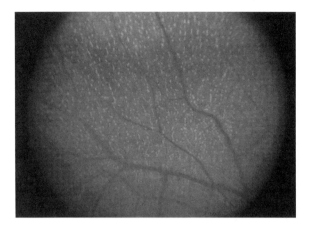

Figure 9.4   Small discrete white-yellow retinal lesions in a patient with fundus albipunctatus. The lesions spare the fovea and are scattered throughout the retina. (From Ref. 96.) (Refer to the color insert.)

flecks in childhood to permanent punctate dots that increase in number over years (52). The optic nerve heads are normal, and there are no apparent abnormality of the retinal vessels.

Although Marmor (52) found that long-term follow-up of patients with fundus albipunctatus showed no progression of dysfunction, Nakazawa et al. (53) have demonstrated that progressive cone dystrophy is frequently observed in elderly patients with fundus albipunctatus. Of the 12 patients with fundus albipunctatus and RDH5 gene mutations studied by Nakazawa, six had progressive cone dystrophy which was most frequently seen in patients over age 40. In another study of 21 patients with fundus albipunctatus, 10 patients had macular dystrophy (54). Therefore, approximately 50% of patients with fundus albipunctatus are likely to have macular dystrophy.

Dark adaptometry or full-field ERG or both are extremely helpful if not essential in the clinical diagnosis of fundus albipunctatus and in differentiating this disorder form other more progressive retinal white dot disorders such as retinitis punctata albescens. Dark adaptometry shows prolonged cone and rod adaptation with delayed cone–rod transition but eventually reaches normal threshold. Rod ERG response after the usual period of 30–40 min of dark-adaptation is reduced (Fig. 9.5). The EOG light-to-dark amplitude ratio is also correspondingly decreased. However, both the rod ERG response and the EOG light-to-dark ratio return to normal with prolonged dark adaptation in as short as 60 min or up to 180 min (51,55). Because scotopic ERG responses normalize after prolonged dark-adaptation, the clinician should alert the ERG laboratory if this disorder is suspected so that appropriately prolonged dark-adapted ERG will be performed. The photopic full-field ERG responses are normal or mildly reduced in fundus albipunctatus patients without macular dystrophy but are significantly reduced in those with macular dystrophy (54).

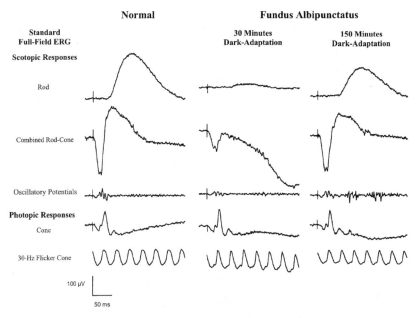

Figure 9.5 Standard full-field ERG responses from the patient with fundus albipunctatus of Fig. 9.4. Note the marked improved scotopic rod and combined rod–cone responses to near normal after prolonged dark adaptation of 150 min as compared to those after 30 min of dark adaptation.

Oguchi Disease

Oguchi disease is a rare autosomal recessive disorder characterized by non-progressive impaired night vision and a yellowish discoloration appearance of the retina, which returns to normal after several hours of dark-adaptation (Mizuo–Nakamura phenomenon) (Fig. 9.6). Visual acuity, color vision, and visual fields are generally unaffected or near normal. The disorder was first reported by Oguchi (56) in Japan in 1907 but occurs also in other ethnic groups. Fuchs et al. (57) have shown that a homozygous 1-base pair deletion (1147delA) of codon 309 in the arrestin gene is a frequent cause of Oguchi disease. Subsequently, Yamamoto et al. (58) found homozygous as well as compound heterozygous mutations in the rhodopsin kinase gene in patients with Oguchi disease whose arrestin gene was normal. Rhodopsin kinase works with arrestin to deactivate rhodopsin after rhodopsin is stimulated by light. Abnormalities of arrestin or rhodopsin kinase produce marked delay in rod sensitivity recovery after light exposure. However, patients with arrestin homozygous 1-base pair deletion (1147delA) may have Oguchi disease or retinitis

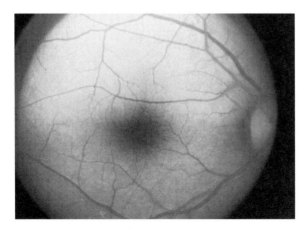

Figure 9.6 Yellowish appearance of the retina in a patient with Oguchi disease. The color of the retina as well as the dark-adapted rod thresholds are restored after very prolonged dark adaptation. (From Ref. 96.) (Refer to the color insert.)

pigmentosa indicating variable expressivity (59,60). In addition, a patient with Oguchi disease and sectoral retinitis pigmentosa has been described (61).

The diagnosis of Oguchi disease is based on the presence of Mizuo–Nakamura phenomenon and ERG findings (Fig. 9.7). Standard full-field ERG in Oguchi disease demonstrates a non-detectable scotopic rod response. Scotopic bright-flash combined rod–cone response shows a reduced a-wave and a severely reduced and prolonged negative b-wave (a-wave amplitude > b-wave amplitude) with correspondingly reduced oscillatory potentials (62). Photopic cone flash and flicker responses are generally normal but may occasionally be mildly reduced. With prolonged dark adaptation of 3–6 h, variable improvement of scotopic responses occurs (63). Dark adaptometry is abnormal although light sensitivity threshold improves with prolonged dark adaptation. Specialized ERG with photopic long-duration flash stimulus is normal, indicating normal ON and OFF responses (63). Likewise, the function of the three types of cones is normal by using

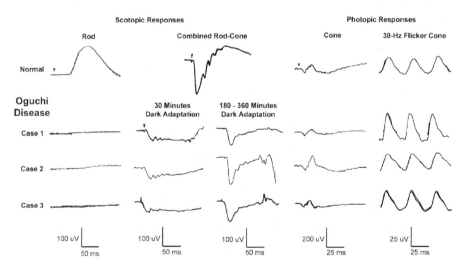

Figure 9.7 Full-field ERG responses of patients with Oguchi disease. Note the marked improved combined rod–cone responses after prolonged dark adaptation of 180–360 min as compared to those after 30 min of dark adaptation. (From Ref. 63 with permission from the Japanese Ophthalmological Society.)

wavelength-specific (i.e., spectral) stimuli (64). Pattern ERG, pattern VEP, and multifocal ERG are normal (60). The EOG light-peak to dark-trough amplitude ratio in Oguchi disease is very reduced (63). Of note, previous findings of normal EOG and normal scotopic a-wave on the combined rod–cone response are contrary to the findings of more recent studies (65,66).

Fleck Retina of Kandori

Kandori et al. (67) described a disorder characterized by early onset non-progressive night vision impairment, relatively large yellow irregular shaped flecks in the peripheral retina, minimal dark adaptation abnormality, and normal visual fields. Although patients with this extremely rare condition may have impaired full-field ERG, EOG and VEP are usually normal, and dark adaptation is only minimally affected (67).

STATIONARY CONE DYSFUNCTION DISORDERS

Hereditary Congenital Color Vision Deficiencies

A normal person requires all three primary colors, red, green, and blue, to match colors within the visible spectrum and is a normal trichromat. However, hereditary congenital color vision deficiency affects approximately 8% of males and 0.5% of females and are often X-linked recessive. Most affected persons are anomalous trichromats who uses abnormal proportions of the three primary colors to match colors in the light spectrum. Those individuals who need only two primary colors for matching colors are designated as dichromats. Persons with red-green deficiencies due to an abnormality of either red-sensitive or green-sensitive cones are said to have protan and deutan defects, respectively, and those with a blue-yellow deficiency due to an abnormality of the blue-sensitive cones have a tritan defect.

Congenital color deficiencies such as anomalous trichromatism are assessed most commonly using color plate tests such as the Ishihara and the Hardy–Rand–Rittler (HRR) tests where colored figures are seen by normal persons but missed by affected persons. Standard white-flash ERG responses are normal for dichromats and anomalous trichromats. However, specialized ERG recordings have demonstrated abnormalities of the early receptor potential (ERP) and responses to color stimuli. For example, in dichromats, the amplitudes of the R_2 wave of the ERP is reduced (68). Abnormal ERG responses to color stimuli have also been found in dichromats and anomalous trichromats (69–71). Further, the x-wave which represents the initial scotopic cone response to red light is reduced in protanopes and protanomalous trichromats but not in deutanopes and deutanomalous trichromats.

Rod Monochromatism (Autosomal Recessive Achromatopsia)

Rod monochromatism is an autosomal recessive congenital disorder characterized by severe or complete cone dysfunction. The condition is also commonly referred to as autosomal recessive achromatopsia, and affected persons are "monochromats" who perceive colors as shades of gray. Many patients with rod monochromatism harbor homozygous or heterozygous mutations of the CNGA3 gene encoding alpha-subunit of cone photoreceptor cGMP-gated channel on choromosome 2 (2q11) or the ACHM3 gene encoding beta-subunit of cone photoreceptor cGMP-gated channel on chromosome 8 (8q21) (72–74). Aside from poor color perception, other clinical features include decreased visual acuity, nystagmus, and light sensitivity. Visual acuity is variable and ranges from 20/40 to 20/400 due to cone dysfunction and the development of early-onset sensory nystagmus. Retinal appearance is usually normal or minimally abnormal with mild non-specific pigmentary changes. "Complete" and "incomplete" forms of rod monochromatism have been designated on the basis of the severity of clinical and ERG findings as well as color-matching tests (Fig. 9.8) (75). Complete rod monochromats have severe disease with markedly impaired visual acuity and non-detectable full-field ERG cone responses while incomplete rod monochromats have better visual acuity and

Stationary Night Blindness and Stationary Cone Dysfunction Disorders **263**

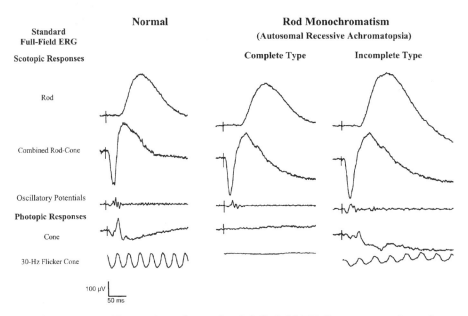

Figure 9.8 Examples of standard full-field ERG responses in rod monochromatism. The photopic cone flash and 30-Hz flicker responses are non-detectable in "complete" rod monochromats and severely reduced in "incomplete" rod monochromats. Similar genotypes are found in complete and incomplete rod monochromats, and members from the same family may have complete or incomplete form of the disease. The ERG responses of rod monochromatism are similar to cone dystrophy and X-linked blue cone monochromatism. These conditions may be differentiated by clinical features and hereditary pattern as well as by specialized ERG and psychophysical testing.

detectable but severely reduced full-field ERG cone responses. However, complete and incomplete forms of rod monochromatism are usually results of variable expressivity. Similar genetic mutations are found in complete and incomplete rod monochromats, and affected members of the same family may have complete or incomplete form of the disease (74).

The diagnosis of rod monochromatism is based on a combination of clinical findings, full-field ERG responses, and genetic analysis. Full-field ERG is a key diagnostic test in rod monochromatism with ERG responses similar to those of cone dystrophy. However, in contrast to cone dystrophy, symptoms of rod monochromatism typically occur in the first years of life with nystagmus. In general, the following is noted on standard full-field ERG in rod monochromatism: (1) scotopic rod flash response—normal or mildly reduced, (2) scotopic combined rod–cone bright-flash response—reduced a-wave and b-wave with variable prolongation, (3) oscillatory potentials—reduced, and (4) photopic cone flash and flicker responses—non-detectable in "complete" rod monochromat and severely reduced in "incomplete" rod monochromat. Of interest, "complete" rod monochromats and blue cone monochromats have similar standard full-field ERG responses but can be differentiated on the basis of hereditary pattern, genetic testing, specialized color testing, and specialized ERG testing (see below).

Blue Cone Monochromatism (X-Linked Incomplete Achromatopsia)

Blue cone monochromatism is a rare X-linked recessive disorder characterized by the absence of functional long-wavelength (L) "red" sensitive cone photoreceptors and medium-wavelength (M) "green" sensitive cone photoreceptors. The function of the short-wavelength (S) "blue" sensitive cone photoreceptors is preserved. Blue cone monochromatism is caused by alterations of the genes encoding the photosensitive pigments of the L- and M-cones, which are arranged in a tandem array with a locus control region on the X chromosome (76,77). Genotypes among persons with blue cone monochromacy or related variants of the disorder are extremely heterogeneous and diverse (78–81). The gene encoding the "blue" photosensitive pigment of the S-cones located on chromosome 7 remains unaffected.

Affected males with blue cone monochromatism have decreased visual acuity of generally 20/80 or worse, myopia, impaired color vision, and congenital nystagmus. These clinical features are similar to those of autosomal recessive rod monochromatism. However, blue cone monochromats of some families with progressive bilateral macular atrophy have been described (76,78,82,83).

Aside from genetic analysis, the differentiation between X-linked blue cone monochromatism and autosomal recessive rod monochromatism is made on the basis of hereditary pattern, specialized color testing, spectral sensitivity testing, or specialized ERG testing. Because the S-cones contribute minimally to the standard full-field ERG, standard white-flash responses of blue cone monochromats and rod monochromats are similar and demonstrate normal or near normal scotopic rod response, reduced scotopic bright-flash rod–cone flash response, and markedly reduced or non-detectable photopic cone response (78). Further, in those blue monochromats with progressive bilateral macular atrophy, the full-field ERG responses and clinical findings would be similar to those with cone dystrophy. However, S-cone full-field ERG response is detectable in blue cone monochromats by using yellow background and blue flash stimulus (84).

In 1983, Berson et al. (85) developed a color test to distinguish patients with blue cone monochromatism from those with rod monochromatism. The test consists of two instructional and four test plates. Each test plate has three identical blue-green arrows and one purple-blue arrow. The test plates differ from one another with respect to the chromaticity of the purple-yellow arrow. Patients with blue cone monochromatis can easily identify the purple-blue arrows on all four test plates but none of the rod monochromats could identify the purple-blue arrows on the test plates. However, the Berson color test may not necessarily differentiate patients with blue cone monochromatism from those with cone dystrophy (86). In terms of more commonly available color tests, blue cone monochromats are much more likely to correctly identify the blue-yellow plates in the HRR color plate test and are unlikely to make any errors along the tritan axis on the Farnsworth D15 panel hue discrimination test (87).

Using spectral sensitivity measurements under light-adapted conditions, blue cone monochromats show a peak sensitivity near light wavelength 440 nm while rod monochromats demonstrate a peak sensitivity near 504 nm (88–90). Spectral sensitivity measurements are made by determining the brightness threshold for light stimuli of various wavelengths. Spectral sensitivity may be obtained through subjective responses of the patient or by ERG so that the minimal luminance of a color stimulus of a specific wavelength that would elicit a response is determined (91).

Female carriers of blue cone monochromatism are generally asymptomatic but may have mild nystagmus and color vision abnormalities (92). The most common full-field ERG finding is a reduced and prolonged 30-Hz flicker cone response although impaired cone flash and scotopic bright-flash rod-cone response may also occur (93,94).

REFERENCES

1. Rosner M, Hefetz L, Abraham FA. The prevalence of retinitis pigmentosa and congenital stationary night blindness in Israel. Am J Ophthalmol 1993; 116:373–374.

2. Heckenlively JR, Marftin DA, Rosenbaum AL. Loss of electro-retinographic oscillatory potentials, optic atrophy and dysplasia in congenital stationary night blindness. Am J Ophthalmol 1983; 96:526–534.

3. Weleber RG, Tongue AC. Congenital stationary night blindness presenting as Leber's congenital amaurosis. Arch Ophthalmol 1987; 105:360–365.

4. Schubert G, Bornschein H. Beitrag zur Analyse des menschlichen Elektroretinogramms. Ophthalmologica 1952; 123: 396–413.

5. Hayakawa M, Imai Y, Wakita M, Kato K, Yanashima K, Miyake Y, Kanai A. A Japanese pedigree of autosomal dominant congenital stationary night blindness with variable expressivity. Ophthalmic Paed Genet 1992; 13: 211–217.

6. Noble KG, Carr RE, Siegel IM. Autosomal dominant congenital stationary night blindness and normal fundus with an electronegative electroretinogram. Am J Ophthalmol 1990; 109:44–48.

7. Miyake Y, Yagasaki K, Horiguchi M, Kawase Y, Kanda T. Congenital stationary night blindness with negative electro-

retinogram: a new classification. Arch Ophthalmol 1986; 104: 1013–1020.

8. Bech-Hansen NT, Naylor MJ, Maybaum TA, Sparkes RL, Koop B, Birch DG, Bergen AAB, Prinsen CFM, Polomeno RC, Gal A, Drack AV, Musarella MA, Jacobson SG, Young RSL, Weleber RG. Mutations in NYX encoding the leucine-rich proteoglycan nyctalopin, cause X-linked complete congenital stationary night blindness. Nat Genet 2000; 26:319–323.

9. Pusch CM, Zeitz C, Brandau O, Pesch K, Achatz H, Feil S, Scharfe C, Maurer J, Jacobi FK, Pinckers A, Andreasson S, Hardcastle A, Wissinger B, Berger W, Meindl A. The complete form of X-linked congenital stationary night blindness is caused by mutations in a gene encoding a leucine-rich repeat protein. Nat Genet 2000; 26:324–327.

10. Miyake Y, Horiguchi M, Suzuki S, Kondo M, Tanikawa A. Complete and incomplete type congenital stationary night blindness (CSNB) as a model of "OFF-retina" and "ON-retina". In: LaVail M, Hollyfield J, Anderson R, eds. Degenerative Retinal Diseases. New York Plenum Press: 1997: 31–41.

11. Scholl HPN, Langrová H, Pusch CM, Wissinger B, Zrenner E, Apfelstedt-Sylla E. Slow and fast rod ERG pathways in patients with X-linked complete stationary night blindess carrying mutations in NYX gene. Invest Ophthalmol Vis Sci 2001; 42:2728–2736.

12. Kim SH, Bush RA, Sieving PA. Increased phase lag of the fundamental harmonic component of the 30 Hz flicker ERG in Schubert–Bornschein complete type CSNB. Vision Res 1997; 37:2471–2475.

13. Young RSL, Chaparro A, Price J, Walters J. Oscillatory potentials of X-linked carriers of congenital stationary night blindness. Invest Ophthalmol Vis Sci 1989; 30:806–812.

14. Bech-Hansen NT, Naylor MJ, Maybaum TA, Pearce WG, Koop B, Fishman GA, Mets M, Musarella MA, Boycott KM. Loss-of-function mutations in a calcium-channel alpha1-subunit gene in Xp11.23 cause incomplete X-linked congenital stationary night blindness. Nat Genet 1998; 19:264–267.

15. Strom TM, Nyakatura G, Apfelstedt-Sylla E, Hellebrand H, Lorenz B, Weber BHF, Wutz K, Gutwillinger N, Rüther K,

Drescher B, Sauer CG, Zrenner E, Meitinger T, Rosenthal A, Meindl A. An L-type calcium-channel gene mutated in incomplete X-linked congenital stationary night blindness. Nat Genet 1998; 19:260–263.

16. Nakamura M, Ito S, Terasaki H, Miyake Y. Novel CACNA1F mutations in Japanese patients with incomplete congenital stationary night blindness. Invest Ophthalmol Vis Sci 2001; 42:1610–1616.

17. Ruether K, Apfelstedt-Sylla E, Zrenner E. Clinical findings in patients with congenital stationary night blindness of the Schubert–Bornschein type. Ger J Ophthalmol 1993; 2: 429–435.

18. Khouri G, Mets MB, Smith VC, Wendell M, Pass AS. X-linked congenital stationary night blindness. Review and report of a family with hyperopia. Arch Ophthalmol 1988; 106: 1417–1422.

19. Pearce WG, Reedyk M, Coupland SG. Variable expressivity in X-linked congenital stationary night blindness. Can J Ophthalmol 1990; 25:3–10.

20. Boycott KM, Pearce WG, Bech-Hansen NT. Clinical variability among patients with incomplete X-linked congenital stationary night blindness and a founder mutation in CACNA1F. Can J Ophthalmol 2000; 35:204–213.

21. Tremblay F, LaRoche RG, De Becker I. The electroretinographic diagnosis of the incomplete form of congenital stationary night blindness. Vision Res 1995; 35:2383–2393.

22. Miyake Y, Yagasaki K, Horiguchi M, Kawase Y. On- and off-responses in photopic electroretinogram in complete and incomplete types of congenital stationary night blindness. Jpn J Ophthalmol 1987; 31:81–87.

23. Quigley M, Roy M-S, Barsoum-Homsy M, Chevrette L, Jacob J-L, Milot J. On- and off-responses in the photopic electroretinogram in complete-type congenital stationary night blindness. Doc Ophthalmol 1996; 92:159–165.

24. Miyake Y, Horiguchi M, Terasuki H, Kondo M. Scotopic threshold response in complete and incomplete types of

congenital stationary night blindness. Invest Ophthalmol Vis Sci 1994; 35:3770–3775.

25. Kamiyanna M, Yamamoto S, Nitta K, Hayasaka S. Undetectable S cone electroretinogram b-wave in complete congenital stationary night blindness. Br J Ophthalmol 1996; 80: 637–639.

26. Terasaki H, Miyake Y, Nomura R, Horiguchi M, Suzuki S, Kondo M. Blue-on-yellow perimetry in the complete type of congenital stationary night blindness. Invest Ophthalmol Vis Sci 1999; 40:2761–2764.

27. Kondo M, Miyake Y, Kondo N, Tanikawa A, Suzuki S, Hortguchi M, Terasaki H. Multifocal ERG findings in complete type congenital stationary night blindness. Invest Ophthalmol Vis Sci 2001; 42:1342–1348.

28. Miyake Y, Kawase Y. Reduced amplitude of oscillatory potentials in female carriers of x-linked recessive congenital stationary night blindness. Am J Ophthalmol 1984; 98: 208–215.

29. Rigaudiere F, Roux C, Lachapelle P, Rosolen SG, Bitoun P, Gay-Duval A, Le Gargasson JF. ERG in female carriers of incomplete congenital stationary night blindness. Doc Ophthalmol 2003; 107:203–212.

30. Ruttum MS, Lewandowski MF, Bateman JB. Affected females in X-linked congenital stationary night blindness. Ophthalmology 1992; 99:747–752.

31. Bech-Hansen NT, Pearce WG. Manifestations of X-linked congenital stationary night blindness in three daughters of an affected male: demonstration of homozygosity. Am J Hum Genet 1993; 52:71–77.

32. Riggs LA. Electroretinography in cases of night blindness. Am J Ophthalmol 1954; 38:70–78.

33. Auerbach E, Godel V, Rowe H. An electrophysiological and psychophysical study of two forms of congenital night blindness. Invest Ophthalmol 1969; 8:332–345.

34. Francois J, Varriest G, de Rouck A, Dejean C. Les fonctions visuelles dans l'hemaralopie essentielle nougarienne. Ophthalmologica 1956; 132:244–257.

35. Dryja TP, Hahn LB, Reboul T, Arnaud B. Missense mutation in the gene encoding the alpha-subunit of rod transducin in Nougaret form of congenital stationary night blindness. Nat Genet 1996; 13:358–360.

36. Sandberg MA, Pawlyk BS, Dan J, Arnaud B, Dryja TP, Berson EL. Rod and cone function in the Nougaret form of stationary night blindness. Arch Ophthalmol 1998; 116:867–872.

37. Rosenberg T, Haim T, Piczenik Y, Simonsen SE. Autosomal dominant stationary night-blindness. A large family rediscovered. Acta Ophthalmol 1991; 69:694–702.

38. Gal A, Orth U, Baehr W, Schwinger E, Rosenberg T. Heterozygous missense mutation in the rod cGMP phosphodiesterase beta-subunit gene in autosomal dominant stationary night blindness. Nat Genet 1994; 7:64–68.

39. Dryja TP, Berson EL, Rao VR, Oprian DD. Heterozygous missense mutation in the rhodopsin gene as a cause of congenital stationary night blindness. Nat Genet 1993; 4:280–283.

40. Sieving PA, Richards JE, Naarendorp F, Bingham EL, Scott K, Alpern M. Dark-light model for night blindness from the human rhodopsin Gly-90-Asp mutation. Proc Natl Acad Sci USA 1995; 92:880–884.

41. al-Jandal N, Farrar GJ, Kiang AS, Humphries MM, Bannon N, Findlay JB, Humphries P, Kenna PF. A novel mutation within the rhodopsin gene (Thr-94-Lle) causing autosomal dominant congenital stationary night blindness. Hum Mutat 1999; 13:75–81.

42. Forsius H, Eriksson AW. Ein neues Augensyndrom mit X-chromosomaler Transmission: eine Sippe mit Fundusalbinismus, Foveahypoplasie, Nystagmus, Myopie, Astigmatismus und Dyschromatopsie. Klin Mbl Augenheilk 1964; 144: 447–457.

43. Hawksworth NR, Headland S, Good P, Thomas NS, Clarks A. Aland island eye disease: clinical and electrophysiological studies of a Walsh family. Br J Ophthalmol 1995; 79:424–430.

44. Barnes CS, Alexander KR, Fishman GA. A distinctive form of congenital stationary night blindness with cone ON-pathway dysfunction. Ophthalmology 2002; 109:575–583.

45. Carr RE, Ripps H, Siegel IM, Weale RA. Rhodopsin and the electrical activity of the retina in congenital night blindness. Invest Ophthalmol Vis Sci 1966; 5:497–507.

46. Krill AE, Martin D. Photopic abnormalities in congenital stationary night blindness. Invest Ophthalmol 1971; 10:625–636.

47. Takahashi Y, Onoe S, Asamizu N, Mori T, Yoshimura Y, Tazawa Y. Incomplete congenital stationary night blindness: electroretinogram c-wave and electrooculogram light rise. Doc Ophthalmol 1988; 70:67–75.

48. Tremblay F, De Becker I, Cheung C, LaRoche R. Visual evoked potentials with crossed asymmetry in incomplete congenital stationary night blindness. Invest Ophthalmol Vis Sci 1996; 37:1783–1792.

49. Yamamoto H, Simon A, Eriksson U, Harris E, Berson EL, Dryja TP. Mutation in the gene encoding 11-*cis* retinal dehydrogenase cause delayed dark adaptation and fundus albipunctatus. Nat Genet 1999; 22:188–191.

50. Wada Y, Abe T, Fuse N, Tamai M. A frequent 1085delC/insGAAG mutation in the RDH5 gene in Japanese patients with fundus albipunctatus. Invest Ophthalmol Vis Sci 2000; 41:1894–1897.

51. Carr R, Ripps H, Siegel IM. Visual pigment kinetics and adaptation in fundus albipunctatus. Doc Ophthalmol Proc Ser 1974; 4:193–204.

52. Marmor MF. Long-term follow-up of the physiologic abnormalities and fundus changes in fundus albipunctatus. Ophthalmology 1990; 97:380–384.

53. Nakazawa M, Hotta Y, Tanikawa A, Terasaki H, Miyake Y. A high association with cone dystrophy in fundus albipunctatus caused by mutations of the RDH5 gene. Invest Ophthalmol Vis Sci 2000; 41:3925–3932.

54. Nakamura M, Skalet J, Miyake Y. RDH5 gene mutations and electroretinogram in fundus albipunctatus with or without macular dystrophy. Doc Ophthalmol 2003; 107:3–11.

55. Margolis S, Siegel I, Ripps H. Variable expressivity in fundus albipunctatus. Ophthalmology 1987; 94:1416–1422.

56. Oguchi C. Über eine Abart von Hemeralopie. Acta Soc Ophtalmol Jpn 1907; 11:123–134.

57. Fuchs S, Nakazawa M, Maw M, Tamai M, Oguchi Y, Gal A. A homozygous 1-base pair deletion in the arrestin gene is a frequent cause of Oguchi disease in Japanese. Nat Genet 1995; 10:360–362.

58. Yamamoto S, Sippel KC, Berson EL, Dryja TP. Defects in the rhodopsin kinase gene in the Oguchi form of stationary night blindness. Nat Genet 1997; 15:175–178.

59. Nakazawa M, Wada Y, Tamai M. Arrestin gene mutations in autosomal recessive retinitis pigmentosa. Arch Ophthalmol 1998; 116:498–501.

60. Yoshi M, Murakami A, Akeo K, Nakamura A, Shimoyama M, Ikeda Y, Kikuchi Y, Okisaka S, Yanashima K, Oguchi Y. Visual function and gene analysis in a family with Oguchi's disease. Ophthalmic Res 1998; 30:394–401.

61. Nakamachi Y, Nakamura M, Fujii S, Yamamoto M, Okubo K. Oguchi disease with sectoral retinitis pigmentosa harboring adenine deletion at position 1147 in the arrestin gene. Am J Ophthalmol 1998; 125:249–251.

62. Kubota Y. The oscillatory potentials of the ERG in Oguchi's disease. Doc Ophthal Proc Ser 1974; 10:317–324.

63. Miyake Y, Horiguchi M, Suzuki S, Kondo M, Tanikawa A. Electrophysiological findings in patients with Oguchi's disease. Jpn J Ophthalmol 1996; 40:511–519.

64. Yamamoto S, Hayashi M, Takeuchi S, Shirao Y, Kita K, Kawasaki K. Normal S cone electroretinogram b-wave in Oguchi's disease. Br J Ophthalmol 1997; 81:1043–1045.

65. Carr RE, Gouras P. Oguchi's disease. Arch Ophthalmol 1965; 73:646–656.

66. Carr RE, Ripps H. Rhodopsin kinetics and rod adaptation in Oguchi's disease. Invest Ophthalmol 1967; 6:426–436.

67. Kandori F, Tamai A, Kurimoto S, Fukunaga K. Fleck retina. Am J Ophthalmol 1972; 73:673–685.

68. Okamoto M, Okajima O, Tanino T. The early receptor potential in the human eye. III. ERP in dichromats. Jpn J Ophthalmol 1982; 26:23–28.

69. Kawasaki K, Yonemura D, Nakazato H, Kawaguchi I. Abnormal spectral sensitivity of the electroretinographic off-response in protanopia and protanomalia. Doc Ophthalmol 1982; 53:51–60.

70. Nakazato H, Hanazaki H, Kawasaki K, Tanabe J, Yonemura D. Electroretinographic off-response in congenital red-green color deficiency and its genetic carrier. Doc Ophthalmol 1986; 63:179–186.

71. Shinzato K, Yokoyama M, Uji Y, Ichikawa H. The electroretinographic characteristics of congenital tritan defects. Doc Ophthalmol 1986; 62:19–24.

72. Kohl S, Baumann B, Broghammer M, Jagle H, Sieving P, Kellner U, Spegal R, Anastasi M, Zrenner E, Sharpe LT, Wissinger B. Mutations in the CNGB3 gene encoding the beta subunit of the cone photoreceptor cGMP-gated channel are responsible for achromatopsia (ACHM3) linked to chromosome 8q21. Hum Mol Genet 2000; 9:2107–2116.

73. Kohl S, Marx T, Giddings I, Jagle H, Jacobson SG, Apfelstedt-Sylla E, Zrenner E, Sharpe S, Wissinger B. Total colour blindness is caused by mutations in the gene encoding the alpha-subunit of the cone photoreceptor cGMP-gated cation channel. Nat Genet 1998; 19:257–259.

74. Wissinger B, Gamer B, Jagle H, Giorda R, Marx T, Tippmann S, Broghammer M, Jurklies B, Rosenberg T, Jacobson SG, Sener EC, Tatlipinar S, Hoyng CB, Castellan C, Bitoun P, Andreasson S, Rudolph G, Kellner U, Lorenz B, Wolff G, Verellen-Dumoulin C, Schwartz M, Cremers FP, Apfelstedt-Sylla E, Zrenner E, Salati R, Sharpe LT, Kohl S. CNGA3 Mutations in hereditary cone photoreceptor disorders. Am J Hum Genet 2001; 69:722–737.

75. Pokorny J, Smith VC, Pinckers AJ, Cozijnsen M. Classification of complete and incomplete autosomal recessive achromatopsia. Graefes Arch Clin Exp Ophthalmol 1982; 219:121–130.

76. Nathans J, Davenport CM, Maumenee IH, Lewis RA, Hejtmanik JF, Litt M, Lovrien E, Weleber R, Bachynski B,

Zwas F, Klingaman R, Fish G. Molecular genetics of human blue cone monochromacy. Science 1989; 245:831–838.

77. Wang Y, Macke JP, Merbs SL, Zack DJ, Klaunberg B, Bennett J, Gearhart J, Nathans J. A locus control region adjacent to the human red and green visual pigment genes. Neuron 1992; 9:429–440.

78. Ayyagari R, Kakuk LE, Bingham EL, Szczesny JJ, Kemp J, Toda Y, Felius J, Sieving PA. Spectrum of color gene deletions and phenotype in patients with blue cone monochromacy. Hum Genet 2000; 107:75–82.

79. Ladekjaer-Mikkelsen AS, Rosenberg T, Jorgensen AL. A new mechanism in blue monochromatism. Hum Genet 1996; 98:403–408.

80. Nathans J, Maumenee IH, Zrenner E, Sadowski B, Sharpe LT, Lewis RA, Hansen E, Rosenberg T, Schwartz M, Heckenlively JR, Traboulsi E, Klingaman R, Bech-Hansen NT, LaRoche RG, Pagon RA, Murphey WH, Weleber RG. Genetic heterogeneity among blue-cone monochromats. Am J Hum Genet 1993; 53:987–1000.

81. Reyniers E, Van Thienen M-N, Meire F, Boulle KD, Devries K, Kestelijn P, Willems PJ. Gene conversion between red and defective green opsin gene in blue cone monochromacy. Genomics 1995; 29:323–328.

82. Ayyagari R, Kakuk LE, Coats CL, Bingham EL, Toda Y, Felius J, Sieving PA. Bilateral macular atrophy in blue cone monochromacy (BCM) with loss of the locus control region (LCR) and part of the red pigment gene. Mol Vis 1999; 5:13.

83. Fleischman JA, O'Donnell REJ. Congenital X-linked incomplete achromatopsia: evidence for slow progression, carrier fundus findings, and possible genetic linkage with glucose-6-phosphate dehydrogenase locus. Arch Ophthalmol 1981; 99:468–472.

84. Gouras P, Mackay CJ, Lewis AL. The blue cone electroretinogram isolated in sex-linked achromat. In: Drum B, Verriest G, eds. Color Vision Deficiencies. Dordrecht: Kluwer, 1989:9:89–93.

85. Berson EL, Sandberg MA, Rosner B, Sullivan PL. Color plates to help identify patients with blue cone monochromatism. Am J Ophthalmol 1983; 95:741–747.

86. Pinckers A. Berson test for blue cone monochromatism. Int Ophthalmol 1992; 16:185–186.

87. Wiess AH, Biersdorf WR. Blue cone monochromatism. J Pediatr Ophthalmol Strabismus 1989; 26:218–223.

88. Alpern M, Lee GB, Maaseidvaag F, Miller SS. Colour vision in blue-cone monochromacy. J Physiol 1971; 212:211–233.

89. Blackwell HR, Blackwell OM. Rod and cone receptor mechanisms in typical and atypical congenital achromatopsia. Vision Res 1961; 1:62–107.

90. Pokorny J, Smith VC, Swartley R. Threshold measurements of spectral sensitivity in a blue monocone monochromat. Invest Ophthalmol 1970; 9:807.

91. Ikeda H, Ripps H. The electroretinogram of the cone monochromat. Arch Ophthalmol 1966; 75:513–517.

92. Gottlob I. Eye movement abnormalities in carriers of blue-cone monochromatism. Invest Ophthalmol Vic Sci 1994; 35:3556–3660.

93. Berson EL, Sandberg MA, Maguire A, Bromley WC, Roderick TH. Electroretinograms in carriers of blue cone monochromatism. Am J Ophthalmol 1986; 102:254–261.

94. Terasaki H, Miyake Y. Japanese family with blue cone monochromatism. Jpn J Ophthalmol 1992; 36:132–141.

95. Sieving PA. Photopic ON- and OFF-pathway abnormalities in retinal dystrophies. Trans Am Ophthalmol Soc 1993; 91:701–703.

96. Lam BL. Hereditary retinal degenerations. In: Parrish R, ed. Bascom Palmer Eye Institute Atlas of Ophthalmology. Philadelphia: Current Medicine, 2000:343–349.

10

Macular Disorders

A number of retinal disorders preferentially involve the macula or have distinct macular characteristics. Electrophysiologically, the multifocal ERG provides topographical information and is a useful objective measure of macular function. Although the focal ERG can also assess macular dysfunction, the popularity and availability of focal ERG are diminished with advances in multifocal ERG. An isolated macular lesion is unlikely to reduce the overall ERG response enough to affect the full-field ERG, but in some "macular" conditions such as cone dystrophy and X-linked retinoschisis, the full-field ERG is still needed diagnostically to determine diffuse retinal abnormalities. The pattern ERG is dominated by macular-related activity but provides no topographical information. Likewise, the VEP is dominated by activity from the central visual field but an impaired VEP may be produced by a deficit anywhere along the visual pathway including the retina, optic nerve, and brain. This chapter discusses the utility of electrophysiologic tests in diseases that may be categorized as "macular disorders." The conditions covered are:

- Age-related macular degeneration
- Macular degeneration—autosomal dominant, recessive
- Central serous chorioretinopathy
- Doyne honeycomb retinal dystrophy/malattia leventinese
- Stargardt macular dystrophy—fundus flavimaculatus
- Best vitelliform macular dystrophy
- Cone dystrophy
- Central cone dystrophy (occult macular dystrophy)
- Peripheral cone dystrophy
- Cone dystrophy with supernormal and delayed rod ERG (supernormal and delayed rod ERG syndrome)
- Sorsby fundus dystrophy
- Pattern dystrophy
- X-linked retinochisis
- Central areolar choroidal dystrophy
- North Carolina macular dystrophy (central areolar pigment epithelial dystrophy)
- Progressive bifocal chorioretinal atrophy
- Fenestrated sheen macular dystrophy
- Familial internal limiting membrane dystrophy

AGE-RELATED MACULAR DEGENERATION

Age-related macular degeneration (AMD), also known as age-related maculopathy or senile macular degeneration, is one of the leading causes of blindness. Age-related macular degeneration usually affects persons over age 50 years and the incidence increases with age. Age-related macular degeneration is more prevalent among Caucasians than ·among blacks. Both environmental and genetic factors are involved in the pathogenesis of AMD. Clinical features include macular drusen, pigmentary changes, and geographic atrophy of the retinal pigment epithelium and choriocapillaris. In addition, the disease may progress with further loss of central vision from neovascular maculopathy characterized by choroidal neovascularization, serous or hemorrhagic detachment of the sensory retina or pigment epithelium, lipid exudates, and subretinal and fibrovascular proliferation with scar formation. The diagnosis of AMD is based on clinical examination with the aid of angiography to assess neovascularization. Treatments include high-dose oral antioxidant, vitamin, and mineral supplementation, focal laser photocoagulation, and photodynamic therapy involving systemic administration of a photosensitizing drug followed by nonthermal laser application.

Electrophysiologic tests are not routinely performed clinically in the setting AMD. Focal macular ERG or multifocal ERG may be helpful to detect macular dysfunction when signs of AMD are mild and not readily apparent or when decrease in visual acuity is out of proportion to retinal appearance and angiographic findings. Because AMD is primarily a macular disease, full-field ERG, EOG, and dark adaptation are generally normal after taking into account the effects of aging (1–3). Mild impaired EOG and full-field ERG in AMD have also been described and are more pronounced in those with greater area of retinal destruction (4,5). In one report, the photopic 30-Hz full-field ERG cone response was found to be reduced in patients with AMD compared to control subjects suggesting extra-foveal involvement at least in some patients (6). Slow rate of dark adaptation and abnormal color matching may occur in eyes whose fellow eye has exudative AMD (7).

Focal macular ERG and multifocal ERG are useful objective measures of macular dysfunction in AMD (Fig. 10.1) (8–13). Reduced foveal ERG amplitude and prolonged latency are found in pre-AMD or early AMD eyes as well as their asymptomatic fellow eyes (13,14). Both focal macular ERG and multifocal ERG have been used as an outcome measure in clinical treatment trials for AMD (15,16). Pattern ERG may also serve as an objective measure of macular function in AMD (8).

MACULAR DEGENERATION—AUTOSOMAL DOMINANT, RECESSIVE

Aside from AMD, distinct autosomal dominant or recessive forms of macular degeneration are recognized. Compared to

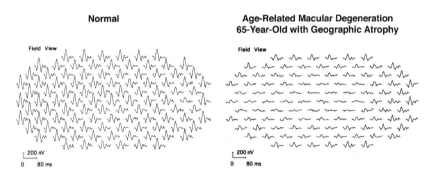

Figure 10.1 Multifocal ERG of a normal subject and a patient with dry AMD. The first-order trace arrays of the right eyes are shown. Note the impaired responses centrally caused by geographic atrophy of the retina.

patients with AMD, these affected patients are generally younger and demonstrate clinical and genetic heterogeneity. For instance, while several mutations of the peripherin/RDS gene are associated with autosomal dominant retinitis pigmentosa, some genotypes (Arg172Trp, Tyr258Stop, Gly167Asp) cause macular dystrophy. Likewise, mutations of the human retinal fascin gene (FSCN2) cause retinitis pigmentosa (RP) or macular degeneration. In patients with autosomal dominant macular degeneration, the full-field ERG cone responses range from normal to reduced and delayed while the rod responses are normal or near normal (17–19).

CENTRAL SEROUS CHORIORETINOPATHY

Central serous chorioretinopathy is a disorder characterized by focal retinal detachment of the macula with focal accumulation of serous fluid between the photoreceptor layer and the retinal pigment epithelium. The focal retinal detachment may be preceded or overlying a smaller retinal pigment epithelium detachment, which is a separation between the retinal pigment epithelium and Bruch's membrane. Fluorescein angiography typically shows focal leakage of fluid at the retinal pigment epithelium into the retinal detachment. Other names for the same disorder include central serous retinopathy and idiopathic central serous chorioretinopathy. Symptoms are usually unilateral and include metamorphopsia, micropsia, and a relative central scotoma. Over weeks to months, the retinal detachment resolves and visual function improves but recurrences are not uncommon. Despite the fact that the symptoms are often unilateral, some retinal pigment epithelium changes are also often seen in the contralateral eye. Pathogenesis is unknown but is more likely to involve broad dysfunction of the retinal pigment epithelium transport system rather than just a focal source of retinal pigment epithelium leakage. The condition affects young or middle-aged adults with men more frequently affected than women. Recent stress and type A personality may be associated with the disorder.

The diagnosis of central serous chorioretinopathy is usually made on the basis of characteristic clinical features and fluorescein angiographic findings. Focal macular ERG or multifocal ERG may be helpful as a measure of retinal function. As expected, focal macular ERG responses are impaired in central serous chorioretinopathy (20–23). Miyake et al. (21) performed focal macular ERG using a 10° size stimulus on 24 patients and found that the a-waves and b-waves were reduced and prolonged in the affected eye as compared to the fellow eye during the active as well as the recovering phases of the disease. B-wave and oscillatory potentials were significantly more deteriorated than a-wave, and the investigators theorized that the disorder may involve functional disturbances in the inner retinal layer as well as the photoreceptors. Using multifocal ERG, Marmor and Tan (20) showed broad retinal function disturbance involving both the affected and unaffected eyes in patients with central serous chorioretinopathy (Fig. 10.2). Furthermore, multifocal ERG impairment was found in areas beyond the zone of the retinal detachment. Although multifocal ERG response amplitudes increased modestly after recovery from the disease, the amplitudes remained statistically subnormal throughout the posterior pole of both eyes (22). These

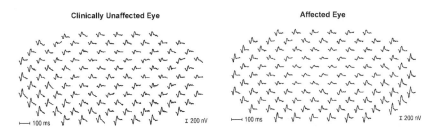

Figure 10.2 Multifocal ERG first-order trace arrays of a 39-year-old woman with central serous chorioretinopathy. For reference, the trace array of a normal subject is shown in Fig. 10.1. Despite unilateral clinical involvement, the multifocal ERG is impaired in the affected eye as well as the unaffected eye. (From Ref. 20 with permission from the American Medical Association.)

investigators concluded that subretinal fluid retention in the disorder is secondary to diffuse pathologic changes in the choroid or retinal pigment epithelium or both, and that multifocal ERG in time may prove to be useful in assessing the degree of susceptibility to central serous chorioretinopathy attacks.

Of interest, patients with resolved central serous chorioretinopathy and those with mild optic neuritis may both report a similar history of a period of visual impairment followed by visual improvement. If the retinal and optic nerve head findings are minimal, the two conditions may be difficult to differentiate, and in such cases, focal macular ERG or multifocal ERG may be helpful to determine the presence of macular dysfunction.

Conventional full-field ERG is typically normal or minimally affected in central serous chorioretinopathy, because a focal macular lesion is unlikely to produce any appreciable reduction of panretinal ERG response. Therefore, the clinical role of full-field ERG in central serous chorioretinopathy is limited except in rare cases. For example, full-field ERG may be of value in a patient with macular pigmentary changes, who cannot provide an accurate ocular history. In such a case, the differential diagnosis may include resolved bilateral central serous chorioretinopathy and cone dystrophy, and full-field ERG may be of value because full-field ERG can detect generalized cone dysfunction due to cone dystrophy.

Visual evoked potential has no established clinical role in central serous chorioretinopathy. Prolonged VEP responses occur in central serous chorioretinopathy and are secondary to the retinal macular dysfunction (24). Since VEP impairment also occurs in patients with optic neuritis, VEP is not helpful in differentiating patients with resolved optic neuritis from central serous chorioretinopathy (25). Sherman et al. (26) recorded pattern-reversal VEP in 10 patients with central serous chorioretinopathy and found that, during the acute stage, 90% of the patients had significant VEP delays in the affected eye while only 30% had significant reduction in amplitude. Six of the 10 patients were re-evaluated after resolution of the disease, and in all six patients, the VEP delays returned to normal. The authors concluded that a VEP delay in isolation of other tests should not be used in the differentiating macular from optic nerve disease.

Lastly, pattern ERG findings were reported on two patients who had systemic lupus erythematosus and associated macular findings that were similar to central serous chorioretinopathy (27). However, the clinical usefulness of pattern ERG in central serous chorioretinopathy is not clear especially in light of the usefulness of focal ERG and multifocal ERG.

DOYNE HONEYCOMB RETINAL DYSTROPHY/MALATTIA LEVENTINESE

In 1899, Doyne (28) described an autosomal dominant disorder characterized by small round drusen-like yellow–white spots at the macula, which were nearly confluent with a honeycomb-like appearance. In 1925, Vogt (29) reported a similar autosomal dominant condition (malattia Leventinese) found in the Leventine valley in Switzerland. Subsequently, Stone et al. (30) discovered that a mutation (Arg345Trp) in the gene EFEMP1 (epithelial growth factor-containing fibrillin-like extracellular matrix protein 1) is the cause of this single disorder. Affected persons with malattia Leventinese/Doyne honeycomb retinal dystrophy usually have visual acuity ranging from 20/20 to 20/100, and subretinal neovascular membrane may rarely occur. The condition may be misdiagnosed as AMD in same cases. Full-field ERG and EOG are generally normal or mildly impaired (31,32). Pattern ERG is usually impaired with reduced P50 and N95 but P50 latency is unaffected (32). Focal and multifocal ERG show near normal to reduced macular responses (31,32). Dark adaptation is prolonged over macular deposits but are normal elsewhere (32).

STARGARDT MACULAR DYSTROPHY— FUNDUS FLAVIMACULATUS

In 1909, Stargardt (33) reported several patients, including siblings, with macular and white fleck-like retinal lesions. The disorder that became known as Stargardt macular dystrophy is an autosomal recessive disorder characterized by bilateral retinal atrophic-appearing foveal lesions and variable number of scattered yellow–white fleck-like lesions. In 1963, Franceschetti (34) used the term "fundus flavimaculatus" for patients with extensive retinal fleck-like lesions with or without a foveal lesion. This attempt to classify patients into two distinct genetic disorders based on retinal appearance alone was not successful because of overlapping clinical and genetic findings between Stargardt macular dystrophy and fundus flavimaculatus. For instance, the degree of macular atrophy and distribution of flecks change over time in many patients. In addition, intrafamilial variation of the disease is common, and within the same family, some siblings can have primarily macular disease while others have only peripheral flecks (35,36). However, the use of Stargardt macular dystrophy and fundus flavimaculatus as distinct clinical phenotypes is still employed by some investigators for describing the natural history and estimating visual prognosis of this condition.

Stargardt macular dystrophy or fundus flavimaculatus affects about 1 in 10,000 people. The atrophic macular lesion may have a "beaten metal" appearance, and the shapes of the fleck-like lesions may be linear, ovoid, or pisciform (fishtail-like). Visible retinal lesions develop in affected persons during the first two decades of life with corresponding moderate to severe progressive deterioration in visual acuity. Visual acuity impairment is variable but usually results in 20/200 vision in 90% of patients over time (37). In the 1970s, and 1980s, diffuse blockage of choroidal filling on fluorescein angiography, the so-called "choroidal silence" or "dark choroids," due in part to the accumulation of lipofuscin-like material in the retinal pigment epithelium was recognized as a feature of Stargardt macular dystrophy (Fig. 10.3) (38–40). The retinal fleck-like lesions was noted to correspond to hypertrophic retinal pigment epithelial cells with extensive accumulation of lipofuscin-like material (39). Despite evidence of widespread accumulation of lipofuscin-like material in the retinal pigment epithelium, peripheral vision is usually relatively well preserved in the disorder.

In 1997, mutations of a gene on chromosome 1, which encodes for a member of the ATP-binding cassette (ABCR)

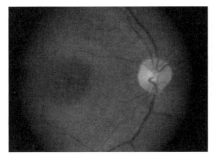 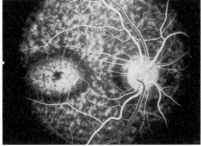

Figure 10.3 *Left*: Fundus appearance of a patient with Stargardt macular dystrophy. Note the macular fleck-like lesions. *Right*: Fluorescein angiography showing numerous retinal fleck-like lesions and diffuse blockage of choroidal filling ("choroidal silence") due in part to the accumulation of lipofuscin-like material in the retinal pigment epithelium. (From Ref. 202.) (Refer to the color insert.)

transporter proteins, were found in patients with Stargardt macular dystrophy and those with fundus flavimaculatus (41). This ATP-binding transporter protein was subsequently designated as ABCA4. The ABCA4 protein is expressed in the outer segments of both rod and cone photoreceptors and is thought to transport vitamin A derivatives across intracellular membranes (42,43). The ABCA4 gene is unusual in many respects when compared to genes of other recessive diseases. First, the gene exhibits a wide degree of sequence variation such that the majority of the unaffected, general population is not homozygous for the consensus ABCR4 sequence (44). Second, in contrast to other autosomal recessive disorders, most affected individuals with disease-causing ABCA4 genotypes are not homozygous but heterozygous and carries at least two variants of the ABCA4 gene (44,45). Third, because of the large number of sequence variations observed in the ABCA4 gene with many possible heterozygous disease-causing genotypes, identifying plausible disease-causing genotypes is difficult in some patients with Stargardt disease. Of interest, clinical as well as electrophysiologic manifestations are variable in Stargardt patients with specific identifiable disease-causing sequence changes in the ABCA4 gene (46). In addition, ABCA4 mutations have also been found in patients with clinical features of cone–rod dystrophy and RP (47,48).

The diagnosis of Stargardt macular dystrophy is based on clinical findings and the presence of choroidal blockage on fluorescein angiography with the support of genetic findings when possible. Electrophysiologic tests may aid in detecting retinal dysfunction and assessing disease progression.

In general, full-field ERG responses are within the normal range in most patients with Stargardt macular dystrophy, but the full-field ERG responses are variable among patients and may demonstrate impaired cone responses as well as impaired rod and cone responses especially in those with more widespread retinal atrophy and fleck-like lesions (Fig. 10.4). Numerous investigators have demonstrated prolonged rod dark adaptation in Stargardt patients, and at least 45 min of dark adaptation are recommended before scotopic

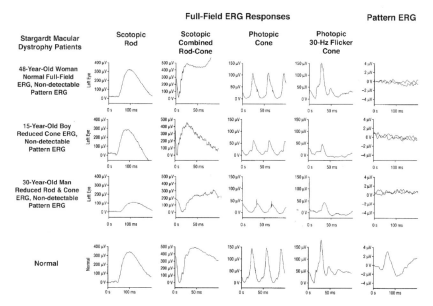

Figure 10.4 Variability of full-field ERG responses in Stargardt macular dystrophy. The full-field ERG responses range from normal to considerable impairment of both cone and rod responses. The pattern ERG is primarily a measure of retinal ganglion cell function and is preferentially affected in macular conditions and is often non-detectable in Stargardt macular dystrophy. (From Ref. 51 with permission from the American Medical Association.)

ERG recordings (49,50). The EOG light-peak to dark-trough amplitude ratios in Stargardt disease may be normal but tend to be reduced in many patients with numerous fleck-like lesions and reduced full-field ERG. By far, the most consistent electrophysiologic abnormalities in Stargardt disease are the focal, multifocal, and pattern ERG responses. The focal and multifocal ERGs show markedly diminished or non-detectable foveal response in almost all patients even in those with good visual acuity, and the pattern ERG response, a measure of ganglion cell activity, is also severely reduced or abolished in almost all patients regardless of visual acuity. This striking, consistent pattern ERG reduction is rather unusual in other macular dystrophies, and the reason for this is unclear (Fig. 10.4) (51).

Noble and Carr (52) found impaired full-field ERG in 27% and reduced EOG responses in 20% in a study of 30 patients with Stargardt macular dystrophy. Itabashi et al. (53) as well as Starvou et al. (54) noted that ERG and EOG abnormalities were common in patients with macular atrophy and diffuse retinal flecks. More recently, using standardized full-field ERG, Lois et al. (51) classified 63 study patients with Stargardt disease into three groups based on full-field ERG responses. Of the total 63 patients, 68% had normal scotopic and photopic full-field ERG amplitudes (group 1), 14% had normal scotopic rod ERG amplitude but reduced photopic cone flash and 30-Hz flicker responses (group 2), and 16% had both reduced scotopic rod and photopic cone responses (group 3) (Fig. 10.4). Using this scheme, only 1 of the 63 patients was not classifiable. Considerable overlap of clinical attributes was noted among the three groups. However, group 1 patients tended to have better visual acuity and more restricted distribution of retinal flecks and atrophy, whereas those in group 3 had the worse visual acuity and consistently demonstrated macular atrophy with more widespread flecks. Pattern ERG and focal foveal ERG were abolished in all patients tested from all three groups even when visual acuity was still good, consistent with similar pattern ERG findings reported earlier by Stavrov et al. (54). Of the patients tested with EOG, 10%, 57%, and 80% in groups 1, 2, and 3, respectively, had impaired EOG light-peak to dark-trough amplitude ratios reflecting, in part, the full-field ERG impairment.

When patients with Stargardt disease are classified by retinal appearance into Stargardt macular dystrophy or fundus flavimaculatus, the prevalence of ERG and EOG abnormalities reported for each clinical subtype is highly variable mostly because of variable expressivity of the disease, differences in recording methodology, and differences in classification criteria (53–59). For instance, Aaberg (55) found impaired scotopic and photopic full-field ERG responses in 24 patients with Stargardt macular dystrophy to be 46%

and 71%, respectively, compared with 44% and 56% for 16 patients classified as fundus flavimaculatus. In contrast, Moloney et al. (59) noted impaired scotopic and photopic full-field ERG responses in 20 patients with Stargardt macular dystrophy to be only 20% and 20%, respectively, compared with only 39% and 21% for 28 patients with fundus flavimaculatus. However, prevalence of EOG abnormalities was similar between the two studies with Aaberg finding reduced EOG light-peak to dark-trough amplitude ratios of 44% and 83% for Stargardt macular dystrophy and fundus flavimaculatus patients, respectively, and Moloney demonstrating similar prevalence of 45% and 61%, respectively. In terms of other reports, Lachepalle et al. (58) noted greater full-field ERG impairment in six fundus flavimaculatus patients compared to nine Stargardt macular dystrophy patients. Klein and Krill (57) found impaired full-field ERG in 83% of their 24 fundus flavimaculatus patients but most of the ERG tests were performed with only 17 min of dark adaptation.

In terms of multifocal ERG, Kretschmann et al. (60) found that 96% of 51 Stargardt patients had markedly reduced or non-detectable macular ERG responses with the area of macular dysfunction usually larger than expected from visual acuity and retinal appearance. Toward more peripheral areas, ERG responses of Stargardt patients approach those of normal, and implicit times are not markedly delayed. Finally, VEP findings in Stargardt disease are rarely reported but are likely to parallel retinal function and show impairment especially in light of impaired pattern ERG and macular dysfunction.

Pedigrees of autosomal dominant Stargardt-like macular dystrophy are rarely found with genetic linkage to 6q14 and 13q34 (61,62). The clinical features of 6q14 dominant Stargardt disease include a well circumscribed, homogenous macular atrophy of the retinal pigment epithelium and choriocapillaris with surrounding yellow fleck-like lesions and temporal pallor of the optic nerve head (63). Full-field ERG for 6q14 Stargardt's disease may be normal or show prolonged b-wave implicit times (61,63). Of interest, fundus flavimaculatus clinical features have been noted in some patients with dominant mutations of the peripherin gene (64).

BEST VITELLIFORM MACULAR DYSTROPHY

Best vitelliform macular dystrophy is an autosomal dominant disorder characterized by early-onset of accumulation of yellowish material within and beneath the retinal pigment epithelium at the macula. Although the first description of the disease is attributed to Friedrich Best in 1905, the first case was likely described by Adams (65) in 1883. The retinal appearance in affected persons is initially normal until a yellowish "egg-yolk-like" foveal lesion develops during the first or second decade of life (Fig. 10.5) (66). In most cases, only a single prominent foveal lesion is present in each eye although rarely multiple yellowish lesions with variable size may also occur near and in the macula. Despite the conspicuous foveal lesion, visual acuity is only mildly affected in the early stages of the disease and is typically 20/25 or better. With time, the yellowish "egg yolk-like" lesion becomes fragmented with a "scrambled egg-like" appearance which gradually progresses to macular atrophy with or without fibrous scarring. Visual acuity tend to worsen with age and is particularly impaired in those with atrophic and fibrotic maculas

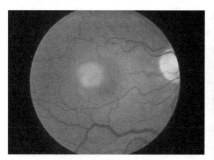 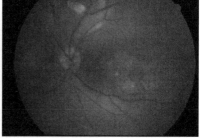

Figure 10.5 Best vitelliform macular dystrophy. *Left*: Foveal yellow egg-yolk-like lesion in a patient with Best vitelliform macular dystrophy. *Right*: Multiple lesions in a patient with Best vitelliform macular dystrophy. (From Ref. 202.) (Refer to the color insert.)

(67). Although visual prognosis is generally favorable, only 20% of Best disease patients older than age 40 have a visual acuity of 20/40 or better in at least one eye (68). Histopathology in early stages of Best disease reveals generalized abnormality of the retinal pigment epithelium with pigmented lipofuscin accumulation as well as lipofuscin within macrophages in the subretinal space and the choroid (69). In more advanced cases, finely granular material is deposited in the inner segments of the degenerating photoreceptors in addition to the retinal pigment epithelial abnormalities (70).

Best vitelliform macular dystrophy is caused by mutations of the gene designated as VMD2 located on chromosome 11 (11q13) (71). The gene encodes a 585-amino-acid protein known as bestrophin which is selectively expressed in the retinal pigment epithelium. Numerous mutations of the VMD2 are found in association with Best disease indicating genetic heterogeneity, and genetic findings suggest that a small fraction of patients with clinical diagnosis of AMD and adult-onset foveomacular vitelliform dystrophy may actually have a late-onset variant of Best disease (72–74).

The diagnosis of Best vitelliform macular dystrophy is based on a combination of clinical features, family history, electrophysiologic testing, and genetic analysis. Electrooculogram is a key diagnostic test and shows marked impairment early even when retinal lesions are not yet visible (75). The EOG light-peak to dark-trough amplitude ratios are typically less than 1.4 (normal ≥ 1.8), reflecting generalized dysfunction of the retinal pigment epithelium (75–80). However, there is no direct correlation between the degree of EOG impairment and visual acuity. Clinical full-field ERG is normal in Best disease so that in contrast to most retinal dystrophies where EOG reductions parallel ERG impairment, Best disease is one of few diseases with a distinct pattern of a normal full-field ERG with a markedly impaired EOG (Fig. 10.6). Although a diagnosis of Best disease may be obvious in a young patient with an "egg-yolk-like" foveal lesion and a positive family history, EOG testing is helpful in confirming the diagnosis. In older patients with atrophic foveal lesions, who are suspected of having Best disease, a combination of full-field

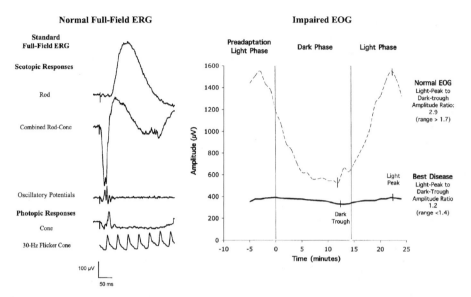

Figure 10.6 Full-field ERG responses and EOG results from a 31-year-old man with Best vitelliform macular dystrophy (fundus appearance shown in Fig. 10.5; left). Note the normal full-field ERG and the strikingly reduced EOG.

ERG and EOG testing will help to confirm Best disease as well as to exclude other retinal dystrophies. Further, reduced EOG amplitude ratios are found in Best dystrophy family members who harbor a VMD2 mutation but have no maculopathy (81).

In general, other electrophysiologic findings in Best disease show retinal pigment epithelium dysfunction as well as localized retinal dysfunction at the macula. Despite normal full-field ERG in Best disease, the full-field ERG c-wave, a measure of retinal pigment epithelium function and not usually assessed in clinical recordings, is reduced in Best disease (82). Focal macular ERG with flicker stimuli is impaired indicating localized retinal dysfunction (83). Likewise, multifocal ERG first-order amplitudes are significantly reduced with normal or slightly increased implicit times for the central and pericentral responses (84,85). Of interest, Weleber (86) noted that despite a dramatically impaired clinical EOG which measures EOG slow oscillation, the EOG fast oscillation, which is not commonly measured, is normal in Best disease even though both fast and slow EOG oscillations are related to retinal pigment epithelium function. In terms of pattern ERG, deterioration of visual acuity and progression of central visual field defects corresponds to decreased ganglion cell activity as measured by reduction in P50 and N95 amplitudes (87).

CONE DYSTROPHY

Cone dystrophy refers to a large group of genetically heterogeneous disorders characterized by progressive diffuse cone dysfunction. Autosomal dominant, autosomal recessive, and X-linked recessive forms have all been reported. Patients with cone dystrophy typically have progressive reduced visual acuity, decreased color vision, and aversion to bright light (88). The onset of symptoms is variable and nystagmus may occasionally occur. Macular appearance is variable and ranges from mild pigmentary mottling to atrophic lesions that may resemble a bull's-eye (Fig. 10.7). Central and pericentral scotomas are present on visual field testing. The genotypes of

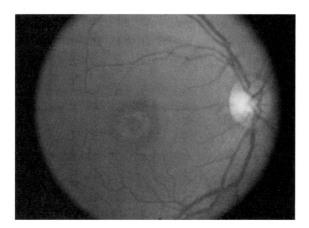

Figure 10.7 "Bull's-eye" macular atrophic lesion in a patient with cone dystrophy. This descriptive pattern of macular atrophy is not specific for cone dystrophy and may occur also in rod–cone dystrophy, chloroquine or hydroxychloroquine retinal toxicity, and Stargardt macular dystrophy. (From Ref. 202.) (Refer to the color insert.)

cone dystrophy are extremely diverse. For example, pedigrees of autosomal dominant forms of cone dystrophy are associated with several genotypes including mutation of the guanylate cyclase activator-1A and mutation mapped to the general area of the recoverin gene. Mutations at codon 172 in the peripherin/RDS gene may also produce a macular dystrophy with primary cone dysfunction and preserved peripheral rod function (89,90). In rare cone dystrophy patients, a greenish-golden tapetal-like sheen of the retina has been observed which returns to normal after several hours of dark adaptation; this Mizuo–Nakamura phenomenon is most commonly encountered with Oguchi disease (91).

Full-field ERG is a key diagnostic test in cone dystrophy and demonstrates diffuse cone dysfunction (Fig. 10.8) (6,92–95). Both interfamilial and intrafamilial variability of clinical features and ERG responses is common (96,97). In general, the standard full-field ERG responses in cone dystrophy are as follows: (1) scotopic rod flash response—normal in early disease and may become impaired in advanced disease, (2) scotopic combined rod–cone bright flash response—mildly to moderately reduced a-wave and b-wave with variable prolongation, (3) oscillatory potentials—reduced, (4) photopic cone flash response—moderately to markedly reduced and prolonged, and (5) photopic cone flicker response—moderately to markedly reduced and prolonged. Because the ERG rod response may be impaired in advanced cases of cone dystrophy, differentiation of such patients from patients with cone–rod dystrophy may be difficult. The reduction of ERG in cone dystrophy correlates with visual field defects and with reduced EOG light rise so reduced EOG is common (93). Further, dark adaptation in cone dystrophy shows abnormal cone adaptation but the final rod sensitivity is normal or only mildly reduced. Of interest, Kellner and Foerster (98) reported two patients with cone dystrophy, who had negative full-field photopic cone flash responses with the a-wave being larger than the b-wave. One of the two patients also had a negative scotopic bright-flash combined rod–cone response. The authors concluded additional inner retinal transmission defects in the cone pathway can occur in cone dystrophy.

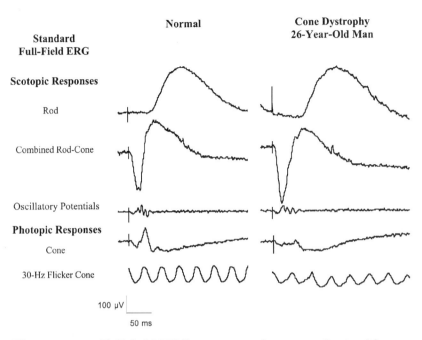

Figure 10.8 Full-field ERG responses from a patient with cone dystrophy. The cone flash and 30-Hz flicker responses are reduced and delayed. The ERG responses of cone dystrophy are similar to incomplete rod monochromatism (autosomal recessive achromatopsia), but the conditions are distinguishable by clinical history and findings.

CENTRAL CONE DYSTROPHY (OCCULT MACULAR DYSTROPHY)

Central cone dystrophy, also called "occult macular dystrophy", is an autosomal dominant or sporadic disorder characterized by progressive bilateral decrease in visual acuity with normal retinal appearance, normal fluorescein angiography, normal EOG, normal full-field ERG, and decreased focal macular ERG response (99–101). The disorder appears to produce impairment of either only the macular cone system or macular cone and rod systems without any other visible abnormality (101). The diagnosis is made by excluding other macular disorders, and reduced macular function is detectable by focal foveal ERG or multifocal ERG (Fig. 10.9). In central cone dystrophy, markedly reduced first-order multifocal ERG amplitudes in the central 7° of the fovea with mild delayed implicit times across the entire central 30° are found (102). Reduced foveal thickness is detected by optical coherence tomography (Fig. 10.9).

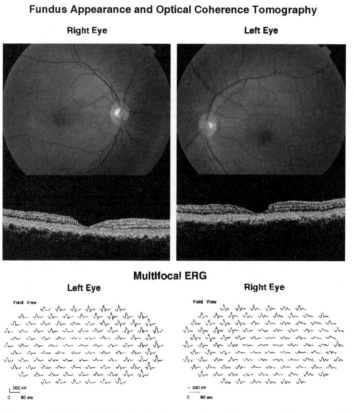

Figure 10.9 Clinical findings of a 31-year-old man with central cone dystrophy (occult macular dystrophy). Photographs showing normal fundus in each eye. Optical coherence tomography demonstrates thinned foveal thickness to 104 and 97 μm (normal ≈ 200 μm) for the right eye and left eye, respectively. The first-order trace arrays of the multifocal ERG reveal impaired responses centrally in each eye. (Refer to the color insert.)

PERIPHERAL CONE DYSTROPHY

Progressive peripheral cone dysfunction with normal central cone function has rarely been reported. Noble et al. (103) documented a 22-year-old man with 20/20 vision and normal Hardy–Rand–Rittler (HRR) and Ishihara color plate testing, who had normal full-field ERG scotopic responses but absent photopic responses. Pearlman et al. (104) in a report of a family with dominant cone dystrophy found an 18-year-old affected man who had 20/20 vision, red–green defect on Hardy–Rand–Rittler color plate testing, and absent full-field photopic flicker ERG response. Kondo et al. (105) reported three patients who had visual acuity ranging from 20/16 to 20/100. The full-field ERG rod responses were normal and the cone responses were significantly reduced. The focal macular cone ERG responses were well preserved in all the three patients, and multifocal ERG in two of the patients showed relatively preserved central responses with decreased responses peripherally. Taken together, these case reports indicate that in progressive cone dysfunction, the peripheral cones may be more affected than central cones in rare cases.

CONE DYSTROPHY WITH SUPERNORMAL AND DELAYED ROD ERG (SUPERNORMAL AND DELAYED ROD ERG SYNDROME)

In 1983, Gouras et al. (106) described two siblings with an unusual retinal dystrophy characterized by decreased visual acuity, decreased color vision, and diminished ERG cone response with supernormal but delayed rod response. Since the initial report, a number of other mostly sporadic or auto-somal recessive cases have been documented. Common features of this rare but distinct disorder include onset of loss of central vision within the first two decades of life with variable progression, variable nyctalopia, and pigmentary disturbance of the macula which may be granular, atrophic or bull's-eye-like. Under standardized clinical ERG conditions, the specific findings include: (1) a delayed but large b-wave on rod response to the scotopic dim flash, (2) a normal or increased a-wave with a delayed but above normal b-wave for the scotopic bright-flash combined rod–cone response, (3) reduced oscillatory potentials, and (4) reduced and delayed cone flash and flicker responses (Fig. 10.10). These clinical ERG findings are explained in part by a delayed rod response that is reduced for very dim flash stimulus but increases above normal for brighter flashes (Fig. 10.11).

A defect of the cGMP cascade of photoreceptors was initially proposed as a mechanism of this disorder and was supported by experiments that showed similar changes in the rod ERG in a cat eye treated with a phosphodiesterase inhibitor to elevate cGMP (107). However, the cGMP hypothesis predicts abnormalities of the scotopic bright-flash rod-dominant a-wave response which have not been consistent noted in this disorder. More recently, Hood et al. (108) studied five affected patients extensively with specialized ERG techniques that included a rod phototransduction activation model, a rod deactivation paradigm, cone "on" and "off" component recordings, and a cone photoreceptor activation model (see Chapter 6). The results indicated that delays in the rod and cone b-waves were not due to the speed or amplification of the phototransduction process and the sites of disease action are beyond the photoreceptor outer segment and involve a delay in the activation of internuclear layer activity. These findings make a defect in the cGMP cascade of the photoreceptor unlikely although a cGMP abnormality beyond the photoreceptor outer segments cannot be completely excluded.

SORSBY FUNDUS DYSTROPHY

In the 1940s, Sorsby described a rare autosomal dominant retinal dystrophy characterized by macular drusen-like deposits, edema, hemorrhages, exudates, and choroidal neovascular membrane followed by macular atrophy with retinal pigment proliferation (109). Other names for the same disorder include pseudoinflammatory macular dystrophy, dominantly inherited disciform macular dystrophy, and hereditary

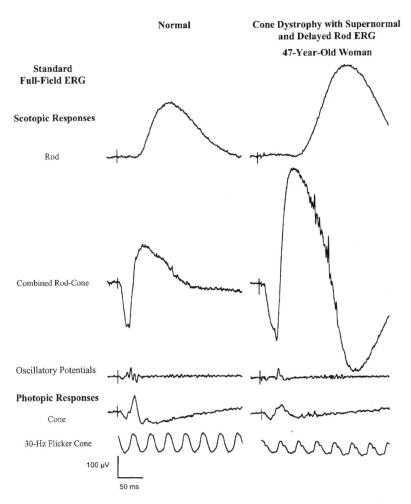

Figure 10.10 Full-field ERG responses from a patient with cone dystrophy with supernormal and delayed rod ERG (supernormal and delayed rod ERG syndrome). Note the characteristic delayed but large b-wave for the scotopic rod and rod–cone responses. The oscillatory potentials are reduced, and the cone flash and flicker responses are reduced and delayed.

hemorrhagic macular dystrophy. In 1994, Weber et al. (110) discovered that Sorsby fundus dystrophy resulted from mutations of the gene encoding tissue inhibitor of metallo-proetinase-3 (TIMP-3). TIMP-3 is expressed in the retinal

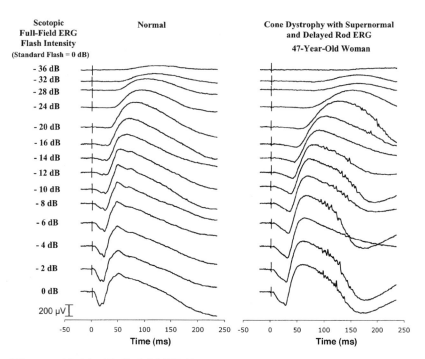

Figure 10.11 Full-field ERG scotopic intensity response series of a patient with supernormal and delayed rod ERG syndrome, whose standard ERG responses are shown in Fig. 10.10. The scotopic ERG responses are reduced compared to normal for very dim flash stimuli. With brighter flashes, the b-wave amplitudes increase above normal but are delayed.

pigment epithelium and the endothelial cells of the choriocapillaris, and its primary roles involve maintaining homeostasis of extracellular matrix and inhibiting angiogenesis (111–113). Histopathologically, eyes with Sorsby fundus dystrophy show deposit within the Bruch's membrane, loss of the outer retinal layers, discontinuous retinal pigment epithelium, and atrophy of the choriocapillaris (114).

Patients with Sorsby fundus dystrophy usually develop night blindness followed by central visual loss between the second and fifth decades of life (115). Bilateral central visual loss due to progressive hemorrhagic macular degeneration occurs simultaneously in both eyes in some patients but decreased central vision in the second eye occasionally may not become noticeable for up to 10 years. Despite the fact that the number of TIMP-3 genotypes associated with Sorsby fundus dystrophy is relatively small, variable intrafamilial expressivity is common (116,117). Several authors have documented abnormal impaired dark adaptation in Sorsby fundus dystrophy (115,118,119). The dark adaptation threshold curves in Sorsby fundus dystrophy and vitamin A deficiency are similar and are prolonged with delayed initial cone dark adaptation followed by a marked prolongation of early rod adaptation ("rod plateaux") but normal final rod threshold is eventually reached (118). Jacobson et al. (120) have shown that high oral vitamin A supplementation of 50,000 IU daily will dramatically alleviate blindness in patients with Sorsby fundus dystrophy. These findings indicate a chronic deprivation vitamin A of the photoreceptors due in part to a thickened Bruch's membrane between the photoreceptors and its blood supply.

The diagnosis of Sorsby fundus dystrophy is based on clinical findings, family history, and genetic analysis. Older Sorsby patients with late-onset of visual symptoms may be misdiagnosed as having AMD. However, Sorsby fundus dystrophy is very rare, and TIMP-3 mutations are generally not found in patients with age-related maculopathy (121). Electrophysiologic tests are helpful in assessing retinal dysfunction.

A wide range of full-field ERG and EOG results ranging from normal to severely abnormal has been reported in patients with Sorsby fundus dystrophy due in part to differences in test methodology as well as to differences in disease severity and expressivity of the patients studied. Because rod dark adaptation is prolonged in Sorsby fundus dystrophy, a prolonged dark adaptation of 50–70 min may be helpful before scotopic ERG recordings. Full-field ERG and EOG responses are generally normal or only mildly impaired in patients with early stages of the disorder (122–124). In addition, Sieving noted normal standardized full-field ERG responses in seven affected members with age range of 35 and 64 years in a family with Sorsby fundus dystrophy from a Ser-181-Cys

TIMP-3 mutation. However, Clarke et al. (125) noted significantly reduced but not prolonged rod and cone full-field ERG responses in four of five Sorsby patients and reduced N30/P50 and P50/N95 amplitudes of the pattern ERG in three of the five patients. Further, Lip et al. (126) performed serial full-field ERG and EOG in a Sorsby patient over a period of 24 years and documented reduced ERG responses, especially the scotopic combined rod–cone response, corresponding to the onset of symptoms; a subsequent standardized full-field showed markedly reduced scotopic rod response with photopic cone flash and flicker responses at the low end of normal. In the same patient, the EOG light-peak to dark-trough amplitude ratio deteriorated to a subnormal level years before any symptoms or clinical evidence of the disease. Likewise, reduced EOG responses in Sorsby patients have also been reported by other authors (115,123,127) Lastly, although not extensively studied, multifocal ERG may be helpful to detect focal macular dysfunction in Sorsby patients, and the VEP is likely reduced in those with notable macular dysfunction.

PATTERN DYSTROPHY

Pattern dystrophy is a descriptive designation of a group of heterogeneous macular disorders characterized by retinal pigment epithelial changes of the macula ranging from pigmentary mottling to patterns of pigmentary clumping (128). Descriptive morphologic subtypes include reticular dystrophy, (129) fundus pulverulentus (130), butterfly dystrophy (131), and macroreticular dystrophy (132). Autosomal dominant inheritance is most common but autosomal recessive cases may occur. Clinical features include gradual progressive loss of central vision with visual acuity typically ranging from 20/20 to 20/70 accompanied by the development of patterns of macular pigmentary alteration. Prognosis is generally favorable, and some older patients with pattern dystrophy are likely to be diagnosed with AMD (133). Expressivity is highly variable and different morphologic subtypes are found even within the same family (134–136). Rarely, different morphologic macular lesions may occur in the same person. For instance, a patient with vitelliform macular dystrophy in one eye and butterfly-shaped pigment dystrophy in the other eye has been reported (137).

Several mutations of the peripherin/RDS gene are associated with autosomal dominant pattern dystrophy (138,139). For example, butterfly-shaped pigment macular dystrophy has been found to be associated with a point mutation in codon 167 in one family and a two base pair deletion in another family (140,141). Further, point mutations at codon 172 of the perihperin/RDS gene are associated with progressive macular atrophy (89,90). Of interest, in a family with a deletion of codon 153 or 154 of the perihperin/RDS gene, Weleber et al. (64) documented wide phenotypic variations including RP, pattern dystrophy, and fundus flavimaculatus. Pattern dystrophy is also associated with a subtype of maternally inherited diabetes and deafness (MIDD) that cosegregates with a mutation of mitochondrial DNA—substitution of guanine for adenine at position 3242 of leucine transfer RNA (142).

Electrophysiologic testing is helpful to distinguish pattern dystrophy from other disorders such as cone dystrophy and cone–rod dystrophy. Full-field ERG is generally normal or only mildly impaired in pattern dystrophy; in contrast, the EOG light-rise to dark-trough amplitude ratio is usually reduced but not always abnormal (134,136,143–148). Central retinal dysfunction can be detected by focal ERG or multifocal ERG. Pattern ERG and pattern VEP are corresponding impaired depending on the disease severity.

X-LINKED RETINOSCHISIS

X-linked retinoschisis is an inherited disorder of retinal development characterized by splitting or schisis of the retinal nerve fiber layer at the macula. X-linked retinoschisis is unrelated to and differs from acquired retinoschsis where the schisis occurs in the middle layers of the sensory retina. In young affected male patients, a cartwheel-shaped cystic formation at the fovea is frequently seen, which progresses to blunted foveal reflex or pigmentary atrophy in older patients. Over 50% of affected persons will develop peripheral retinoschisis, most commonly in the inferotemporal quadrant. Decrease of visual acuity begins in the first decade of life with variable progression. Visual acuity is usually decreased to between 20/50 to 20/100, ranging from 20/20 to light perception (149). Prognosis is generally good, but further deterioration of vision from macular atrophy occurs in the fourth and fifth decades of life. In addition, serious sight-threatening complications such as vitreous hemorrhage and retinal detachment occur in approximately 20% of patients (150). Of interest, a golden fundus light reflex that simulating Mizuo phenomenon of Oguchi disease may occur rarely in X-linked retinoschisis patients and may disappear after surgical removal of the posterior vitreous surface (151,152).

The disorder is caused by mutations of the X-linked retinoschisis gene, XLRS1, which encodes a protein expressed in rod and cone photoreceptor cells but not in the inner retina (153). The protein sequence contains a highly conserved discoidin domain that is implicated in phospholipid binding and cellular adhesion. Missense genetic mutations are not distributed randomly but are clustered in the discoidin domain. However, despite the genetic findings, histologic studies have suggested that the defect is located in Müller cells (154).

The full-field ERG is a key diagnostic test in X-linked retinoschisis because the ERG has characteristic findings and fluorescein angiography is often normal. The most striking ERG finding is a selective impairment of the b-wave responses presumably due to functional deficit of the inner retinal layers (155–157). However, mild impairment of the a-wave also occurs implying some photoreceptor dysfunction (158). On standard full-field ERG, patients with X-linked retinoschisis are typically found to have impaired scotopic rod response and a selective reduced and prolonged b-wave for the scotopic combined rod–cone response such that the b- to a-wave amplitude ratio is less than 1.0 and a "negative

ERG" pattern is produced (Fig. 10.12). Oscillatory potentials are also reduced. The severity of the ERG impairment does not correlate with specific genetic mutation and is often variable in affected males of the same family, (158,159). Further, Sieving et al. (160) have reported that patients with Arg213Trp mutation of the XLRS1 gene may have a relative normal ERG without reduced scotopic b-wave. Therefore, a normal ERG does not absolutely exclude the diagnosis of X-linked retinoschisis but ERG is still of significant diagnostic value in the vast majority of X-linked retinoschisis cases. In terms of other electrophysiologic tests, patients with X-linked retinoschisis usually have normal EOG light-peak to dark-trough ratios (156). Not surprisingly, pattern

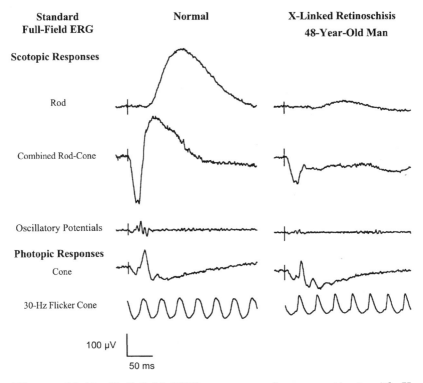

Figure 10.12 Full-field ERG responses from a patient with X-linked juvenile retinoschisis. Note the selectively reduced b-wave of the scotopic combined rod–cone response.

ERG and VEP may show abnormalities presumably secondary to retinal dysfunction. With time, in addition to macular
pigmentary atrophy, some patients may develop a diffuse pigmentary retinal degeneration with atrophy and pigment
clumping that may simulate RP. At this stage, marked
impairment of the ERG a-wave and b-wave may occur along
with reduced EOG ratio. Of note, aside from genetic analysis,
no clinical, electrophysiologic, or psychophysical abnormalities are found consistently in heterozygous carriers of
X-linked retinoschisis (161).

Results form specialized ERG techniques indicate that
there is a considerable impairment of the ON-bipolar cell
pathway in X-linked retinoschisis. Shinoda et al. (162)
using long-duration ERG light stimulus assessed the ON-
and OFF-responses of the photopic ERG and demonstrated
considerable impairment of the ON-pathway in 11 patients
with XLRS1 genetic mutations. No significant correlation
was found between the ERG responses and the locus of
the mutation, and the authors postulated that the defect
of the on-responses is due to ON-bipolar cell dysfunction
or possibly secondary to Müller cell abnormality. In addition, Alexander et al. (163) studied the photopic cone
ERG response of patients with X-linked retinoschisis with
various flicker frequencies and found that the amplitudes
of the ERG response were significantly reduced for frequencies of 32 Hz or higher. The impaired response at
higher flicker frequencies stems in part from a predominant attenuation of the ON-bipolar cell contribution to
the flicker ERG.

The multifocal ERG responses are more impaired in the
central than peripheral retina in X-linked retinoschisis
(164,165). Multiple areas of reduced amplitude may be present with significant reduction at the fovea (165). Delayed
first-order responses and reduced second-order responses
are found across the entire field suggesting a widespread dysfunction of the cone system (164).

The occurrence of foveal retinoschisis without X-linked
pedigree is occasionally encountered. Such patients have
disorders that are genetically distinct from X-linked

retinoschisis. For example, Lewis et al. (166) reported three female patients with familial foveal retinoschisis with mildly impaired ERG responses without a selective impairment of the b-wave. Noble et al. (167) noted foveal retinoschisis associated with rod–cone dystrophy in a brother and sister born of a consanguinous marriage. Shimazaki and Matsubashi (168) reported a mother and daughter with presumably dominant retinoschisis with a selective impairment of the b-wave and a "negative" ERG pattern. In another report, peripheral retinoschsis without foveal retinoschisis was found in a father and daughter with mildly impaired ERG responses without a selective impairment of the b-wave (169).

CENTRAL AREOLAR CHOROIDAL DYSTROPHY

Central areolar choroidal dystrophy refers to a heterogeneous group of disorders that is autosomal dominant or autosomal recessive and characterized by progressive loss of central vision associated with the development of a demarcated area of macular retinal and choroidal atrophy (170,171). Central areolar choroidal dystrophy has been associated with mutations of the peripherin/RDS gene (172). In addition, Lotery et al. (173,174) examined a large 3 generation kindred with autosomal dominant central areolar choroidal dystrophy and established linkage of the disease in this family to chromosome 17p. Clinical features include decreased color vision and decreased visual acuity with central visual field defect corresponding to the area of the atrophic lesion. Dark adaptation is either normal or near normal.

The diagnosis is based on clinical features, and a positive family history is helpful for autosomal dominant cases. In general, full-field ERG responses in patients with central areolar choroidal dystrophy demonstrate normal or near normal responses except for mildly impaired photopic cone responses (175–177). Progressive loss of cone b-wave amplitude parallels disease progression (178). However, in some cases of central areolar choroidal dystrophy, generalized decrease in both scotopic and photopic full-field ERG is found (172,176). In the large autosomal dominant family with 17p-linked central areolar choroidal dystrophy described by Lotery et al. (179), standard full-field ERG was performed in seven of eight affected persons, and impaired scotopic and photopic responses were encountered. Four of the eight affected persons had impaired EOG. Lastly, multifocal ERG, pattern ERG, and pattern VEP are all sensitive but non-specific objective tests of macular dysfunction in central areolar choroidal dystrophy (175,179).

NORTH CAROLINA MACULAR DYSTROPHY (CENTRAL AREOLAR PIGMENT EPITHELIAL DYSTROPHY)

North Carolina macular dystrophy or central areolar pigment epithelial dystrophy is a mildly progressive macular autosomal dominant disorder initially described by Lefler et al. (180) in 1971. The disorder was subsequently called North Carolina macular dystrophy because many affected persons in the United States live in North Carolina and are descendants of three Irish brothers who settled in North Carolina in the 1830s. Genealogy investigations eventually revealed that patients who were previously diagnosed with central areolar pigment epithelial dystrophy were also descendants of this large North Carolina kindred (181–183). Patients with North Carolina macular dystrophy now reside in other areas, and affected families in Europe, South America, and Asia, who have no known relationship with the North Carolina kindred, have also been described (184–186). The disorder is linked to the same locus located on chromosome 6q16 for all affected families, and evidence for genetic heterogeneity is lacking (187–189).

Visual acuity in North Carolina macular dystrophy ranges from 20/20 to 20/200. The most prominent clinical feature is the bilateral macular lesions that range from tiny flat yellow flecks with mild pigment irregularity to large oval area of marked colobomatous-like atrophy of the retinal pigment epithelium and choroid (190,191). Peripheral retinal drusen may also occur. The clinical course is generally stable with mild progression in some affected persons (192). Other clinical findings include decreased color vision and central visual field defects. EOG and full-field ERG responses are generally normal or rarely, midly reduced (180–182,185,187,193). Multifocal ERG, pattern ERG, and pattern VEP are likely to be impaired due to macular dysfunction but these tests have not been studied in detail in this disorder.

PROGRESSIVE BIFOCAL CHORIORETINAL ATROPHY

Progressive bifocal chorioretinal atrophy, first reported by Douglas et al. (194), is a rare autosomal dominant chorioretinal dystrophy characterized by congenital, progressive macular and nasal chorioretinal atrophic lesions. Visual loss is severe, and nystagmus and myopia are present in affected persons. The disorder is genetically linked to chromosome 6q (195). Full-field ERG rod and cone responses are markedly reduced (194,196). Light rise response of EOG is absent (196).

FENESTRATED SHEEN MACULAR DYSTROPHY

Fenestrated sheen macular dystrophy, first described by O'Donnell and Welch (197) in 1979, is a rare autosomal dominant disorder characterized by the early development of a yellowish refractive sheen with fenestrations within the sensory retina at the macula. Red-free photograph accentuates the appearance of the fenestrations. By the third decade of life, an annular area of hypopigmentation appears around the area of the sheen and progressively enlarges forming a bull's-eye-like appearance. Visual acuity is normal or mildly reduced and prognosis is generally favorable (197–200). Peripheral retinal pigment epithelial granularity also develops (200). Full-field ERG responses may be normal or demonstrate mild photopic response impairment (197). However, markedly reduced rod and cone full-field ERG responses may occur in older patients with more advanced disease (200). The EOG light-peak to dark-trough amplitude ratio is normal or near the low end of normal range in patients with mild to moderate disease (197).

FAMILIAL INTERNAL LIMITING MEMBRANE DYSTROPHY

Familial internal limiting membrane dystrophy described by Polk et al. (201) is a rare autosomal dominant disorder characterized by a diffuse glistening of the inner retinal surface. Cystoid macular edema and localized retinal detachment may also occur. Histopathology demonstrates areas of diffuse irregular, thickened internal limiting membrane with superficial retinal schisis cavities, and cystoid spaces in the inner nuclear layer. Visual acuity does not occur until after the fifth decade. Full-field ERG demonstrates a selective reduction of the b-wave on the scotopic bright-flash combined rod–cone response. The full-field ERG rod and cone responses may be reduced and prolonged in more advanced cases. The EOG light-peak to dark-trough amplitude ratio is normal or mildly impaired.

REFERENCES

1. Holopigian K, Seiple W, Greenstein V, Kim D, Carr RE. Relative effects of aging and age-related macular degeneration on peripheral visual function. Optom Vis Sci 1997; 74:152–159.

2. Sunness JS, Massof RW, Johnson MA, Finkelstein D, Fine SL. Peripheral retinal function in age-related macular degeneration. Arch Ophthalmol 1985; 103:811–816.

3. Sunness JS, Massof RW. Focal electro-oculogram in age-related macular degeneration. Am J Optom Physiol Opt 1986; 63:7–11.

4. Henkes HE. ERG in circulatory disturbances of the retina. III. ERG in cases of senile degeneration of the macular area. Arch Ophthalmol 1954; 51:54–66.

5. Walter P, Widder RA, Luke C, Konigsfeld P, Brunner R. Electrophysiological abnormalities in age-related macular degeneration. Graefes Arch Clin Exp Ophthalmol 1999; 237:962–968.

6. Ladewig M, Kraus H, Foerster MH, Kellner MD. Cone dysfunction in patients with late-onset cone dystrophy and age-related macular degeneration. Arch Ophthalmol 2003; 121:1557–1561.

7. Eisner A, Stoumbos VD, Klein ML, Fleming SA. Relations between fundus appearance and function. Eyes whose fellow eye has exudative age-related macular degeneration. Invest Ophthalmol Vis Sci 1991; 32:8–20.

8. Birch DG, Anderson JL, Fish GE, Jost F. Pattern-reversal electroretinographic follow-up of laser photocoagulation for subfoveal neovascular lesions in age-related macular degenerations. Am J Ophthalmol 1993; 116:148–155.

9. Falsini B, Serrao S, Fadda A, Iarossi G, Porrello G, Cocco F, Merendino E. Focal electroretinograms and fundus appearance in nonexudative age-related macular degeneration. Quantitative relationship between retinal morphology and function. Graefes Arch Clin Exp Ophthalmol 1999; 237: 193–200.

10. Falsini B, Fadda A, Iarossi G, Piccardi M, Canu D, Minnella A, Serrao S, Scullica L. Retinal sensitivity to flicker modulation: reduced by early age-related maculopathy. Invest Ophthalmol Vis Sci 2000; 41:1498–1506.

11. Heinemann-Vernaleken B, Palmowski AM, Allgayer R, Ruprecht KW. Comparison of different high resolution multifocal electroretinogram recordings in patients with age-related maculopathy. Graefes Arch Clin Exp Ophthalmol 2001; 239:556–561.

12. Huang S, Wu D, Jiang F, Ma J, Wu L, Liang J, Luo G. The multifocal electroretinogram in age-related maculopathies. Doc Ophthalmol 2000; 101:115–124.

13. Li J, Tso MO, Lam TT. Reduced amplitude and delayed latency in foveal response of multifocal electroretinogram in early age related macular degeneration. Br J Ophthalmol 2001; 85:287–290.

14. Sandberg MA, Miller S, Gaudio AR. Foveal cone ERGs in fellow eyes of patients with unilateral neovascular age-related macular degeneration. Invest Ophthalmol Vis Sci 1993; 34:3477–3480.

15. Falsini B, Piccardi M, Iarossi G, Fadda A, Merendino E, Valentini P. Influence of short-term antioxidant supplementation on macular function in age-related maculopathy. Ophthalmology 2003; 110:51–61.

16. Palmowski AM, Allgayer R, Heinemann-Vernaleken B, Rulprecht KW. Influence of photodynamic therapy in choroidal neovascularization on focal retinal function assessed with the multifocal electroretinogram and perimetry. Ophthalmology 2002; 109:1788–1792.

17. Wada Y, Abe T, Itabashi T, Sato H, Kawamura M, Tamai M. Autosomal dominant macular degeneration. Arch Ophthalmol 2003; 121:1613–1620.

18. Wroblewski JJ, Wells JA III, Eckstein A, Fitzke F, Jubb C, Keen TJ, Inglehearn C, Bhattacharya S, Arden GB, Jay M. Macular dystrophy associated with mutations at codon 172 in the human retinal degeneration slow gene. Ophthalmology 1994; 101:12–22.

19. Nakazawa M, Wada Y, Tamai M. Macular dystrophy associated with monogenic Arg172Trp mutation of the peripherin/RDS gene in a Japanese family. Retina 1995; 15:518–523.

20. Marmor MF, Tan F. Central serous chorioretinopathy: bilateral multifocal electroretinographic abnormalities. Arch Ophthalmol 1999; 117:184–188.

21. Miyake Y, Shiroyama N, Ota I, Horiguchi M. Local macular electroretinographic responses in idiopathic central serous chorioretinopathy. Am J Ophthalmol 1988; 106:546–550.

22. Chappelow AV, Marmor MF. Multifocal electroretinogram abnormalities persist following resolution of central serous chrioretinopathy. Arch Ophthalmol 2000; 118:1211–1215.

23. Zhang W, Zhao K. Multifocal electroretinography in central serous chorio-retinopathy and assessment of the reproducibility of the multifocal electroretinography. Doc Ophthalmol 2003; 106:209–213.

24. Folk JC, Thompson HS, Han DP, Brown CK. Visual function abnormalities in central serous retinopathy. Arch Ophthalmol 1984; 102:1299–1302.

25. Han DP, Thompson HS, Folk JC. Differentiation between recently resolved optic neuritis and central serous retinopathy. Arch Ophthalmol 1985; 103:394–396.

26. Sherman J, Bass SJ, Noble KG, Nath S, Sutija V. Visual evoked potential delays in central serous choroidopathy. Invest Ophthalmol Vis Sci 1986; 27:214–221.

27. Eckstein MB, Spalton DJ, Holder G. Visual loss from central serous retinopathy in systemic lupus erythematosus. Br J Ophthalmol 1993; 77:607–609.

28. Doyne RW. A peculiar condition of choroiditis occurring in several members of the sma family. Trans Ophthal Soc UK 1899; 19:71.

29. Vogt A. Die Ophthalmoskopie, im rotfreien Licht. In: Graefe A, Saemisch T, eds. Handbuch der gesammten Augenheikunde. Untersuchungsmethoden. Berlin: Verlag von Wilhelm Engelman, 1925:1–118.

30. Stone EM, Lotery AJ, Munier FL, Heon E, Guymer RH, Vandenburgh K, Cousin P, Nishimura D, Swiderski RE, Silvestri G, Mackey DA, Hageman GS, Bird AC, Sheffield VC, Schorderet DF. A single EFEMP1 mutation associated with both malattia Leventinese and Doyne honeycomb retinal dystrophy. Nat Genet 1999; 22:199–202.

31. Gerber DM, Niemeyer G. Ganzfeld and multifocal electroretinography in Malattia Leventinese and Zermatt macular dystrophy. Klin Monatsbl Augenheikd 2002; 219: 206–210.

32. Halmovici R, Wroblewski J, Piguet B, Fitzke FW, Holder GE, Arden GB, Bird AC. Symptomatic abnormalities of dark adaptation in patients with EFEMP1 retinal dystrophy (Malattia Leventinese/Doyne honeycomb retinal dystrophy). Eye 2002; 16:7–15.

33. Stargardt DK. Über familiäre, progressive Degeneration in der Makulagegend des Auges. Albrecht von Graefes Arch Ophthalmol 1909; 71:534–550.

34. Franceschetti A. Ueber tapeto-retinale Degenerationen in Kindesalter. In: Sautter H, ed. Entwicklung und Fortschritt in der Augenheikunde. Stuttgart: Enke Verlag, 1963: 107–120.

35. Isashiki Y, Ohba N. Fundus flavimaculatus: polymorphic retinal change in siblings. Br J Ophthalmol 1985; 69: 522–524.

36. Lois N, Holder GE, Fitzke FW, Plant C, Bird AC. Intrafamilial variation of phenotype in Stargardt macular dystrophy-fundus flavimaculatus. Invest Ophthalmol Vis Sci 1999; 40: 2668–2675.

37. Armstrong JD, Meyer D, Xu S, Elfervig JL. Long-term follow-up of Stargardt's disease and fundus flavimaculatus. Ophthalmology 1998; 105:448–457.

38. Bonnin M-P. Le signe du silence choroïdien dans les dégénér-escences tapéto-rétiniennes centrales examinées sous fluores-céine. Bul Soc Ophtalmol Fr 1971; 71:348–351.

39. Eagle RC, Lusier AC, Bernardino VB, Yanoff M. Retinal pigment abnormalities in fundus flavimaculatus: a light and electron microscopic study. Ophthalmology 1980; 87: 1189–1200.

40. Fish G, Grey R, Sehmi KS, Bird AC. The dark choroid in posterior retinal dystrophies. Br J Ophthalmol 1981; 65: 359–363.

41. Allikmets R, Singh N, Sun H, Shroyer NF, Hutchinson A, Chidambaram A, Gerrard B, Baird L, Stauffer D, Peiffer A, Rattner A, Smallwood P, Li B, Anderson KL, Lewis RA, Nathans J, Leppert M, Dean M, Lupski JR. A photoreceptor cell-specific ATP-binding trasporter gene (ABCR) is mutated in recessive Stargardt macular dystrophy. Nat Genet 1997; 15:236–246.

42. Molday LL, Rabin AR, Molday AS. ABCR expression in foveal cone photoreceptors and its role in Stargardt macular dystro-phy. Nat Genet 2000; 25:257–158.

43. Sun H, Nathans J. Stargardt's ABCR is localized to the disc membrane of retinal rod outer segments. Nat Genet 1997; 17:15–16.

44. Webster AR, Heon E, Lotery AJ, Vandenburgh K, Casavent TL, Oh KT, Beck G, Fishman GA, Lam BL, Levin A, Heckenlively JR, Jacobson SG, Weleber RG, Sheffield VC, Stone EM. An analysis of allelic variation in the ABCA4 gene. Invest Ophthalmol Vis Sci 2001; 42:1179–1189.

45. Briggs CE, Rucinski D, Rosenfeld PJ, Hirose T, Berson EL, Dryja TP. Mutations in ABCR (ABCR (ABCA4) in patients with Stargardt macular degeneration or cone–rod degeneration. Invest Ophthalmol Vis Sci 2001; 42:2229–2236.

46. Fishman GA, Stone EM, Grover S, Derlacki DJ, Haines HL, Hockey RR. Variation of clinical expression in patients with Stargardt dystrophy and sequence variations in the ABCR gene. Arch Ophthalmol 1999; 117:504–510.

47. Cremers FP, van de Pol TH, van Driel M, den Hollander AI, van Haren FJ, Tijmes N, Bergen AA, Rohrschneider K, Blankenagel A, Pinckers AJ, Deutman AF, Hoyng CB. Autosomal recessive retinitis pigmentosa and cone–rod dystrophy caused by splice site mutations in Stargardt's disease gene. Hum Mol Genet 1998; 7:355–362.

48. Klevering BJ, Maugeri A, Wagner A, Go SL, Vink C, Cremers FPM, Hoyng CB. Three families displaying the combination of Stargardt's disease with cone–rod dystrophy or retinitis pigmentosa. Ophthalmology 2004; 111:546–553.

49. Fishman GA, Farbman JS, Alexander KR. Delayed rod dark adaptation in patients with Stargardt's disease. Ophthalmology 1991; 98:957–962.

50. Krill AE, Klein BA. Flecked retina syndrome. Arch Ophthalmol 1974; 74:496–508.

51. Lois N, Holder GE, Bunce C, Fitzke FW, Bird AC. Phenotypic subtypes of Stargardt macular dystrophy-fundus flavimaculatus. Arch Ophthalmol 2001; 119:359–369.

52. Noble KG, Carr RE. Stargardt's disease and fundus flavimaculatus. Arch Ophthalmol 1979; 97:1281–1285.

53. Itabashi R, Katsumi O, Mehta M, Wajima R, Tamai M, Hirose T. Stargardt's disease/fundus flavimaculatus: psychophysical and electrophysiologic results. Graefes Arch Clin Exp Ophthalmol 1993; 231:555–562.

54. Stavrou P, Good PA, Misson GP, Kritzinger EE. Electrophysiological findings in Stargardt's-fundus flavimaculatus disease. Eye 1998; 12:953–958.

55. Aaberg TM. Stargardt's disease and fundus flavimaculatus: evolution of morphologic progression and intrafamilial coexistence. Trans Am Ophthal Soc 1986; 84:453–487.

56. Hadden OB, Gass JDM. Fundus flavimaculatus and Stargardt's disease. Am J Ophthalmol 1976; 82:527–539.

57. Klein BA, Krill AE. Fundus flavimaculatus. Am J Ophthalmol 1967; 64:3–23.

58. Lachepalle P, Little JM, Roy MS. The electroretinogram in Stargardt's disease and fundus flavimaculatus. Doc Ophthalmol 1989; 73:395–404.

59. Moloney JBM, Mooney DJ, O'Connor MA. Retinal function in Stargardt's disease and fundus flavimaculatus. Am J Ophthalmol 1983; 96:57–65.

60. Kretschmann U, Seeliger M, Ruether K, Usui T, Apfelstedt-Sylla E, Zrenner E. Multifocal electroretinography in patients with Stargardt's macular dystrophy. Br J Ophthalmol 1998; 82:267–275.

61. Stone EM, Nichols BE, Kimura AE, Weingeist TA, Drack A, Sheffield VC. Clinical features of a Stargardt-like dominant progressive macular dystrophy with genetic linkage to chromosome 6q. Arch Ophthalmol 1994; 112:765–772.

62. Zhang K, Bither PP, Park R, Donoso LA, Seidman JG, Seidman CE. A dominant Stargardt's maculopathy dystrophy locus maps to chromosome 13q34. Arch Ophthalmol 1994; 112:759–764.

63. Edwards AO, Miedziak A, Vrabec T, Verhoeven J, Acott TS, Weleber RG, Donoso LA. Autosomal dominant Stargardt-like macular dystrophy: 1. clinical characterization, longitudinal follow-up, and evidence for a common ancestry in families linked to chromosome 6q14. Am J Ophthalmol 1999; 127:426–435.

64. Weleber RG, Carr RE, Murphey WH, Sheffield VC, Stone EM. Phenotypic variations including retinitis pigmentosa, pattern dystrophy, and fundus flavimaculatus in a single family with

a deletion of codon 153 or 154 of the peripherin/RDS gene. Arch Ophthalmol 1993; 111:1531–1542.

65. Adams JE. Case showing peculiar changes in the macula. Trans Ophthalmol Soc UK 1883; 3:113–114.

66. Barricks ME. Vitelliform lesions developing in normal fundi. Am J Ophthalmol 1977; 83:324–327.

67. Mohler CW, Fine SL. Long-term evaluation of patients with Best's vitelliform dystrophy. Ophthalmology 1981; 88:688–692.

68. Fishman GA, Baca W, Alexander KR, Derlacki DJ, Glenn AM, Viana M. Visual acuity in patients with Best vitelliform macular dystrophy. Ophthalmology 1993; 100:1665–1670.

69. Weingeist TA, Kobrin JL, Watzke RC. Histopathology of Best's macular dystrophy. Arch Ophthalmol 1982; 100:1108–1114.

70. Frangieh GT, Green WR, Fine SL. A histopathologic study of Best's macular dystrophy. Arch Ophthalmol 1982; 100: 1115–1121.

71. Petrukhin K, Koisti MJ, Bakall B, Li W, Xie G, Marknell T, Sandgren O, Forseman K, Holmgreen G, Andreasson S, Vujic M, Bergen AAB, McGarty-Dugan V, Figuerosa D, Austin CP, Metzker ML, Caskey CT, Wadelius C. Identification of the gene responsible for Best macular dystrophy. Nat Genet 1998; 19:241–247.

72. Eksandh L, Bakall B, Bauer B, Wadelius C, Andreasson S. Best's vitelliform macular dystrophy caused by a new mutation (Val89Ala) in the VMD2 gene. Ophthalmic Genet 2001; 22:107–115.

73. Lotery AJ, Munier FL, Fishman GA, Weleber RG, Jacobson SG, Affatigato LM, Nichols BE, Schorderet DF, Sheffield VC, Stone EM. Allelic variation in the VMD2 gene in Best disease and age-related macular degeneration. Invest Ophthalmol Vis Sci 2000; 41:1291–1296.

74. Seddon JM, Afshari MA, Sharma S, Bernstein PS, Chong S, Hutchinson A, Petrukhin K, Allikmets R. Assessment of mutations in the Best macular dystrophy (VMD2) gene in patients with adult-onset foveomacular vitelliform dystrophy,

age-related maculopathy, and bull's-eye maculopathy. Ophthalmology 2001; 108:2060–2067.

75. Deutman AF. Electro-oculography in families with vitelliform dystrophy of the fovea: detection of carrier state. Arch Ophthalmol 1969; 81:305–316.

76. François J. Vitelliform macular degeneration. Ophthalmologica 1971; 163:312–324.

77. François J, de Rouck A, Fernandez-Sasso D. Electro-oculography in vitelliform degeneration of the macula. Arch Ophthalmol 1967; 77:726–733.

78. Sabates R, Pruett RC, Hirose T. The electroretinogram in 'vitelliform' macular lesions. Doc Ophthal Proc Ser 1983; 37:93–103.

79. Schwartz LJ, Metz HS, Woodward F. Electrophysiologic and fluorescein studies in vitelliform macular degeneration. Arch Ophthalmol 1972; 87:636–641.

80. Thorburn W, Nordstrom S. EOG in a large family with hereditary macular degeneration. (Best's vitelliform macular dystrophy) identification of gene carriers. Acta Ophthalmol (Copenh) 1978; 56:455–464.

81. Seddon JM, Sharma S, Chong S, Hutchinson A, Allikmets R, Adelman RA. Phenotype and genotype correlations in two Best families. Invest Ophthalmol Vis Sci 2003; 110: 1724–1731.

82. Nilsson SE, Skong KO. The ERG c-wave in vitelliform macular degeneration (VMD). Acta Ophthalmol 1980; 58:659–666.

83. Falsini B, Porciatti V, Porrello G, Merendino E, Minnella A, Cermola S, Buzzonetti L. Macular flicker electroretinograms in Best vitelliform dystrophy. Curr Eye Res 1996; 6: 638–646.

84. Scholl HPN, Schuster AM, Vonthein R, Zrenner E. Mapping of retinal function in Best macular dystrophy using multifocal electroretinography. Vis Res 2002; 42:1053–1061.

85. Palmowski AM, Allgayer R, Heinemann-Vernaleken B, Scherer V, Ruprecht KW. Detection of retinal dysfunciton

in vitelliform macular dystrophy using the multifocal ERG (MF-ERG). Doc Ophthalmol 2003; 106:145–152.

86. Weleber RG. Fast and slow oscillations of the electro-oculogram in Best's macular dystrophy and retinitis pigmentosa. Arch Ophthalmol 1989; 107:530–537.

87. Jarc-Vidmar M, Pepovic P, Hawlina M, Brecelj J. Pattern ERG and psychophysical functions in Best's disease. Doc Ophthalmol 2001; 103:47–61.

88. Goodman G, Ripps H, Siegel IM. Cone dysfunction syndromes. Arch Ophthalmol 1963; 70:214–231.

89. Downes SM, Fitzke FW, Holder GE, Payne AM, Bessant DA, Bhattacharya SS, Bird AC. Clinical features of codon 172 RDS macular dystrophy: similar phenotype in 12 families. Arch Ophthalmol 1999; 117:1373–1383.

90. Wroblewski HJ, Wells JA, III, Eckstein A, Fitzke F, Jubb C, Keen TJ, Inglehearn C, Bhattacharya S, Arden GB, Jay M, Bird AC. Macular dystrophy associated with mutations at codon 172 in the human retinal degeneration slow gene. Ophthalmology 1994; 101:12–22.

91. Heckenlively JR, Weleber RG. X-linked recessive cone dystrophy with tapetal-like sheen: a newly recognized entity with Mizuo–Nakamura phenomenon. Arch Ophthalmol 1986; 104:1322–1328.

92. Berson EL, Gouras P, Gunkel RD. Progressive cone degeneration, dominantly inherited. Arch Ophthalmol 1968; 80:77–83.

93. Kellner U, Klein-Hartlage P, Foerster MH. Cone dystrophies: clinical and electrophysiological findings. Ger J Ophthalmol 1992; 1:105–109.

94. Krill AE, Deutman AF. Dominant macular degenerations: the cone dystrophies. Am J Ophthalmol 1972; 73:352–369.

95. Krill AE, Deutman AF, Fishman M. The cone degenerations. Doc Ophthalmol 1973; 35:1–80.

96. Francois J, de Rouck A, de Laey JJ. Progressive cone dystrophies. Ophthalmologica 1976; 173:81–101.

97. Ripps H, Noble KG, Greenstein VC, Siegel IM, Carr RE. Progressive cone dystrophy. Ophthalmology 1987; 94:1401–1409.

98. Kellner U, Foerster MH. Cone dystrophies with negative photopic electroretinogram. Br J Ophthalmol 1993; 77: 404–409.

99. Mathews GP, Sandberg MA, Berson EL. Foveal cone electroretinograms in patients with central visual loss of unexplained etiology. Am J Ophthalmol 1992; 110:1568–1570.

100. Miyake Y, Ichikawa H, Shiose Y, Kawase Y. Hereditary macular dystrophy without visible fundus abnormalities. Am J Ophthalmol 1989; 108:292–299.

101. Miyake Y, Horiguchi M, Tomita N, Kondo M, Tanikawa A, Takahashi H, Suzuki S, Terasaki H. Occult macular dystrophy. Am J Ophthalmol 1996; 112:644–653.

102. Piao CH, Kondo M, Tanikawa A, Terasaki H, Miyake Y. Multifocal electroretinogram in occult macular dystrophy. Invest Ophthalmol Vis Sci 2000; 41:513–517.

103. Noble KG, Siegel IM, Carr RE. Progressive peripheral cone dysfunction. Am J Ophthalmol 1988; 106:557–560.

104. Pearlman JT, Owen WG, Brounley DW. Cone dystrophy with dominant inheritance. Am J Ophthalmol 1974; 77:293–303.

105. Kondo M, Miyake Y, Kondo N, Ueno S, Takakuwa H, Terasaki H. Peripheral cone dystrophy. A variant of cone dystrophy with predominant dysfunction in the peripheral cone system. Ophthalmology 2004; 111:732–739.

106. Gouras P, Eggers HM, Mckay CJ. Cone dystrophy, nyctalopia, and supernormal rod responses. Arch Ophthalmol 1993; 101:718–724.

107. Pawlyk BS, Sandberg MA, Berson EL. Effects of IBMX on the rod ERG of the isolated perfused cat eye: antagonism with light calcium or l-cis-diltiazem. Vis Res 1991:1093–1097.

108. Hood DC, Cideciyan AV, Halevy DA, Jacobson SG. Sites of disease action in a retinal dystrophy with supernormal and delayed rod electroretinogram b-wave. Vis Res 1996; 36:889–901.

109. Sorsby S, Mason MEJ. A fundus dystrophy with unusual features. Br J Ophthalmol 1949; 33:67–97.

110. Weber BHF, Vogt G, Pruett RC, Stöhr H, Felbor U. Mutations in the tissue inhibitor of metaliproteinase-3 (TIMP3) in patients with Sorsby's fundus dystrophy. Nat Genet 1994; 8:352–356.

111. Anand-Apte B, Pepper MS, Voest E, Montesano R, Olsen B, Murphy G, Apte SS, Zetter B. Inhibition of angiogenesis by tissue inhibitor of metalloproteinase-3. Invest Ophthalmol Vis Sci 1997; 38:817–823.

112. Clark AF. New discoveries on the roles of matrix metalloproteinases in ocular cell biology and pathology. Invest Ophthalmol Vis Sci 1998; 39:2514–2516.

113. Steen B, Sejersen S, Berglin L, Seregard S, Kvanta A. Matrix metalloproteinases and metalloproteinase inhibitors in choroidal neovascular membranes. Invest Ophthalmol Vis Sci 1998; 39:2194–2200.

114. Capon MR, Marshall J, Kraft JI, Alexander RA, Hiscott PS, Bird AC. Sorsby's fundus dystrophy—a light and electron microscopic study. Ophthalmology 1989; 96:1769–1777.

115. Capon MRC, Polkingborne PJ, Fitzke FW, Bird AC. Sorsby's pseudoinflammatory macula dystrophy-Sorsby's fundus dystrophies. Eye 1988; 2:114–122.

116. Felbor U, Berkowitz C, Klein ML, Greenberg J, Gregory CY, Weber BHF. Sorsby fundus dystrophy: reevaluation of variable expressivity in patients carrying a TIMP3 founder mutation. Arch Ophthalmol 1997; 115:1569–1571.

117. Polkingborne PJ, Capon MRC, Berninger T, Lyness AL, Sehmi K, Bird AC. Sorsby's fundus dystrophy: a clinical study. Ophthalmology 1989; 96:1763–1768.

118. Cideciyan AV, Pugh EN, Lamb TD, Huang Y, Jacobson SG. Rod plateaux during dark adaptation in Sorsby's fundus dystrophy and viatamin A deficiency. Invest Ophthalmol Vis Sci 1997; 38:1786–1794.

119. Steinmetz RL, Polkinghorne PC, Fitzke FW, Kemp CM, Bird AC. Abnormal dark adaptation and rhodopsin kinetics in

Sorsby's fundus dystrophy. Invest Ophthalmol Vis Sci 1992; 33:1633–1636.

120. Jacobson SG, Cideciyan AV, Regunath G, Rodriguez FJ, Vandenburgh K, Sheffield VC, Stone EM. Night blindness in Sorsby's fundus dystrophy reversed by vitamin A. Nat Genet 1995; 11:27–32.

121. De La Paz MA, Pericak-Vance MA, Lennon F, Haines JL, Seddon JM. Exclusion of TIMP3 as a candidate locus in age-related macular degeneration. Invest Ophthalmol Vis Sci 1997; 38:1060–1065.

122. Carrero-Valanzuela RD, Klein ML, Weleber RG, Murphey WH, Litt M. Sorsby fundus dystrophy: a family with the Ser181Cys mutation of the tissue inhibitor of metalloproteinase 3. Arch Ophthalmol 1996; 114:737–738.

123. Hamilton WK, Ewing CC, Ives EJ, Caruthers JD. Sorsby's fundus dystrophy. Ophthalmology 1989; 96:1755–1762.

124. Hoskin A, Sehmi K, Bird AC. Sorsby's pseudoinflammatory macular dystrophy. Br J Ophthalmol 1981; 65:859–865.

125. Clarke MP, Mitchell KW, McDonnell S. Electroretinographic findings in macular dystrophy. Doc Ophthalmol 1997; 92: 325–339.

126. Lip P-L, Good PA, Gibson JM. Sorsby's fundus dystrophy: a case report of 24 years follow-up with electrodiagnostic tests and indocyanine green angiography. Eye 1999; 13:16–25.

127. Saperstein DA. Advances in macular dystrophies. Int Ophthalmol Clin 1995; 35:19–35.

128. Marmor MF, Byers B. Pattern dystrophy of the pigment epithelium. Am J Ophthalmol 1977; 84:32–44.

129. Sjögren H. Dystrophia reticularis laminae pigmentossae retinae. Acta Ophthalmol 1950; 28:279–295.

130. Slezak H, Hommer K. Fundus pulverulentis. Albrecht von Graefes Arch Klin Exp Ophthalmol 1969; 178:177–182.

131. Deutman AF, van Blommestein JD, Henkes HE, Waardenburg PJ, Solleveld-van Driest E. Butterfly-shaped pigment dystrophy of the fovea. Arch Ophthalmol 1970; 83:558–569.

132. Mesker BP, Oosterhuis JA, Delleman JW. A retinal lesion resembling Sjögren's dystrophia reticularis laminae pigmentossae retinae. In: Winkelman P, Crone R, eds. Perspectives in Ophthalmology. Amsterdam: Excerpta Medica Foundation Vol. 2, 1970:40–45.

133. Marmor MF, McNamara J. Pattern dystrophy of the retinal pigment epithelium and geographic atrophy of the macula. Am J Ophthalmol 1996; 122:382–392.

134. de Jong PT, Delleman JW. Pigment epithelial pattern dystrophy. Four different manifestations in a family. Arch Ophthalmol 1982; 100:1416–1421.

135. Giuffre G. Autosomal dominant pattern dystrophy of the retinal pigment epithelium. Intrafamilial variability. Retina 1988; 8:169–173.

136. Hsieh RC, Fine BS, Lyons JS. Pattern dystrophies of the retinal pigment epithelium. Arch Ophthalmol 1977; 95:429–435.

137. Gutman I, Walsh JB, Henkind P. Vitelliform macular dystrophy and butterfly-shaped epithelial dystrophy: a continuum? Br J Ophthalmol 1982; 66:170–173.

138. Kim RY, Dollfus H, Keen TJ, Fitzke FW, Arden GB, Bhattacharya SS, Bird AC. Autosomal dominant pattern dystrophy of the retina associated with a 4-base pair insertion at codon 140 in the peripherin/RDS gene. Arch Ophthalmol 1995; 113:451–455.

139. Sears JE, Aaberg TA Sr, Daiger SP, Moshfeghi DM. Splice site mutation in the peripherin/RDS gene associated with pattern dystrophy of the retina. Am J Ophthalmol 2001; 132:693–699.

140. Nichols BE, Sheffield VC, Vandenburgh K, Drack AV, Kimura AE, Stone EM. Butterfly-shaped pigment dystrophy of the fovea caused by a point mutation in codon 167 of the RDS gene. Nat Genet 1993; 3:202–207.

141. Nichols BE, Drack AV, Vandenburgh K, Kimura AE, Sheffield VC, Stone EM. A 2-base pair deletion in the RDS gene associated with butterfly-shaped pigment dystrophy of the fovea. Hum Mol Genet 1993; 2:601–603.

142. Massin P, Virally-Monod M, Vialettes B, Paques M, Gin H, Porokhov B, Caillat-Zucman S, Froguel P, Paquis-Fluckinger V, Gaudric A, Guillausseau P-J. Prevalence of macular pattern dystrophy in maternally inherited diabetes and deafness, GEDIAM GROUP. Ophthalmology 1999; 106: 1821–1827.

143. Daniele S, Carbonara A, Daniele C, Restagno G, Orcidi R. Pattern dystrophies of the retinal pigment epithelium. Acta Ophthalmol Scand 1996; 74:51–55.

144. Duinkerke-Eerola, K U, Pinckers A, Cruysberg JR. Pattern dystrophy of the retinal pigment epithelium. Int Ophthalmol 1987; 11:65–72.

145. Kingham JD, Fenzi RE, Willerson D, Aaberg TM. Reticular dystrophy of the retinal pigment epithelium. A clinical and electrophysiologic study of three generations. Arch Ophthalmol 1978; 96:1177–1184.

146. O'Donnell FE, Schatz H, Reid P, Green WR. Autosomal dominant dystrophy of the retinal pigment epithelium. Arch Ophthalmol 1979; 97:680–683.

147. Shiono T, Ishikawa A, Hara S, Tamai M. Pattern dystrophy of the retinal pigment epithelium. Retina 1990; 104:251–254.

148. Watzke RC, Folk JC, Lang RM. Pattern dystrophy of the retinal pigment epithelium. Ophthalmology 1982; 89: 1400–1406.

149. Forsius H, Krause U, Helve J, Vuopala V, Mustonen E, Vainio-Mattila B, Fellman J, Eriksson AW. Visual acuity in 183 cases of X-chromosomal retinoschisis. Can J Ophthalmol 1973; 8:385–393.

150. George NDL, Yates JRW, Moore AT. Clinical features in affected males with X-linked retinoschisis. Arch Ophthalmol 1996; 114:274–280.

151. de Jong PT, Zrenner E, van Meel GJ, Keunen JE, van Norren D. Mizuo phenomenon in X-linked retinoschisis: pathogenesis of the Mizuo phenomenon. Arch Ophthalmol 1991; 109:1104–1108.

152. Miyake Y, Terasaki H. Golden tapetal-like fundus reflex and posterior hyaloid in a patient with X-linked juvenile retinoschisis. Retina 1999; 19:84–86.

153. Sauer CG, Gehrig A, Warneke-Wittstock R, Marquardt A, Ewing CC, Gibson A, Lorenz B, Jurklies B, Weber BH. Positional cloning of the gene associated with X-linked juvenile retinoschisis. Nat Genet 1997; 17:164–170.

154. Condon GP, Brownstein S, Wang NS, Kearns JA, Ewing CC. Congenital hereditary (juvenile X-linked) retinoschisis. Histologic and ultrastructural findings in three eyes. Arch Ophthalmol 1986; 104:576–583.

155. Kellner U, Brümmner S, Foerster MH, Wessing A. X-linked congenital retinoschisis. Graefes Arch Clin Exp Ophthalmol 1990; 228:432–437.

156. Peachey NS, Fishman GA, Derlacki DJ, Brigell MG. Psychophysical and electroretinographic findings in X-linked juvenile retinoschisis. Arch Ophthalmol 1987; 105: 513–516.

157. Tanino T, Katsumi O, Hirose T. Electrophysiological similarities between two eyes with X-linked recessive retinoschisis. Doc Ophthalmol 1985; 60:149–161.

158. Bradshaw K, George N, Moore A, Trump D. Mutations of the XLRS1 gene cause abnormalities of the photoreceptor as well as inner responses of the ERG. Doc Ophthalmol 1999; 98:153–173.

159. Eksandh LC, Ponjavic V, Ayyagari R, Bingham BA, Hirlyanna KT, Andréasson S, Ehinger B, Sieving PA. Phenotypic expression of juvenile X-linked retinoschisis in Swedish families with different mutations in the XLRS1 gene. Arch Ophthalmol 2000; 118:1098–1104.

160. Sieving PA, Bingham EL, Kemp J, Richards J, Hiriyanna K. Juvenile X-linked retinoschisis from XLRS1 Arg213Trp mutation with preservation of the electroretinogram scotopic b-wave. Am J Ophthalmol 1999; 128:179–184.

161. Arden GB, Gorin MB, Polkinghorne PL, Jay M, Bird AC. Detection of the carrier state of X-linked retinoschisis. Am J Ophthalmol 1988; 105:590–595.

162. Shinoda K, Ohde H, Mashima Y, Inoue R, Ishida S, Inoue M, Kawashima S, Oguchi Y. On- and off-responses of the photopic electroretinograms in X-linked juvenile retinoschisis. Am J Ophthalmol 2001; 131:489–494.

163. Alexander KR, Fishman GA, Grover S. Temporal frequency deficits in the electroretinogram of the cone system in X-linked retinoschisis. Vis Res 2000; 40:2861–2868.

164. Piao CH, Kondo M, Nakamura M, Terasuki H, Miyake Y. Multifocal electroretinograms in x-linked retinoschisis. Invest Ophthalmol Vis Sci 2003; 44:4920–4930.

165. Huang S, Wu D, Jiang F, Luo G, Liang J, Wen F, Yu M, Long S, Wu L. The multifocal electroretinogram in X-linked juvenile retinoschisis. Doc Ophthalmol 2003; 106:251–255.

166. Lewis RA, Lee GB, Martonyi CL, Barnett JM, Falls HF. Familial foveal retinoschisis. Arch Ophthalmol 1977; 95:1190–1196.

167. Noble KG, Carr RE, Siegel IM. Familial foveal retinoschisis associated with a rod–cone dystrophy. Am J Ophthalmol 1978; 85:551–557.

168. Shimazaki J, Matsubashi M. Familial retinoschisis in female patients. Doc Ophthalmol 1987; 65:393–400.

169. Yamaguchi K, Hara S. Autosomal juvenile retinoschisis ithout foveal retinoschisis. Br J Ophthalmol 1989; 73: 470–473.

170. Sorsby A, Crick RP. Central areolar choroidal schlerosis. Br J Ophthalmol 1953; 37:129–139.

171. Waardenburg PJ. Angio-schlerose familiale de la choroide. J Genet Hum 1952; 1:83–93.

172. Yanagihashi S, Nakazawa M, Kurotaki J, Sato M, Miyagawa Y, Ohguro H. Autosomal dominant central areolar choroidal dystrophy and a novel Arg195Leu mutation in the peripherin/RDS gene. Arch Ophthalmol 2003; 121:1458–1461.

173. Hughes AE, Lotery AJ, Silvestri G. Fine localisation of the gene for central areolar choroidal dystrophy on chromosome 17p. J Med Genet 1998; 35:770–772.

174. Lotery AJ, Einnis K, Silvestri G, Nicholl S, McGibbon D, Collins AD, Hughes AE. Localisation of a gene for central areolar choroidal dystrophy to chromosome 17p. Hum Mol Genet 1996; 5:705–708.

175. Adachi-Usami E, Murayama K, Yamamoto Y. Electroretinogram and pattern visually evoked cortical potentials in central areolar choroidal dystrophy. Doc Ophthalmol 1990; 75:33–40.

176. Carr RE. Central areolar choroidal dystrophy. Arch Ophthalmol 1965; 73:32–35.

177. Noble K. Central areolar choroidal dystrophy. Am J Ophthalmol 1977; 84:310–318.

178. Ponjavic V, Andreasson S, Ehinger B. Full-field electroretinograms in patients with central areolar choroidal dystrophy. Acta Ophthalmol (Copenh) 1994; 72:537–544.

179. Lotery AJ, Silvestri G, Collins AD. Electrophysiology findings in a large family with central areolar choroidal dystrophy. Doc Ophthalmol 1999; 97:103–119.

180. Lefler WH, Wadsworth JA, Sidbury JB Jr. Hereditary macular degeneration and aminoaciduria. Am J Ophthalmol 1971; 71:224–230.

181. Fetkenhour CL, Gurney N, Dobbie JG, Choromokos E. Central areolar pigment epithelial dystrophy. Am J Ophthalmol 1976; 81:745–753.

182. Frank HR, Landers MBI, Willems RJ, Sidbury JB Jr. A new dominant progressive foveal dystrophy. Am J Ophthalmol 1974; 78:903–916.

183. Small KW, Hermsen V, Gurney N, Fetkenhour CL, Folk JC. North Carolina macular dystrophy and central areolar pigment epithelial dystrophy: one family, one disease. Arch Ophthalmol 1992; 110:515–518.

184. Rabb M, Mullen L, Yelchitis S, Udar N, Small KW. A North Carolina macular dystrophy phenotype in a Belizean family maps to the MCDR1 locus. Am J Ophthalmol 1998; 125: 502–508.

185. Rohrschneider K, Blankenagel A, Kruse FE, Fendrich T, Volcker HE. Macular function testing in a German pedigree with North Carolina macular dystrophy. Retina 1998; 18:453–459.

186. Small KW, Puech B, Mullen L, Yelchitis S. North Carolina macular dystrophy phenotype in France maps to the MCDR1 locus. Mol Vis 1997; 3:1–6.

187. Reichel MB, Kelsell RE, Fan J, Gregory CY, Evans K, Moore AT, Hunt DM, Fitzke FW, Bird AC. North Carolina macular dystrophy family linked to chromosome 6q. Br J Ophthalmol 1998; 82:1162–1168.

188. Small KW, Weber JL, Roses A, Lennon F, Vance JM, Pericak-Vance MA. North Carolina macular dystrophy is assigned to chromosome 6. Genomics 1992; 13:681–685.

189. Small KW. North Carolina macular dystrophy: clinical features, genealogy, and genetic linkage analysis. Trans Am Ophthalmol Soc 1998; 96:925–961.

190. Small KW. North Carolina macular dystrophy. Revisited. Ophthalmology 1989; 96:1747–1754.

191. Voo I, Glasgow BJ, Flannery J, Udar N, Small KW. North Carolina macular dystrophy: clinicopathologic correlation. Am J Ophthalmol 2001; 132:933–935.

192. Small KW, Killian J, McLean WC. North Carolina's dominant progressive foveal dystrophy: how progressive is it. Br J Ophthalmol 1991; 75:401–406.

193. Hermsen VM, Judisch GF. Central areolar pigment epithelial dystrophy. Ophthalmologica 1984; 189:69–72.

194. Douglas AA, Waheed I, Wyse CT. Progressive bifocal chorioretinal atrophy: a rare familial disease of the eyes. Br J Ophthalmol 1968; 52:742–751.

195. Kelsell RE, Godley BF, Evans K, Tiffin PA, Gregory CY, Plant C, Moore A, Bird AC, Hunt DM. Localization of the gene for progressive bifocal chorioretinal atrophy (PBVRA) to chromosome 6q. Hum Mol Genet 1995; 4:1653–1656.

196. Godley BF, Tiffin P, Evans K, Kelsell RE, Hunt DM, Bird AC. Clinical features of progressive bifocal chorioretinal atrophy:

a retinal dystrophy linked to chromosome 6q. Ophthalmology 1996; 103:893–898.

197. O'Donnell FE, Welch RB. Fenestrated sheen macular dystrophy. A new autosomal dominant maculopathy. Arch Ophthalmol 1979; 97:1292–1296.

198. Daily MJ, Mets MB. Fenestrated sheen macular dystrophy. Arch Ophthalmol 1984; 102:855–856.

199. Slagsvold JE. Fenestrated sheen macular dystrophy. A new autosomal dominant maculopathy. Acta Ophthalmol (Copenh) 1981; 59:683–688.

200. Sneed SR, Sieving PA. Fenestrated sheen macular dystrophy. Am J Ophthalmol 1991; 112:1–7.

201. Polk TD, Gass JD, Green WR, Novak MA, Johnson MW. Familial internal limiting membrane dystrophy. A new sheen retinal dystrophy. Arch Ophthalmol 1997; 115:878–885.

202. Lam BL. Hereditary retinal degenerations. In: Parrish R, ed. Bascom Palmer Eye Institute Atlas of Ophthalmology. Philadelphia: Current Medicine, 2000:343–349.

11

Chorioretinal Disorders

Progressive degenerations of the retina and the choroid are the common feature of chorioretinal disorders. The electrophysiologic findings of this group of disorders are not diagnostic but may be helpful to rule out other retinal dystrophies as well as to assess retinal function. Chorioretinal degenerations involving primarily the macula such as central areolar choroidal dystrophy are discussed in Chapter 10. The outline of this chapter is:

- Choroideremia
- Gyrate atrophy
- Hereditary choroidal atrophy
- Helicoid peripapillary chorioretinal degeneration
- Pigmented paravenous retinochoroidal atrophy (PPRCA)

CHOROIDEREMIA

Choroideremia is a X-linked recessive dystrophy characterized by progressive early-onset atrophy of the retina and choroid. The disorder was first described in the 19th century and is now known to be produced by mutations of the gene encoding component A of Rab geranylgeranyl transferase called Rab escort protein-1 (REP-1) (1). The enzyme attaches geranylgeranyl lipid groups to selected intracellular proteins called Rab proteins. Rab proteins control cellular secretory and endocytic pathways. Choroideremia is a disease confined to the retina, because there are two Rab escort proteins, REP-1 and REP-2. In choroideremia patients, REP-1 is defective but REP-2 is functional. Retinal cells need both REP-1 and REP-2 to function properly but most cells elsewhere function adequately with only REP-2. Several different mutations of the REP-1 gene are found in association with choroideremia, and variable symptoms and features are frequently encountered. A recent histologic, immunocytochemistry study suggests rod photoreceptors as a primary site of pathology in choroideremia (2).

Affected males with choroideremia usually have poor night vision and decreased peripheral vision within the first two decades of life. Bilateral progressive degeneration of the retina and choroid occurs with initial sparing of the fovea. Areas of granularity and depigmentation are first visible in the peripheral regions of the retina, but bone-spicule-like pigmentary clumping and severe retinal vascular attenuation as seen in retinitis pigmentosa are not typical (Fig. 11.1). Visual acuity is minimally affected early but as the retinal degeneration progresses, central vision deteriorates gradually with generally favorable prognosis for visual acuity until the seventh decade of life (3). In contrast, female carriers of choroideremia are commonly asymptomatic with preserved visual function. However, patchy areas of peripheral retinal depigmentation, granularity, or pigmentary clumping are found in as high as 96% of female carriers (4).

The diagnosis of choroideremia is arrived on the basis of ocular history, characteristic clinical features, and genetic analysis if available. Examination of the mother of the suspected affected male and other possible female carriers within the family for patchy peripheral areas of retinal pigmentary disturbance is extremely helpful. A family history of X-linked retinal disease may or may not be present. Genetic analysis, if

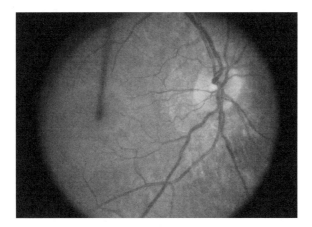

Figure 11.1 Chorioretinal degeneration in a patient with choroideremia. (From Ref. 29.) (Refer to the color insert.)

available, will not only determine whether the patient has choroideremia but will also identify female carriers. Demonstrating the absence of REP-1 protein in peripheral blood samples with immunologic technique will identify affected individuals but not female carriers (5).

A useful measure of retinal function in affected males with choroideremia is the full-field ERG. But it has very low sensitivity in detecting female carriers (Fig. 11.2). The ERG is marked impaired early in the disease with reduced and prolonged rod and cone responses. During the early stage, the rod response is more impaired than the cone response, and ERG reductions are usually easily apparent even when symptoms are minimal. Only very rarely are normal ERG amplitudes observed in young patients with very early stage of disease (6). With further disease progression, all components of the ERG responses deteriorate and become non-detectable. Sieving and associates (4) reviewed the full-field ERG records of 47 affected males and 26 carrier females with choroideremia. The rod response was markedly reduced or non-detectable in all affected males, and in those whom the cone response was still detectable, the cone implicit times were delayed even when cone amplitudes were in the normal range. Of the 26 females carriers, only four (15%) had

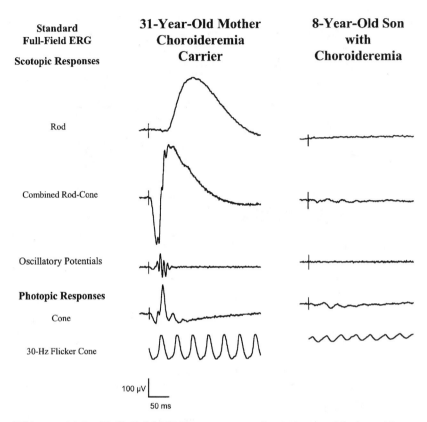

Figure 11.2 Full-field ERG responses of a 31-year-old choroideremia carrier and her 8-year-old affected son. Note the normal ERG responses in the carrier and the markedly impaired responses of the affected son with non-detectable rod response and severely impaired cone responses.

abnormal ERG. EOG impairment parallels ERG reductions, and EOG is normal in carriers (7). Likewise, VEP findings parallel ERG impairment.

GYRATE ATROPHY

Gyrate atrophy is an autosomal recessive dystrophy involving the retina and choroid, caused by mutations of the gene encoding ornithine aminotransferase, a vitamin B6 (pyridoxal phosphate) dependent mitochondrial enzyme which catalyzes the conversion of ornithine to glutamate and proline (8). The ornithine aminotransferase gene is located on chromosome 10, and mutations producing gyrate atrophy show a high degree of heterogeneity with more than 50 mutations identified. In addition, even among subjects who harbor the same single mutation, the symptoms and findings vary widely (9). The systemic defect results in elevated serum ornithine level as well as hypolysinemia and hyperornithinuria.

In general, patients with gyrate atrophy start to experience poor night vision and impaired peripheral vision between the age of 20 and 40 years. Multiple, bilateral discrete areas of chorioretinal atrophy occur initially in the peripheral and midperipheral regions of the fundus (Fig. 11.3). Over time, the lesions coalesce and progress toward the macula with corresponding progressive impairment of night vision, peripheral vision, and central vision. Myopia and posterior capsular lens opacities are common. Two subtypes of gyrate atrophy are distinguished based on response to vitamin B6 supplementation. Patients responsive to vitamin B6 supplementation have less severe disease, and serum ornithine level falls substantially with therapy (10). Specific

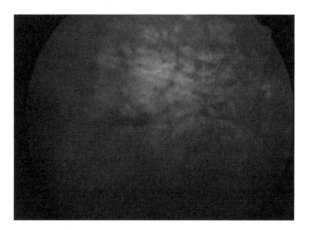

Figure 11.3 Chorioretinal atrophy lesions in a patient with gyrate atrophy. (From Ref. 29.)

identifiable genotypes are found in patients' response to vitamin B6 supplementation (11,12). Low arginine diets also reduce serum ornithine level in some patients with gyrate atrophy (13). However, the effect of dietary therapies on the progression of retinal degeneration is conflicting, perhaps due in part to the genetic heterogeneity and variable expressivity of the disease. Berson and associates (14,15) found no visual improvement in patients treated with vitamin B6 or low arginine diets. Likewise, progressive visual loss in affected children treated with low arginine diet was reported by Vannas-Sulonen and colleagues (16). In contrast, Kaiser-Kupfer and colleagues (17) noted only modest progressive visual loss in their group of affected children treated with low arginine diet.

   The diagnosis of gyrate atrophy is based on characteristic clinical findings, elevated serum ornithine level, and genetic analysis if available. Full-field rod and cone ERG responses are typically markedly reduced or non-detectable at the time of diagnosis. Accordingly, ERG plays a supportive role in the diagnosis of the disorder. However, when the disease is not advanced and ERG responses are still detectable, ERG can serve as a measure of retinal function (14). In such cases, the amplitudes of the rod and cone responses are moderately to severely reduced, the implicit times are mildly to moderately prolonged, and the a-wave and b-wave components are equally affected (18). The degree of retinal involvement produces corresponding reductions in EOG and VEP. Interestingly, clinical and ERG findings similar to gyrate atrophy have been found in patients without elevated serum ornithine, some of whom have dominant disease (19). These patients with gyrate-atrophy-like findings have normal ornithine aminotransferase activity and by definition, do not have gyrate atrophy.

HEREDITARY CHOROIDAL ATROPHY

Aside from X-linked recessive choroideremia, other autosomal dominant and recessive forms of choroidal atrophy are found.

The choroidal atrophy may be more localized, located centrally or in the peripapillary region, or more diffuse. Krill and Archer (20) proposed a clinical classification of choroidal atrophy based on the extent of involvement, regional vs. diffuse, and whether choriocapillaris atrophy occurs with or without atrophy of the large choroidal vessels. However, regional choroidal atrophy may progress to diffuse involvement in some individuals and different clinical patterns of choroidal may occur within the same pedigree due to variable expressivity. The degree of involvement on clinical examination generally parallels ERG b-wave amplitudes, and the implicit times are less affected (Fig. 11.4) (20). Reduced EOG light-peak to dark-trough amplitudes ratios are common (20). Central areolar choroidal dystrophy discussed in chapter10.

HELICOID PERIPAPILLARY CHORIORETINAL DEGENERATION

Helicoid peripapillary chorioretinal degeneration is a rare bilateral dominant dystrophy characterized by well-demarcated, wing-shaped peripapillary atrophic areas of retinal pigmented epithelium and choroid radiating from the optic nerve head. The disorder was first reported by Sveinsson in 1939 as "chorioditis areata," and received its current name from Francescetti in 1962 (21,22). The disease occurs mostly in European and Icelandic pedigrees and is linked to chromosome 11p15 (23). Dysfunction of the affected retinal areas produces variable decrease in vision, which becomes severe if the macula is involved. The diagnosis is made on clinical ophthalmoscopic appearance and positive family history.

Results of electrophysiology testing in helicoid peripapillary chorioretinal degeneration are rarely reported. However, Eysteinsson and associates (24) studied 17 affected members of a family and found the full-field ERG to be highly variable. Of the 17 patients, 5 had normal ERG, 6 had reduced photopic and scotopic responses with normal implicit times, and 6 had marked reduced scotopic and photopic a-wave and b-wave

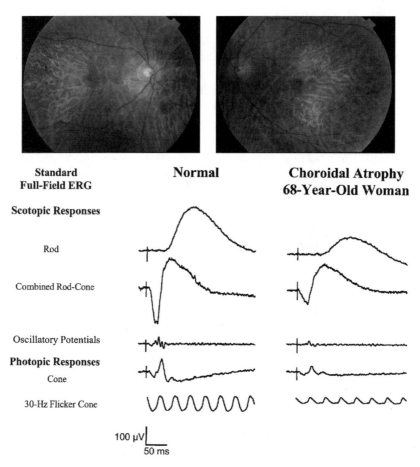

Figure 11.4 *Top (left and right)*: Diffuse choroidal atrophy in a 68-year-old woman who reported progressive worsening of vision for 1 year. In contrast to pigmentary retinal degeneration, the retinal arterioles are not significantly attenuated. *Bottom*: Note the reduced, mildly prolonged full-field ERG responses. (Refer to the color insert.)

amplitudes with prolonged b-wave. Interestingly, a-wave implicit times were normal in all patients. Of the 17 patients, 3 had normal light-peak to dark-trough EOG ratios and 14 had reduced EOG ratios. These results suggest that dysfunction of the retinal pigment epithelium is greater than that of the sensory retina. The findings of VEP have not been extensively studied and are likely to parallel the degree of retinal involvement.

PIGMENTED PARAVENOUS RETINOCHOROIDAL ATROPHY

Pigmented paravenous retinochoroidal atrophy (PPRCA) is a rare bilateral progressive condition diagnosed solely by the prominent perivascular retinal pigment epithelium disturbance. The disorder was first described in 1937 by Brown as "retino-choroiditis radiata" (25). The cause of PPRCA is likely numerous. Most reported cases are sporadic, but a few familial occurrences including dominant pedigrees are also observed (26). Interestingly, in a report of monozygotic twins, only one twin had the disease, implicating that the cause may not always be genetic or that the expressivity of the disease is highly variable (27).

Reports of ERG responses in PPRCA are scarce. Full-field ERG is variable depending on the extent of the disease. Mild to severe reduction of photopic and scotopic responses is found and selective reduction of b-wave amplitude may occur (26). Focal areas of retinal dysfunction produced by the perivascular atrophy are apparent on multifocal ERG. In general, EOG and VEP responses parallel ERG responses (26,28).

REFERENCES

1. Seabra MC, Brown MS, Goldstein JL. Retinal degeneration in choroideremic: deficiency of RAb geranylgeranyl transferase. Science 1993; 259:377–381.

2. Syed N, Smith JE, John SK, Seabra MC, Aquirre GD, Milam AH. Evaluation of retinal photoreceptors and pigment epithelium in a female carrier of choroideremia. Ophthalmology 2001; 108:711–720.

3. Roberts MF, Fishman GA, Roberts DK, Heckenlively JR, Weleber RG, Anderson RJ, Grover S. Retrospective, longitudinal, and cross sectional study of visual acuity impairment in choroideraemia. Br J Ophthalmol 2002; 86:658–662.

4. Sieving PA, Niffenegger JH, Berson EL. Electroretinographic findings in selected pedigrees with choroideremia. Am J Ophthalmol 1986; 101:361–367.

5. MacDonald IM, Mah DY, Ho YK, Lewis RA, Seabra MC. A practical diagnostic test for choroideremia. Ophthalmology 1998; 1998:1637–1640.

6. Fishman GA, Birch DG, Holder GE, Brigell MG. Choroideremia. Electro-physiologic Testing in Disorders of the Retina, Optic Nerve, and Visual Pathway. San Francisco: The Foundation of the American Academy of Ophthalmology, 2001:66–68.

7. Pinckers A, van Aarem A, Brink H. The electrooculogram in heterozygote carriers of Usher syndrome, retinitis pigmentosa, neuronal ceroid lipofuscinosis, senior syndrome and choroideremia. Ophthalmic Genet 1994; 15:25–30.

8. Mashima Y, Murakami A, Weleber RG, Kennaway NG, Clarke L, Shiono T, Inana G. Nonsense-codon mutations of the ornithine aminotransferase gene with decreased levels of mutant mRNA in gyrate atrophy. Am J Hum Genet 1992; 51:81–91.

9. Peltola KE, Nanto-Salonen K, Heinonen OJ, Jääskeläinen S, Heinänen K, Simell O, Nikoskelainen E. Ophthalmologic heterogeneity in subjects with gyrate atrophy of choroid and retina harboring the L402P mutation of ornithine aminotransferase. Ophthalmology 2001; 108:721–729.

10. Weleber RG, Kennaway NG. Clinical trial of vitamin B6 for gyrate atrophy of the choroid and retina. Ophthalmology 1981; 88:316–324.

11. Dougherty KM, Swanson DA, Brody LC, Valle D. Molecular basis of ornithine aminotransferase deficiency in B-6-responsive and -nonresponsive forms of gyrate atrophy. Proc Natl Acad Sci USA 1988; 85:3777–3780.

12. Mashima Y, Weleber RG, Kennaway NG, Inana G. Genotype–phenotype correlation of a pyridoxine-responsive form of gyrate atrophy. Ophthalmic Genet 1999; 20:219–224.

13. Valle D, Walser M, Brusilow SW, Kaiser-Kupfer MI, Takki K. Gyrate atrophy of the choroid and retina: amino acid metabolism and correction of hyperornithinemia with an arginine-deficient diet. J Clin Invest 1980; 65:371–378.

14. Berson EL, Shih VE, Sullivan PL. Ocular findings in patients with gyrate atrophy on pyridoxine and low-protein, low-arginine diets. Ophthalmology 1981; 88:311–315.

15. Berson E, Hanson AHI, Rosner B, Shih VE. A two year trial of low protein, low arginine diets or vitamin B6 for patients with gyrate atrophy. Birth Defects 1982; 18:209–218.

16. Vannas-Sulonen K, Simell O, Sipila I. Gyrate atrophy of the choroid and retina: the ocular disease progresses in juvenile patients despite normal or near normal plasma ornithine concentration. Ophthalmology 1987; 1987:1428–1433.

17. Kaiser-Kupfer MI, Caruso RC, Valle D. Gyrate atrophy of the choroid and retina: long-term reduction of ornithine slows retinal degeneration. Arch Ophthalmol 1991; 109:1539–1548.

18. Raitta C, Carlson S, Vannas-Sulonen K. Gyrate atrophy of the choroid and retina: ERG of the neural retina and the pigment epithelium. Br J Ophthalmol 1990; 74:363–367.

19. Kellner U, Weleber RG, Kennaway NG, Fishman GA, Foerster MH. Gyrate atrophy-like phenotype with normal plasma ornithine. Retina 1997; 17:403–413.

20. Krill AE, Archer D. Classification of the choroidal atrophies. Am J Ophthalmol 1971; 72:562–585.

21. Francescetti A. A curious affection of the fundus oculi: helicoidal peripapillar chorioretinal degeneration: its relation to pigmentary paravenous chorioretinal degeneration. Doc Ophthalmol 1962; 16:81–110.

22. Sveinsson K. Choroiditis areata. Acta Ophthalmol 1939; 17:73–80.

23. Fossdal R, Magnussion L, Weber JL, Jensson O. Mapping the focus of atrophia areata, a hellicoid peripapillary chorioretinal degeneration with autosomal dominant inheritance, to chromosome 11p15. Hum Mol Genet 1995; 4:479–483.

24. Eysteinsson T, Jónasson F, Jónsson V, Bird AC. Helicoidal peripapillary chorioretinal degeneration: electrophysiology and psychophysics in 17 patients. Br J Ophthalmol 1998; 82:280–285.

25. Brown TH. Retino-choroiditis radiata. Br J Ophthalmol 1936; 21:645–648.

26. Skalka HW. Hereditary pigmented paravenous retinochoroidal atrophy. Am J Ophthalmol 1979; 87:286–291.

27. Small KW, Anderson WB. Pigmented paravenous retinochoroidal atrophy. Discordant expression in monozygotic twins.
Arch Ophthalmol 1991; 109:1408–1410.

28. Parafita M, Diaz A, Torrijos IG, Gomez-Ulla F. Pigmented
paravenous retinochoroidal atrophy. Optom Vis Sci 1993;
70:75–78.

29. Lam BL. Hereditary retinal degenerations. In: Parrish R, ed.
Bascom Palmer Eye Institute Atlas of Ophthalmology.
Philadelphia: Current Medicine, 2000:343–349.

12

Vitreoretinal Disorders

Diseases exhibiting prominent clinical retinal and vitreous abnormalities are categorized as "vitreoretinal" disorders. Electrophysiologic responses typically reflect the degree of retinal involvement in this group of rare conditions. X-linked retinoschisis previously considered as a vitreoretinal disorder is due to genetic mutations involving a protein expressed mostly in photoreceptors and is discussed in Chapter 10. Goldmann–Favre syndrome, a disorder that also demonstrates retinal and vitreous abnormalities, has similar ERG and genotypes as enhanced S-cone syndrome and is covered in Chapter 8. The outline of this chapter is as follows:

- Stickler syndrome
- Wagner vitreoretinopathy
- Familial exudative vitreoretinopathy
- Autosomal dominant vitreoretinochoroidopathy
- Autosomal dominant neovascular inflammatory vitreoretinopathy

STICKLER SYNDROME

Stickler syndrome is an autosomal dominant disorder caused by mutations of the gene encoding type II collagen, COL2A1, which is located on chromosome 12 (1). The syndrome was described by Stickler et al. (2) in 1965 and termed "hereditary progressive arthro-ophthalmopathy." Common ocular features include high myopia, vitreous syneresis, and rhegmatogenous retinal detachment with a high risk of multiple and giant retinal tears. Other ocular findings include cataract and retinal perivascular pigmentary clumping (Fig. 12.1). Common systemic features include arthropathy, cleft palate, sensorineural hearing loss, and midfacial hypoplasia. Genetic mutations producing Stickler syndrome show a high degree of heterogeneity, and clinical expression is highly variable both between and within families. Variations of the vitreous syneresis are associated with different genotypes (3). Stickler syndrome is categorized into two subtypes, the more common ocular Stickler syndrome (type 1) and "non-ocular" Stickler syndrome (type 2). Type 2 is associated with mutations on another collagen gene, COL11A1.

Full-field ERG is generally normal in Sticker syndrome but the associated high myopia may produce mild to moderate reduction of scotopic and photopic b-wave amplitudes

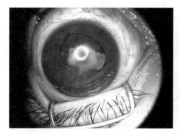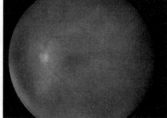

Figure 12.1 Stickler syndrome. Photographs of a 14-year-old boy showing significant cataract in the right eye (*left*). The view of the retina of the left eye (*right*) is obscured by cataract and vitreous syneresis, and shows myopic and perivascular pigmentary changes.

corresponding to the degree of the myopic retinal degeneration. The ERG responses are also impaired if retinal detachment occurs with the amount of impairment relating to the size and chronicity of the retinal detachment. In addition, if associated cataract is present, mild ERG a-wave and b-wave reduction with prolonged implicit time may occur. In general, EOG and VEP findings parallel ERG responses.

WAGNER VITREORETINOPATHY

Wagner vitreoretinopathy is a rare autosomal dominant disorder characterized by high myopia, vitreous strands, and occasional rhegmatogenous retinal detachment. Funduscopic findings are variable and include vitreous avascular strands or condensed bands, retinal pigmentary epithelium and choroidal atrophy, retinal perivascular pigmentary clumping, optic nerve atrophy, and situs inversus of the optic nerve head vessels. The disease was described by Wagner (4) in 1938 in a Swiss family and has no associated systemic features. In the past, Wagner vitreoretinopathy and Stickler syndrome have been confused with one another, and affected persons have been reported as having the same disorder. Wagner vitreoretinopathy is genetically heterogeneous. A frame shift mutation of the gene encoding type II collagen, COL2A1, was found to be associated with Wagner vitreoretinopathy in one kindred (5). Mutations of COL2A1 are also associated with Stickler syndrome. However, in other kindreds, Wagner vitreoretinopathy is genetically linked to chromosome 5q14, a region which contains genes encoding two extracellular macromolecules, link protein (CRTL1) and versican (CSPG2), which are important in binding hyaluronan, a component of the vitreous (6,7).

In Wagner disease, ERG may be normal but both the a-wave and the b-wave may be impaired if retinal and choroidal atrophy is present (8). In addition, the associated high myopia may produce mild to moderate reduction of scotopic and photopic b-wave amplitudes corresponding to the degree of the myopic retinal degeneration. If retinal detachment occurs, the ERG responses are impaired with the amount of impairment depending on the size and chronicity of the retinal detachment. The EOG and VEP findings parallel ERG responses, but the VEP may be impaired further if associated optic atrophy is present.

FAMILIAL EXUDATIVE VITREORETINOPATHY

Familial exudative vitreoretinopathy commonly called "FEVR" is a rare dominant or X-linked hereditary disorder with variable expressivity (9–11). Clinical manifestation of FEVR ranges from subtle termination of retinal vessels in the peripheral temporal equatorial region to vitreal fibrovascular mass with marked traction of the retina and optic nerve head (Fig. 12.2). Clinical findings of FEVR may mimic residual changes of retinopathy of prematurity and may lead to misdiagnosis in some patients.

In FEVR, ERG and EOG findings are related to the degree of retinal involvement and correlates with visual function. The ERG is generally normal in mildly affected persons and becomes impaired or even non-detectable with severe disease (12–14). The VEP findings parallel ERG responses.

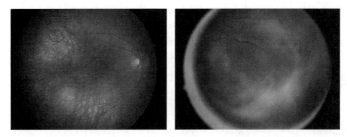

Figure 12.2 Familial exudative vitreoretinopathy. *Left*: Right eye of a 5-year-old boy with mild temporal retinal atrophic changes. *Right*: Right eye of an unrelated 4-year-old boy with severe fibrovascular proliferation and retinal detachment.

AUTOSOMAL DOMINANT VITREORETINOCHOROIDOPATHY

Autosomal dominant vitreoretinochoroidopathy (ADVIRC) is a very rare hereditary disorder found in a few families in the United States and Germany. Characteristic feature is the circumferential chorioretinal hypopigmentary or hyperpigmentary disturbance between the vortex veins and the ora serrata (15–18). In this zone, there are a discrete posterior boundary, preretinal punctate white opacities, retinal arteriolar narrowing and occlusion, and occasional choroidal atrophy. Other findings include retinal neovascularization, vitreous abnormalities, macular edema, vitreous hemorrhage, and early cataract. Histopathology reveals a retinal pigment epithelial response with marked intraretinal migration and extracellular matrix deposition (19,20).

Han and Lewandowski (21) performed EOG and full-field ERG on four affected patients with ADVIRC and found reduced EOG Arden light-peak to dark-trough ratios of 1.1–1.5 (normal ≥ 1.8) despite full-field ERG consisting of mildly affected rod function and normal cone function. However, Kellner et al. (22) noted reduced full-field ERG with a normal EOG in an affected patient, but the patient's affected mother had normal full-field ERG and EOG. Therefore, the expression of the disease may be variable within the same family, and a reduced EOG is not a typical sign for all affected persons (22). The VEP response in ADVIRC has not been extensively studied but is likely related to ERG impairment.

AUTOSOMAL DOMINANT NEOVASCULAR INFLAMMATORY VITREORETINOPATHY

Autosomal dominant neovascular inflammatory vitreoretinopathy (ADNIV) is a very rare hereditary disorder reported in a large kindred in the United States. The disorder is characterized by peripheral retinal scarring and pigmentation, peripheral arteriolar closure, and neovascularization of the peripheral retina at the ora serrata (23). Neovascularization of the optic disc, vitreous hemorrhage, tractional retinal detachment, cystoid macular edema, and neovascular glaucoma may also occur. The disease is linked to chromosome 11q13 (24).

Affected patients are asymptomatic in early adulthood but have vitreous cells and a selective reduced ERG b-wave response that is most apparent under dark-adapted condition (23). With progression of the disease, the ERG is further impaired and may become non-detectable. The EOG and VEP findings have not been extensively studied but are likely to parallel reduction in ERG responses.

REFERENCES

1. Ahmad NN, Ala-Kokko L, Knowlton RG, Jimenez SA, Weaver EJ, Maguire JI, Tasman W, Prockop DJ. Stop codon in the procollagen II gene (COL2A1) in a family with the Stickler syndrome (arthro-ophthalmopathy). Proc Natl Acad Sci USA 1991; 88:6624–6627.

2. Stickler GB, Belau PG, Farrell FJ. Hereditary progressive arthro-ophthalmopathy. Mayo Clin Proc 1965; 40:433–455.

3. Richards AJ, Baguley DM, Yates JR, Lane C, Nicol M, Harper PS, Scott JD, Snead MP. Variation in the vitreous phenotype of Stickler syndrome can be caused by different amino acid substitutions in the X-position of the type II collagen Gly-X-Y triple helix. Am J Hum Genet 2000; 67:1083–1094.

4. Wagner H. Ein bisher unbekanntes Erbleiden des Auges (Degeneratio hyaloideoretinalis hereditaria). Beobachter im Känton Zürich. Klin Monatsbl Augenheilkd 1938; 100: 840–857.

5. Gupta SK, Leonard BC, Damji KF, Bulman DE. A frame shift mutation in tissue-specific alternatively spliced exon of Collagen 2A1 in Wagner's vitreoretinal degeneration. Am J Ophthalmol 2002; 133:203–210.

6. Brown DM, Graemiger RA, Hergersberg M, Schinzel A, Messmer EP, Niemeyer G, Schneeberger SA, Streb LM, Kimura AE, Weingeist TA, Sheffield VC, Stone EM. Genetic

linkage of Wagner disease and erosive vitreoretinopathy to chromosome 5 q13–14. Arch Ophthalmol 1995; 113:671–675.

7. Perveen R, Hart-Holden N, Dixon MJ, Wiszniewski W, Fryer AE, Brunner HG, Pinkners AJ, van Beersum SE, Black GC. Refined genetic and physical localization of the Wagner disease (WGN1) locus and the genes CRTL1 and CSPG2 to a 2- to 2.5-cM region of chromosome 5q14.3. Genomics 1999; 57:219–226.

8. Hirose T, Lee KY, Schepens CL. Wagner's hereditary vitreoretinal degeneration and retinal detachment. Arch Ophthalmol 1973; 89:176–185.

9. Criswick VG, Schepens CL. Familial exudative vitreoretinopathy. Am J Ophthalmol 1969; 68:578–594.

10. Plager DA, Orgel IK, Ellis FD, Hartzer M, Trese MT, Shastry BS. X-linked recessive familial exudative vitreoretinopathy. Am J Ophthalmol 1992; 114:145–148.

11. Muller B, Orth U, Van Noubuys CE, Duvigneau C, Fuhrmann C, Scheinger E, Laqua H, Gal A. Mapping of the autosomal dominant exudative vitreoretinopathy locus (EVR1) by multipoint linkage analysis in four families. Genomics 1994; 20:317–319.

12. Feldman EL, Norris JL, Cleasby GW. Autosomal dominant exudative vitreoretinopathy. Arch Ophthalmol 1983; 101: 1532–1535.

13. Ohkubo H, Tamino T. Electrophysiological findings in familial exudative vitreoretinopathy. Doc Ophthalmol 1987; 65: 461–469.

14. Van Noubuys CE. Dominant exudative vitreoretinopathy and other vascular developmental disorders of the peripheral retina. Doc Ophthalmol 1982; 54:1–414.

15. Blair NP, Goldberg MR, Fishman GA, Salzano T. Autosomal dominant vitreoretinochoroidopathy. Br J Ophthalmol 1984; 68:2–9.

16. Kaufman SJ, Goldberg MR, Orth DH, Fishman GA, Tessler HH, Mizuno K. Autosomal dominant vitreoretinochoroidopathy. Arch Ophthalmol 1982; 100:272–278.

17. Roider J, Frisch E, Hoerauf H, Heide W, Laqua H. Autosomal dominant vitreoretinochoroidopathy. Retina 1997; 17:294–299.

18. Traboulsi EI, Payne JW. Autosomal dominant vitreoretinochoroidopathy: report of the third family. Arch Ophthalmol 1993; 111:194–196.

19. Goldberg MR, Lee FL, Tso MO, Fishman GA. Histopathologic study of autosomal dominant vitreoretinochoroidopathy: peripheral annular pigmentary dystrophy of the retina. Ophthalmology 1989; 96:1736–1746.

20. Han DP, Burke JM, Blair JR, Simons KB. Histopathologic study of autosomal dominant vitreoretinochoroidopathy in a 26-year-old woman. Arch Ophthalmol 1995; 113:1561–1566.

21. Han DP, Lewandowski MF. Electro-oculography in autosomal dominant vitreoretinochoroidopathy. Arch Ophthalmol 1992; 110:1563–1567.

22. Kellner U, Jandeck C, Kraus H, Foerster MH. Autosomal dominant vitreoretinochoroidopathy with normal electrooculogram in a German family. Graefes Arch Clin Exp Ophthalmol 1998; 236:109–114.

23. Bennett SR, Folk JC, Kimura AE, Russell SR, Stone EM, Raphtis EM. Autosomal dominant neovascular inflammatory vitreoretinopathy. Ophthalmology 1990; 97:1135–1136.

24. Stone EM, Kimura AE, Folk JC, Bennett SR, Nichols BE, Streb LM, Sheffield VC. Genetic linkage of autosomal dominant neovascular inflammatory vitreoretinopathy to chromosome 11q13. Hum Mol Genet 1992; 1:685–689.

13

Inflammatory and Immune-Related Ocular Disorders

Inflammatory and immune-related ocular disorders encompass a wide spectrum of conditions. Electrophysiological testing may serve as a measure of retinal function in this group of diseases and has a critical diagnostic role in disorders such as paraneoplastic retinopathies. The topics covered in this chapter are:

Inflammatory retinal disorders:

- Uveitis (non-specific intraocular inflammation)
- Presumed ocular histoplasmosis syndrome (POHS) and toxoplasmosis retinopathy
- Behçet disease
- Vogt–Koyanagi–Harada disease
- Sympathetic ophthalmia
- Acute posterior multifocal placoid pigment epitheliopathy (APMPPE)
- Serpiginous choroiditis

- Birdshot retinochoroidopathy (vitiligenous chorio-retinitis)
- Diffuse unilateral subacute neuroretinitis (DUSN)

Zonal inflammatory retinal disorders:

- Acute zonal occult outer retinopathy (AZOOR)
- Multiple evanescent white-dot syndrome (MEWDS)
- Acute macular neuroretinopathy (AMN)
- Multifocal choroiditis
- Punctate inner choroidopathy (PIC)

Paraneoplastic and immune-related retinopathies:

- Cancer-associated retinopathy (CAR)
- Recoverin-associated retinopathy and autoimmune retinopathy without cancer
- Melanoma-associated retinopathy (MAR)
- CRMP-5 paraneoplastic retinopathy and optic neuropathy

INFLAMMATORY RETINAL DISORDERS

Uveitis (Non-Specific Intraocular Inflammation)

In acute iridocyclitis, or anterior uveitis, the ERG is normal because the retina is not involved (1).

In patients with pars planitis or intermediate uveitis, Cantrill et al. (2) found selective prolonged scotopic and photopic b-wave responses and reduced oscillatory potentials in a study of 13 patients. In contrast, Tetsuka and colleagues (3) performed ERG in nine patients with pars planitis and noted that the a-wave and b-wave were equally impaired without a selective effect on the b-wave. In the same study, the ERG responses varied from supernormal, due to early active retinal inflammation, to non-detectable from late chronic severe diffuse retinal degeneration. The EOG light-peak to dark-trough ratios were also reduced.

In posterior uveitis, the ERG is normal with vitreous inflammation and minimal retinal involvement (1). However, when retinal vasculitis is present, impaired ERG responses correlate directly with the degree of vasculitis on fluorescein angiography (4). When intraocular inflammation produces cystoid macular edema, the foveal focal ERG and multifocal ERG are impaired due to localized retinal dysfunction but the full-field ERG is normal or only mildly impaired since the foveal region may contribute only about 10% of the full-field cone ERG response. Because the ERG impairment in cystoid macular edema is non-specific, fluorescein angiography and optical coherence tomography are more useful in determining any active macular inflammation. Reduced EOG light-peak to dark-trough ratios parallel ERG reductions, but the EOG ratio may be mildly supernormal in early uveitis presumably due to the acute inflammatory response (4). The VEP findings parallel ERG responses but may be further reduced when secondary optic nerve head inflammation occurs as part of the posterior uveitis.

Presumed Ocular Histoplasmosis Syndrome (POHS) and Toxoplasmosis Retinopathy

Focal lesions of the choroid and retina from presumed histoplasmosis and toxoplasmosis cause local areas of retinal dysfunction that rarely produce significant reduction on full-field ERG unless the lesions are extensive. However, areas of localized retinal dysfunction may be detected with multifocal ERG technique.

Behçet Disease

Behçet disease, described in 1937, is a generalized vasculitis syndrome of unknown origin characterized by intraocular inflammation and ulcers of the mouth and genitals. Other manifestations of the vasculitis include retinal vasculitis, ischemic optic neuropathy, cerebrovascular occlusion, gastrointestinal bleed, and arthralgia. Behçet disease is rare in most countries, but is much more common in the Middle and Far East. Factor V Leiden mutation is found at an increased frequency in Behçet patients with retinal vascular occlusions (5).

The diagnosis of Behçet disease is made on clinical findings. The ERG is variable in Behçet disease and correlates with the severity of retinal involvement. Cruz et al. (6) performed full-field ERG and pattern VEP on 12 patients with posterior uveitis from Behçet disease. Marked reduction of ERG oscillatory potentials was noted early in the disease with subsequent impairment of a-wave and b-wave. Significant prolongation of the VEP response was also found when the ERG responses were impaired. These impaired ERG responses from Behçet disease were confirmed by other authors, some of whom found a selective reduction of the ERG b-wave presumably due to retinal ischemia (7–9). However, in a comparison of 16 Behçet patients and 11 patients with non-specific posterior uveitis by Hatt and Niemeyer (10), the scotopic full-field ERG responses were found to be more impaired than photopic responses in both groups, and no characteristic ERG changes for Behçet disease were encountered. Therefore, in Behçet disease ERG is helpful to assess retinal function although the ERG findings are variable and non-specific. The EOG and VEP in Behçet disease have not been extensively studied but are likely to parallel ERG responses.

Vogt–Koyanagi–Harada Disease

Vogt–Koyanagi–Harada disease is a granulomatous inflammatory disorder due to autoimmune response associated with melanocytes (11). The disease is more common in more pigmented ethnic groups. Ocular manifestations include bilateral diffuse choroiditis, serous retinal detachment, pigmentary retinopathy, vitritis, and optic disc hyperemia. Systemic findings include meningismus, alopecia, poliosis, and vitiligo.

Reports of electrophysiological findings in Vogt–Koyanagi–Harada disease are scarce. Degree of ERG impairment correlates with retinal involvement.

Sympathetic Ophthalmia

Sympathetic ophthalmia is a rare form of uveitis in which intraocular inflammation occurs in both eyes after penetrating trauma or ocular surgery in one eye (12). Aside from penetrating ocular trauma, sympathetic ophthalmia may follow intraocular procedures such as paracentesis, iridectomy, lysis of iris adhesions, cyclodialysis, cataract extraction, evisceration, retinal detachment repair, and pars plana vitrectomy. In addition, sympathetic ophthalmia may rarely follow nonpenetrating ocular procedures such as cyclocryotherapy, laser cyclotherapy, proton beam irradiation, and helium ion therapy for choroidal melanoma. The fellow eye to the injured or operated eye is referred to as the sympathizing eye. The onset of blurred vision and photophobia typically occurs between 3 weeks and 6 months following the inciting trauma or surgery. Clinical features include iridocyclitis and diffuse, focal, or multifocal granulomatous choroiditis. The etiology of sympathetic ophthalmia is unknown but an autoimmune response to ocular antigens is suspected. The risk of sympathetic ophthalmia is reduced if the injured, exciting eye is promptly enucleated after the trauma.

The diagnosis of sympathetic ophthalmia is made based on history and clinical features. Reports of electrophysiological findings in sympathetic ophthalmia are scarce. Degree of ERG impairment correlates with retinal involvement.

Acute Posterior Multifocal Placoid Pigment Epitheliopathy

Acute posterior multifocal placoid pigment epitheliopathy commonly called "APMPPE" is characterized by multiple flat gray-white subretinal lesions involving the retinal pigment epithelium. The disease is typically bilateral and the cause is unknown. Affected persons are often young adults who develop blurred vision over days and may have had a recent flu-like illness. In early APMPPE, fluorescein angiography shows early blockage by lesions that become diffusely stained in mid- and late-phases. The lesions fade over several days, and visual recovery occurs over weeks to months. Visual prognosis is good with final visual acuities of 20/30 or better in most patients. Recurrences are infrequent. Occasionally, APMPPE patients may have concomitant central nervous system vasculitis. The diagnosis of APMPPE is based on clinical features and fluorescein angiographic findings.

During the acute phase of APMPPE, the ERG and EOG are variably impaired and are related to the degree of ocular involvement. Fishman et al. (13) documented a patient who initially had reduced EOG and full-field ERG, and with recovery, the ERG normalized but the EOG remained impaired, suggesting persistent dysfunction of the retinal pigment epithelium. However, Smith et al. (14) reported a patient who initially had minimally reduced full-field ERG and a notably reduced EOG amplitude ratio of 1.55 which normalized three weeks later. More recently, Vianna et al. (15) reviewed the records of 42 APMPPE patients. The EOG was performed on 36 affected eyes, and 21 (58%) eyes had reduced light-peak to dark-trough amplitude ratios of less than 1.8. In the same series, full-field ERG was available in 30 eyes, and reduced ERGs were found in only three (10%) patients. Taken together, although both variable ERG and EOG impairments may occur during the acute phase of APMPPE, the EOG is more likely to be abnormal. Both ERG and EOG improve with disease recovery, but EOG impairments are more likely to persist. Reports of VEP in AMPPE are rare; the VEP is likely to parallel ERG findings and macular function.

Serpiginous Choroiditis

Serpiginous choroiditis is a rare, acute, and chronically recurrent disorder characterized by demarcated geographic zones of gray-white discoloration of the retinal pigment epithelium, followed by atrophy of the retinal pigment epithelium and choroid. Other names for the same disorder include geographic choroiditis and helicoid peripapillary choroidopathy. The cause is unknown and young or middle-aged adults are typically affected. Acute onset of central scotoma in one eye is common, and sequential involvement of the contralateral eye is common. The lesions usually occur initially in the peripapillary region and tend to spread over months to years to involve the macula and the peripheral retina. The diagnosis is made on clinical features.

The ERG and EOG are variably impaired and are related to the severity of the condition. In general, the EOG is more likely to be abnormal than the full-field ERG. Chisholm et al. (16) reviewed the full-field ERG and EOG records of 26 eyes with serpiginous choroiditis. The ERG was abnormal in three (12%) eyes, all had severe disease, and the EOG light-peak to dark-trough ratios were markedly reduced to less than 1.45 in eight (37%) eyes. Multifocal ERG would be more likely to pick up focal retinal dysfunction produced by focal areas of choroiditis. The VEP is likely to parallel ERG findings and macular function.

Birdshot Retinochoroidopathy (Vitiligenous Chorioretinitis)

Birdshot retinochoroidopathy is a rare, chronic, bilateral, ocular inflammatory disease characterized by vitritis, retinal vasculitis, and the presence of multiple, scattered, discrete, cream-colored depigmented fundus lesions, which appear to be at the level of the choroid and the retinal pigment epithelium (Fig. 13.1). The commonly used term "birdshot retinochoroidopathy" was first coined by Ryan and Maumenee

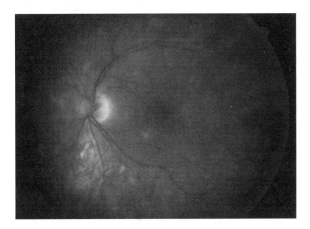

Figure 13.1 Retinal appearance of the left eye of a 52-year-old woman with birdshot retinochoroidopathy. Note the multiple scattered lesions. The patient was positive for HLA-A29.

(17) in 1980 because the fundus lesions have a pattern which resembles the scatter from a shotgun. Other less popular terms such as salmon patch choroidopathy and vitiligenous chorioretinitis have also been used to describe the same disorder. Other possible clinical features include epiretinal membrane, retinal neovascularization, subretinal neovascular membrane, cystoid macular edema, and optic nerve head edema or atrophy. Symptoms include decreased visual acuity, impaired peripheral visual field, floaters, photopsia, and nyctalopia. The pathogenesis of birdshot retinochoroidopathy is unclear but appears to be autoimmune in origin. The disease is strongly associated with HLA-A29, and persons with this human leukocyte antigen are at a much higher risk of developing the disorder (18). Middle-aged white persons of northern European descent are most commonly affected, and there is a higher prevalence in women.

The diagnosis of birdshot retinochoroidopathy is typically arrived on the basis of characteristic clinical features, a positive serum HLA-A29, and characteristic fluorescein angiographic findings of the fundus lesions and retinal vasculitis. The relatively unique but not completely specific ERG pattern may be useful in the diagnosis of birdshot retinochoroidopathy or as a measure of retinal function during follow-up.

The amount of ERG alteration in birdshot retinochoroidopathy is related not only to severity but also to variable expression of the disease, and this may in part explain the variability of results among studies. Although Hirose et al. (19) in their study of 15 patients reported supranormal ERG responses in some patients during the initial phase of the disorder, this is an extremely rare finding presumably due to acute retinal inflammation and have not been consistently confirmed by other investigators. More characteristically, patients with birdshot retinochoroidopathy have the following on standardized full-field ERG (Fig. 13.2): (1) scotopic rod flash response—reduced and prolonged b-wave, (2) scotopic combined rod–cone bright flash response—reduced a-wave and b-wave with variable prolongation with a possible greater selective decrease in the b-wave amplitude as compared to the a-wave, but usually not to such an extent as to produce a

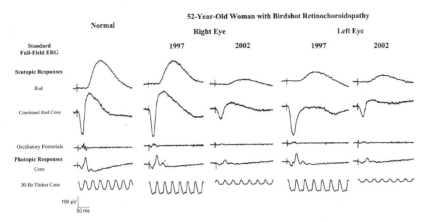

Figure 13.2 Full-field ERG responses of a patient with birdshot retinochoroidopathy. The retinal appearance of the left eye of this patient is shown in Fig. 13.1. Note the progressive deterioration of ERG responses from 1997 to 2002 for both eyes. The relatively selective impairment of b-wave is most apparent on the 1997 scotopic combined rod–cone response for the left eye. In general, the scotopic responses are more affected than the photopic responses.

negative pattern (i.e., the reduced b-wave is still higher than the baseline), (3) oscillatory potentials—reduced, (4) photopic cone flash response—reduced a-wave and b-wave with variable prolongation with a more selective decrease in the b-wave amplitude, and (5) photopic cone flicker response— reduced and prolonged b-wave (19–22).

In general, the scotopic responses are more affected than the photopic responses, and the degree of selective impairment of b-wave is somewhat variable among studies. For example, Priem et al. (22) in their study of 16 patients found a very striking selective impairment of the b-wave with a well-preserved a-wave. In contrast, Gasch et al. (23) in their report of 22 patients found that the selective impairment of b-wave to be less prominent with some impairment of the a-wave in all study patients. This relative selective effect on the b-wave in birdshot retinochoroidopathy implies greater dysfunction in the inner retina in some cases despite the fact that the clinical lesions appear to be deep at the level of the choroid or the retinal pigment epithelium.

In general, ERG indices decrease over time in patients with birdshot retinochoroidopathy, indicating the progressive nature of the condition (Fig. 13.2) (24). In one study, abnormalities of the scotopic bright-flash rod–cone amplitude and photopic 30-Hz flicker implicit time were found to be associated with recurrence of inflammation as immunosuppressive therapy was tapered (25).

The EOG and VEP in birdshot retinochoroidopathy tend to parallel the ERG response, and reduced EOG light-peak to dark-trough ratio and delayed VEP response are common (19,21–23,26). Moreover, optic atrophy when present may also be a source of VEP impairment.

Diffuse Unilateral Subacute Neuroretinitis

Diffuse unilateral subacute neuroretinitis commonly called "DUSN" is caused by nematodes that wander in the subretinal space producing visual loss due to vitritis, retinal vasculitis, optic nerve inflammation, recurrent evanescent gray-white outer retinal lesions, and diffuse pigmentary degeneration (27).

Depending on the extent of retinal involvement, moderate to severe impaired ERG is typical in the DUSN eye as compared to responses of the normal, unaffected eye. Gass and Scelfo (28) reviewed findings in 37 DUSN patients, 36 of whom underwent full-field ERG. Moderate to marked impaired rod and cone responses were found in all but two patients who initially had responses in the normal range, which subsequently worsened. In general, the b-wave was more severely affected than the a-wave, and none of the patients had a non-detectable ERG. In the same series, EOG was performed on 29 patients, and 16 had impaired EOG. The VEP has not been extensively studied in DUSN but is likely to parallel the extent of the retinal as well as optic nerve involvement.

ZONAL INFLAMMATORY RETINAL DISORDERS

In 1993, "acute zonal occult outer retinopathy" was described by Gass (29) who proposed that this rare retinopathy is part of the spectrum of a single disorder which includes multiple evanescent white-dot syndrome, acute idiopathic blind spot enlargement syndrome, acute macular neuroretinopathy, multifocal choroiditis, and punctate inner choroidopathy. The validity of this hypothesis is not clearly established. Regardless, these rare disorders share some common features such as zonal inflammatory retinopathy and occasional occurrence of enlarged blind spot on visual field testing.

Acute Zonal Occult Outer Retinopathy

Acute zonal occult outer retinopathy commonly referred to as "AZOOR" is characterized by: (1) acute loss of one or more large zones of outer retinal function with photophobia and photopsia, (2) minimal or no fundus changes initially with normal fluorescein angiography, (3) ERG abnormalities, and (4) permanent visual field loss often associated with late development of atrophic or pigmentary retinal changes and narrowing of the retinal vessels in the affected zones. The diagnosis of AZOOR is given to patients with these clinical features; however, the term "AZOOR," as mentioned, has also been used to encompass other disorders in this category including multiple evanescent white-dot syndrome, acute idiopathic blind spot enlargement syndrome, acute macular neuroretinopathy, and multifocal choroiditis (29). Visual acuity is usually mildly affected although the visual acuity may be as worse as 20/400. The disorder affects one or both eyes of predominantly young women. However, of the 13 patients initially reported by Gass, three were men. In addition, one of the 13 patients was as young as 13 years and another was as old as 63 years. In a subsequent long-term follow-up study of 51 patients with AZOOR (37 women and 14 men, median follow-up 96 months), Gass et al. (30) found that AZOOR was present in one eye of 12 (24%) patients and both eyes of 39 (76%) patients. Residual visual field defects were present in all patients, and ERG was essential for early diagnosis.

In AZOOR, the full-field ERG is usually abnormal but may occasionally be near normal in some cases (Fig. 13.3). Of the 13 patients initially reported by Gass (29), the full-field

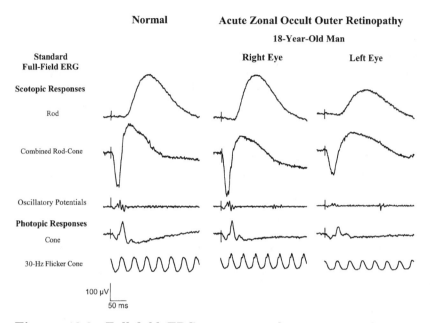

Figure 13.3 Full-field ERG responses of a patient with acute zonal occult outer retinopathy (AZOOR) involving the left eye. Full-field ERG responses are highly variable in AZOOR, and the responses are often asymmetric between the two eyes.

ERG was abnormal in 17 out of 21 affected eyes. Most of the affected eyes showed only mild to moderate reduction in rod and cone amplitudes. In a few eyes, the responses were within the lower range of normal but were notably lower than in the unaffected eye. Jacobson et al. (31) examined a group of 24 patients with "AZOOR," a term that they used to encompass patients with multiple evanescent white-dot syndrome, acute idiopathic blind spot enlargement syndrome, acute macular neuroretinopathy, and multifocal choroiditis. The investigators found that full-field ERG was significantly asymmetric between the two eyes in this group of patients, and that visual field area correlated well with ERG a-wave amplitude, suggesting that the visual dysfunction was photoreceptor in origin. Multifocal ERG may also be useful in determining retinal dysfunction and in documenting the location of retinal dysfunction in AZOOR (32). In the long-term follow-up study of AZOOR by Gass et al. (30), the full-field or multifocal ERG amplitudes were diminished in all 51 patients. The EOG and VEP abnormalities are also reported but are thought to be related to retinal dysfunction. Taken together, the diagnosis of AZOOR is based on clinical findings and ERG is important for early diagnosis. The ERG abnormalities are often asymmetric, and the degree of impaired of ERG impairment is variable among patients.

Multiple Evanescent White-Dot Syndrome

Multiple evanescent white-dot syndrome, commonly referred to as "MEWDS," is a rare, acute, usually unilateral ocular inflammatory disease characterized by the presence of small discrete white dots at the level of the outer retina or retinal pigment epithelium during the acute phase of the disorder. The syndrome was described by Jampol et al. (33) in 1984, and the cause is unknown. The disease often affects young to middle-age women, but men as well older persons may also be affected (34). Patients with MEWDS typically experience an acute onset of unilateral visual loss, which gradually improves over several weeks. Visual prognosis is generally favorable with the majority recovering to normal or near normal vision, and recurrences and bilateral involvement are rare (35). Aside from the characteristic retinal lesions during the acute phase, other findings include vitritis, retinal vascular sheathing, foveal granularity, and optic disc edema. In addition, an enlarged blind spot on visual field testing may occur and persists even after visual acuity recovery (36,37).

Of the 11 patients in the initial report of MEWDS by Jampol and associates, the full-field ERG was found to have profound diffuse impairment of both rod and cone responses, with greater rod impairment, during the acute phase of the disease (38). However, complete or almost complete ERG recovery occurred over weeks during clinical resolution of the disorder. In the same study, early receptor potential, an early ERG component due to bleaching of the photosensitive photoreceptor pigments, was assessed in two of the patients, and the R1 and R2 portions of the early receptor potential were reduced but returned to normal with clinical recovery. Based on these findings, the investigators concluded that during the acute phase of MEWDS, diffuse retinal dysfunction occurs and that both rod and cone photoreceptor pigment densities are likely to be decreased with prolonged regeneration of the light-sensitive visual pigments. Subsequent case reports of MEWDS patients during the active phase indicate that focal and multifocal ERG amplitudes are markedly reduced in the retinal area corresponding to the visual field defect and are also moderately reduced in other retinal regions (39,40). The VEP impairment in patients with MEWDS is also found and is related in part to the reduced ERG response, although optic nerve involvement such as disc edema may also be a source of VEP impairment.

During the acute phase of MEWDS, diagnosis is arrived based on clinical features and characteristic funduscopic findings. The ERG reductions may lend support to the diagnosis. However, MEWDS is much more difficult to diagnose in patients in the recovered phase. An enlarged blind spot may be present on visual field testing, but an ERG may have improved and may not necessarily be helpful. Interestingly, patients with acute idiopathic blind spot enlargement syndrome are found to have impaired ERG responses relative to the other eye, and this has led to the proposal that MEWDS and acute idiopathic blind spot enlargement syndrome may be related disorders. Further, as mentioned, Gass has proposed that MEWDS and acute idiopathic blind spot enlargement syndrome may belong to a spectrum of a single disorder encompassed by AZOOR (29). Lastly, with specialized techniques, the ERG response of the short-wavelength-sensitive cone (S-cone) system is more impaired than those of the long- and medium-wavelength-sensitive cone (L- and M-cone) systems (41).

Acute Macular Neuroretinopathy

Acute macular neuroretinopathy is a rare disorder characterized by gray to reddish brown petal-shaped macular lesions (Fig. 13.4). Visual acuity is typically reduced mildly to

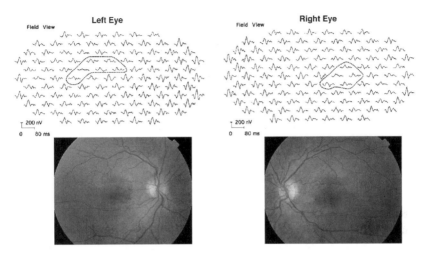

Figure 13.4 Multifocal ERG responses and retinal appearance of a 20-year-old woman with acute macular neuroretinopathy. The impaired focal responses (*circled*) correlate with the gray-reddish petal-shaped macular abnormality in each eye (*bottom left*: right eye; *bottom right*: left eye). Visual acuity was 20/20 in each eye. (Refer to the color insert.)

20/40 or better. The onset may be preceded by a flu-like illness, and similar macular lesions are encountered in some patients with multiple evanescent white-dot syndrome and acute idiopathic blind spot enlargement syndrome. Multifocal ERG identifies focal areas of retinal dysfunction (Fig. 13.4). The full-field ERG responses may be asymmetric (31).

Multifocal Choroiditis

Multifocal choroiditis is a clinical syndrome described initially by Nozik and Dorsch (42) in 1973 and is characterized by vitreous and anterior chamber inflammation and multiple chorioretinal scars similar to those of patients with presumed ocular histoplasmosis syndrome (POHS). In contrast to POHS patients, patients with multifocal choroiditis have negative histoplasmin skin test and have no calcified granulomas on chest x-ray. In addition, patients with POHS do not typically have vitreous inflammation. Other names for multifocal choroiditis include "pseudo-POHS," and "multifocal choroiditis with panuveitis."

Dreyer and Gass (43) reviewed 28 cases of multifocal choroiditis and found that female outnumbered male patients 3:1 and nearly 80% of the cases were bilateral. Multiple etiologies were likely, and occasional unilateral cases may have similar retinal appearance to diffuse unilateral subacute neuroretinitis. In the same series, 29 affected eyes of 16 patients underwent full-field ERG with 16 (55%) eyes as having normal or borderline responses. Of the remaining 13 (45%) eyes which had moderately to severely reduced responses, all except two eyes from one patient, showed both impaired rod and cone responses. EOG light-peak to dark-trough ratios appear to parallel ERG responses (43,44). The VEP has not been extensively studied but is also likely to parallel ERG responses. Of interest, acute enlargement of the blind spot may occur in multifocal choroiditis (45,46), and as mentioned, in 1993 Gass (29) proposed multifocal choroiditis may belong to a spectrum of a single disorder encompassed by AZOOR.

Punctate Inner Choroidopathy

Punctate inner choroidopathy (PIC), described by Watzke et al. (47) in 1984, is a rare disorder characterized by numerous, scattered, often macular, small discrete yellow lesions that appear to be at the level of the retinal pigment epithelium and choroid. With time, the lesions become atrophic chorioretinal scars. Other manifestations include serous retinal detachment, choroidal neovascularization, optic nerve head edema or hyperemia, and enlarged blind spot on visual field testing (48). The condition is more commonly seen in young women and is often bilateral. The cause is unknown, and prognosis is variable but generally favorable (49).

Reddy et al. (48) noted full-field ERG in the normal range in seven PIC patients, three of whom had mild asymmetry in b-wave amplitudes between the two involved eyes, correlating with differences in the number of lesions. Focal retinal dysfunction from PIC is more likely to be detectable by Multifocal ERG. Reports of EOG and VEP in PIC are very scarce.

PARANEOPLASTIC AND IMMUNE-RELATED RETINOPATHIES

Autoimmune retinopathy occurs when antibodies are produced against antigens expressed in retinal cells. Autoimmune retinopathy may occur with or without the presence of cancer. In paraneoplastic syndromes, autoimmune retinopathy is produced by the effect of immune responses initiated by antigens expressed in cancer cells. Antibodies against these antigens may recognize similar antigens expressed in normal neuronal tissue including the retina and the optic nerve. Only a small proportion of cancer patients will develop paraneoplastic syndromes associated mostly with small-cell lung carcinoma, melanoma, thymoma, breast carcinoma, colon carcinoma, breast carcinoma, prostate carcinoma, or gynecological tumors.

Cancer-Associated Retinopathy

Cancer-associated retinopathy (CAR) describes a paraneoplastic disorder that is often associated with small-cell carcinoma of the lung and characterized by antibodies against retinal cells, producing rod and cone dysfunction (50). This retinopathy may be produced by autoimmune reactions to retinal antigens including recoverin, 75-kDa heat shock cognate protein 70, and possibly enolase. The CAR associated with antirecoverin antibody is the most extensively studied. Recoverin is a 23-kDa retinal photoreceptor calcium-binding protein that regulates rhodopsin phosphorylation and is involved in light and dark adaptation (51,52). Aside from small-cell carcinoma, CAR is also rarely associated with endometrial, cervical, ovarian, and breast carcinomas.

Symptoms of CAR include bilateral diminished vision, impaired color vision, nyctalopia, and photopsias occurring over days to weeks. The symptoms may appear before or after the diagnosis of the carcinoma. Mild vitreous inflammation and retinal vascular attenuation may be evident on examination, but in the early stages, the retina may appear normal. Patients with CAR, in general, suffer progressive visual loss. Therapies such as systemic corticosteroids, intravenous immunoglobulin, and plasmophoresis have not consistently yielded favorable results.

Early in CAR, ERG is markedly impaired even when the retina appears normal and, therefore, is a key diagnostic test (Fig. 13.5). Virtually, all ERG parameters including scotopic and photopic a-wave and b-wave responses are severely diminished and prolonged early in the disease even when the retina appears normal (53,54). With further progression of the disease, the ERG responses become non-detectable. The EOG and VEP findings parallel ERG responses. For instance, pattern VEP is also severely impaired early in the disease secondary to the retinal dysfunction (53).

Recoverin-Associated Retinopathy and Autoimmune Retinopathy without Cancer

Not all patients with retinopathy associated with autoantibodies to recoverin are found to have cancer and, therefore, do not have cancer-associated retinopathy (55). Whitcup et al.

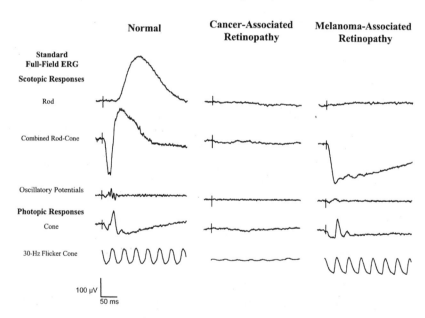

Figure 13.5 Examples of full-field ERG responses in cancer-associated retinopathy (CAR) and melanoma-associated retinopathy (MAR). The ERG responses are impaired early in CAR even when the retina appears normal. The ERG responses in MAR are similar to those of congenital stationary night blindness.

(56) reported a patient with recoverin autoantibodies with similar findings as cancer-associated retinopathy but no cancer was found after 3 years of investigation. Heckenlively et al. (57) documented antirecoverin immunoreactivity in 10 patients with retinitis pigmentosa and no systemic malignancy (57). This suggests that autoimmune retinopathy may have clinical features similar to retinitis pigmentosa or that in some retinitis pigmentosa cases, there may be an autoimmune component exacerbating the underlying disease. A diagnosis of autoimmune retinopathy without cancer should be made with caution as cancer-associated retinopathy may occur before the diagnosis of cancer, and occult malignancy may be present in patients with autoimmune retinopathy. Regardless, the ERG findings in recoverin-associated retinopathy are similar to those in cancer-associated retinopathy with early impairment of ERG components even when the retina appears normal.

Melanoma-Associated Retinopathy

Melanoma-associated retinopathy (MAR) is a paraneoplastic disorder that occurs usually in patients with an established diagnosis of cutaneous melanoma. Visual symptoms include flickering shimmering photopsias, nyctalopia, and diminished vision. The symptoms progress over months and are typically but not always associated with metastatic disease. As in cancer-associated retinopathy, the retina in MAR may have a normal appearance in the early stage of the disease.

In MAR, ERG is a key diagnostic test not only because it is impaired early in the disorder even when the retina appears normal but also because of its characteristic pattern of selective impaired b-wave (Fig. 13.5) (58–60). Patients with MAR are found to have the following on standardized full-field ERG: (1) scotopic rod flash response—reduced and prolonged, (2) scotopic combined rod–cone bright flash response—mildly reduced a-wave with a marked selective decrease in the b-wave amplitude resulting in a negative pattern (i.e., b-wave to a-wave amplitude ratio <1.0 with the peak of the b-wave not reaching baseline), (3) oscillatory potentials—reduced, (4) photopic cone flash response—normal or mildly reduced, and (5) photopic cone flicker response—normal in amplitude with or without mildly prolonged. Focal foveal ERG may be reduced and prolonged depending on foveal function (60).

Taking together, the full-field ERG responses in MAR are similar to those of congenital stationary night blindness (58). Dysfunction of the on-response in MAR has been found with specialized ERG techniques, consistent with the finding on immunofluorescence microscopy that human retinal bipolar cells are bound by labeled antibodies from serum of MAR patients, thus implicating that bipolar cells may be the targets of the paraneoplastic antibody in MAR (60,61).

CRMP-5 Paraneoplastic Retinopathy and Optic Neuropathy

Paraneoplastic autoantibody specific for type 5 collapsin response-mediator protein (CRMP-5), a neuronal cytoplasmic protein expressed in central and peripheral neurons, may be associated with bilateral vitritis, retinopathy, and optic neuropathy (62). Of the 116 CRMP-5-seropositive patients reported by Yu et al. (63), lung carcinoma, mostly small-cell, was found in 77% and thymoma in 6%. Among CRMP-5-seropositive patients, multifocal neurologic signs are common, but bilateral retinopathy and optic neuropathy may occur as the predominant features of this paraneoplastic syndrome (62). Both the scotopic and the photopic full-field ERG responses may be impaired in this condition (62).

REFERENCES

1. Algvere P. Electroretinographic studies on posterior uveitis. Acta Ophthalmol 1967; 45:299–313.

2. Cantrill HL, Ramsay RC, Knobloch WH, Purple RL. Electrophysiologic changes in chronic pars planitis. Am J Ophthalmol 1981; 91:505–512.

3. Tetuka S, Katsumi O, Mehta MC, Tetsuka H, Hirose T. Electrophysiological findings in peripheral uveitis. Ophthalmologica 1991; 203:89–98.

4. Ikeda H, Franchi A, Turner G, Shilling J, Graham E. Electroretinography and electro-oculography to localize abnormalities in early-stage inflammatory eye disease. Doc Ophthalmol 1989; 73:387–394.

5. Verity DH, Vaughan RW, Madanat W, Kondeatis E, Zureikat H, Fayyad F, Knanwati CA, Ayesh I, Stanford MR, Wallace GR. Factor V Leiden mutation is associated with ocular involvement in Behçet
    disease. Am J Ophthalmol 1999; 128:352–356.

6. Cruz RD, Adachi-Usami E, Kakisu Y. Flash electroretinogram and pattern visually-evoked cortical potentials in Behçet disease. Jpn J Ophthalmol 1990; 34:142–148.

7. Kubota Y, Kubota S. ERG of Behçet disease and its diagnostic significance. Doc Ophthalmol Proc Ser 1980; 23:91–93.

8. Adachi E, Chiba Y, Kanaizuka D, Kubota Y. The ERG in uveitis. Acta Soc Ophthalmol Jpn 1970; 74:1557–1560.

9. Kozousek V. ERG und Behçet-Uveitis. Ophthalmologica 1970; 161:196–201.

10. Hatt M, Niemeyer G. Electroretinography in connection with Behcet's disease. Graefes Arch Clin Exp Ophthalmol 1976; 198:113–120.

11. Read RW, Holland GN, Rao NA, Tabbara KF, Ohno S, Arellanes-Garcia L, Pivetti-Pezzi P, Tessler HH, Usui M. Revised diagnostic criteria for Vogt–Koyanagi–Harada disease: report of an international committee on nomenclature. Am J Ophthalmol 2001; 131:647–652.

12. Rao NA. Sympathetic ophthalmia. In: Ryan S, ed. Retina. Vol. 2. St. Louis: CV Mosby Co, 1989:715–721.

13. Fishman GA, Rabb MF, Kaplan J. Acute posterior multifocal placoid pigment epitheliopathy. Arch Ophthalmol 1974; 92:173–177.

14. Smith VC, Pokorny J, Ernest JT, Starr SJ. Visual function in acute posterior multifocal placoid pigment epitheliopathy. Am J Ophthalmol 1978; 85:192–199.

15. Vianna R, van Egmond J, Priem H, Kestelyn P. Natural history and visual outcome in patients with APMPPE. Bull Soc Belge Ophthalmol 1995; 248:73–76.

16. Chisholm IH, Gass JDM, Hutton WL. The late stage of serpiginous (geographic) choroiditis. Am J Ophthalmol 1976; 82:343–351.

17. Ryan SJ, Maumenee AE. Birdshot retinochoroidopathy. Am J Ophthalmol 1980; 89:31–45.

18. Nussenblatt RB, Mittal KK, Ryan S, Green WA, Maumenee AE. Birdshot retinochoroidopathy associated with HLA-A29 antigen and immune responsiveness to retinal S-antigen. Am J Ophthalmol 1982; 94:147–158.

19. Hirose T, Katsumi O, Pruett RC, Sakaue H, Mehta M. Retinal function in birdshot retinochoroidopathy. Acta Ophthalmol 1991; 69:327–337.

20. Fuerst DJ, Tessler HH, Fishman GA, Yokoyana MM, Wykinny GJ, Vyantas CM. Birdshot retinochoroidopathy. Arch Ophthalmol 1984; 102:214–219.

21. Kaplan HJ, Aaberg TM. Birdshot retinochoroidopathy. Am J Ophthalmol 1980; 90:773–782.

22. Priem HA, Rouck A, De Laey J-J, Bird AC. Electrophysiologic studies in birdshot chorioretinopathy. Am J Ophthalmol 1988; 106:430–436.

23. Gasch AT, Smith JA, Whitcup SM. Birdshot retinochoroidopathy. Br J Ophthalmol 1999; 83:241–249.

24. Oh KT, Christmas NJ, Folk JC. Birdshot retinochoroiditis: long term follow-up of a chronically progressive disease. Am J Ophthalmol 2002; 133:622–629.

25. Zacks DN, Samson CM, Loewenstein J, Foster CS. Electroretinograms as an indicator of disease activity in birdshot retinochoroidopathy. Graefes Arch Clin Exp Ophthalmol 2002; 240:601–607.

26. Priem HA, Oosterhuis JA. Birdshot chorioretinopathy: clinical characteristics and evolution. Br J Ophthalmol 1988; 72:646–659.

27. Gass JDM, Braunstein RA. Further observations concerning the diffuse unilateral subacute neuroretinitis syndrome. Arch Ophthalmol 1983; 101:1689–1697.

28. Gass JDM, Scelfo R. Diffuse unilateral subacute neuro-retinitis. J R Soc Med 1978; 71:95–111.

29. Gass JDM. Acute zonal occult outer retinopathy. J Clin Neuroophthalmol 1993; 13:79–97.

30. Gass JD, Agarwal A, Scott IU. Acute zonal occult outer retinopathy: a long-term follow-up study. Am J Ophthalmol 2002; 134:329–339.

31. Jacobson SG, Morales DS, Sun XK, Feuer WJ, Cideciyan AV, Gass JDM, Milam AH. Pattern of retinal dysfunction in acute zonal occult outer retinopathy. Ophthalmology 1995; 102:1187–1198.

32. Arai M, Nao-i N, Sawada A, Hayashida T. Multifocal electrore-tinogram indicates visual field loss in acute zonal occult outer retinopathy. Am J Ophthalmol 1998; 126:466–469.

33. Jampol LM, Sieving PA, Pugh D, Fishman GA, Gilbert H. Multiple evanescent white dot syndrome: I. Clinical findings. Arch Ophthalmol 1984; 102:671–674.

34. Lim JI, Kokame GT, Douglas JP. Multiple evanescent white-dot syndrome in older patients. Am J Ophthalmol 1999; 127:725–728.

35. Aaberg TM, Campo RV, Joffe L. Recurrences and bilaterality in the multiple evanescent white-dot syndrome. Am J Ophthalmol 1985; 100:29–37.

36. Hamed LM, Glaser JS, Gass JDM, Schatz NJ. Protracted enlargement of the blind spot in multiple evanescent white dot syndrome. Arch Ophthalmol 1989; 107:194–198.

37. Kimmel AS, Folk JC, Thompson HS, Strnad LS. The multiple evanescent white-dot syndrome with acute blind spot enlarge-ment. Am J Ophthalmol 1989; 107:425–426.

38. Sieving PA, Fishman GA, Jampol LM, Pugh D. Multiple eva-nescent white dot syndrome: II. Electrophysiology of the photoreceptors during retinal pigment epithelial disease. Arch Ophthalmol 1984; 102:675–679.

39. Horiguchi M, Miyake Y, Nakamura M, Fujii Y. Focal electrore-tinogram and visual field defect in multiple evanescent white dot syndrome. Br J Ophthalmol 1993; 77:452–455.

40. Huang H-J, Yamazaki H, Kawabata H, Ninomiya T, Adachi-Usami E. Multifocal electroretinogram in multiple evanescent white dot syndrome. Doc Ophthalmol 1997; 92:301–309.

41. Yamamoto S, Hayashi H, Tsuruoka M, Yamamoto T, Tsukahara I, Takeuchi S. S-cone electroretinograms in multiple evanescent white dot syndrome. Doc Ophthalmol 2003; 106:117–120.

42. Nozik RA, Dorsch W. A new chorioretinopathy associated with anterior uveitis. Arch Ophthalmol 1984; 76:758–762.

43. Dreyer RF, Gass JDM. Multifocal choroiditis and panuveitis: a syndrome that mimics ocular histoplasmosis. Arch Ophthalmol 1984; 102:1776–1784.

44. Morgan CM, Schatz H. Recurrent multifocal choroiditis. Ophthalmology 1986; 93:1138–1147.

45. Holz FG, Kim RY, Schwartz SD, Harper CA, Wroblewski HJ, Arden GB, Bird AC. Acute zonal occult outer retinopathy (AZOOR) associated with multifocal choroidopathy. Eye 1994; 8:77–83.

46. Khorram KD, Jampol LM, Rosenberg MA. Blind spot enlarge-ment as a manifestation of multifocal choroiditis. Arch Ophthalmol 1991; 109:1403–1407.

47. Watzke RC, Packer AJ, Folk JC, Benson WE, Burgess D, Ober RR. Punctate inner choroidopathy. Am J Ophthalmol 1984; 98:572–584.

48. Reddy CV, Brown J Jr, Folk JC, Kimura AE, Gupta S, Walker J. Enlarged blind spots in chorioretinal inflammatory disor-ders. Ophthalmology 1996; 103:606–617.

49. Brown JJ, Folk JC, Reddy CV, Kimura AE. Visual prognosis of multifocal choroiditis, punctate inner choroidopathy, and the diffuse subretinal fibrosis syndrome. Ophthalmology 1996; 103:1100–1105.

50. Keltner JL, Thirkill CE. Cancer-associated retinopathy vs recoverin-associated retinopathy. Am J Ophthalmol 1998; 126:296–302.

51. Maeda T, Maeda A, Maruyama I, Ogawa KI, Kuroki Y, Sahara H, Sato N, Ohguro H. Mechanisms of photoreceptor cell death in cancer-associated retinopathy. Invest Ophthalmol Vis Sci 2001; 42:705–712.

52. Thirkill CE, Tait RC, Tyler NK, Roth AM, Keltner JL. The cancer-associated retinopathy antigen is a recoverin-like protein. Invest Ophthalmol Vis Sci 1992; 33:2768–2772.

53. Matsui Y, Mehta MC, Katsumi O, Brodie SE, Hirose T. Electrophysiological findings in paraneoplastic retinopathy. Graefes Arch Clin Exp Ophthalmol 1992; 230:324–328.

54. Jacobson DM, Thirkill CE, Tipping SJ. A clinical triad to diagnose paraneoplastic retinopathy. Ann Neurol 1990; 28:162–167.

55. Mizener JB, Kimura AE, Adamus G, Thirkill CE, Goeken JA, Kardon RH. Autoimmune retinopathy in the absence of cancer. Am J Ophthalmol 1997; 123:607–618.

56. Whitcup SM, Vistica BP, Milam AH, Nussenblatt RB, Gery I. Recoverin-associated retinopathy: a clinically and immunologically distinctive disease. Am J Ophthalmol 1998; 126:230–237.

57. Heckenlively JR, Fawzi AA, Oversier JJ, Jordan BL, Aptsiauri N. Autoimmune retinopathy: patients with antirecoverin immunoreactivity and panretinal degeneration. Arch Ophthalmol 2000; 118:1525–1533.

58. Berson EL, Lessell S. Paraneoplastic night blindness with malignant melanoma. Am J Ophthalmol 1988; 106:307–311.

59. Kim RY, Retsas S, Fitzke FW, Arden GB, Bird AC. Cutaneous melanoma-associated retinopathy. Ophthalmology 1994; 101:1837–1843.

60. Potter M, Thirkill CE, Dam OM, Lee AS, Milam AH. Clinical and immunocytochemical findings in a case of melanoma-associated retinopathy. Ophthalmology 1999; 106:2121–2125.

61. Alexander KR, Fishman GA, Peachey NS, Marchese AL, Tso MO. 'On' response defect in paraneoplastic night blindness

with cutaneous malignant melanoma. Invest Ophthalmol Vis Sci 1992; 33:447–483.

62.   Cross SA, Salomao DR, Parisi JE, Bradely EA, Mines JA, Lam BL, Lennon VA. A paraneoplastic syndrome of combined optic neuritis and retinitis defined serologically by CRMP-5-IgG. Ann Neurol 2003; 54:38–50.

63.   Yu Z, Kryzer TJ, Griesmann GE, Kim K-K, Benarroch EE, Lennon VA. CRMP-5 neuronal autoantibody: marker of lung cancer and thymoma-related autoimmunity. Ann Neurol 2001; 49:146–154.

14

Ocular Vascular Disorders

The electrophysiologic findings of ocular vascular disorders caused by vascular occlusion and neovascular proliferation are summarized in this chapter. The ERG is particularly useful in determining retinal damage from vascular occlusion when acute clinical signs are no longer present (Fig. 14.1). In addition, the ERG is helpful to assess the risk of neovascular development in central retinal vein occlusion. Retinal vasculitis disorders such as Behçet disease are discussed in Chapter 13. The outline of this chapter is as follows:

Vascular occlusions:
- Ophthalmic artery occlusion
- Central retinal artery occlusion
- Branch retinal artery occlusion
- Central retinal vein occlusion
- Branch retinal vein occlusion

Other proliferative neovascular disorders:
- Retinopathy of prematurity
- Diabetes retinopathy
- Sickle cell retinopathy

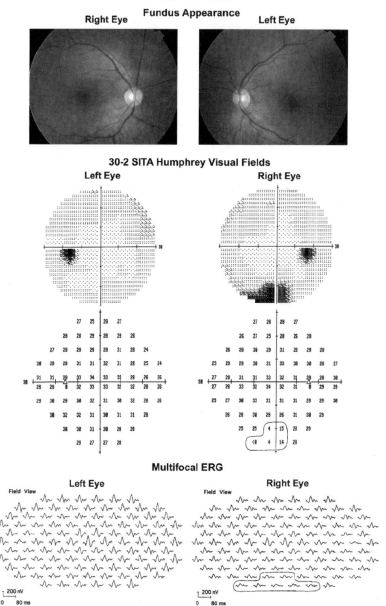

Figure 14.1 (*Caption on facing page*)

Other ocular vascular disorders:
- Hypertensive retinopathy
- Idiopathic polypoidal choroidal vasculopathy

VASCULAR OCCLUSIONS

The ophthalmic artery is a branch of the internal carotid artery and gives rise to the ciliary arteries and the central retinal artery. The ciliary arteries, in turn, give rise to the choroidal arteries and the choriocapillaris, a network of capillaries adjacent to the Bruch's membrane and the retinal pigment epithelium. The choriocapillaris supplies the retinal pigment epithelium and the outer layers of the retina including the photoreceptor layer, outer plexiform layer, and the outer portion of the inner nuclear layer (see Chapter 1). The central retinal artery, which is visible at the optic nerve head, provides circulation to the inner layers of the retina including the nerve fiber layer, ganglion cell layer, inner plexiform layer, and the inner portion of the inner nuclear layer. The venous drainage from these inner retinal layers is provided by the central retinal vein. The ERG components such as the b-wave and oscillatory potentials have their origins in the inner retinal layers and are more likely to be selectively impaired when the retinal circulation provided by the central retinal artery and vein is disrupted. In contrast, the ERG a-wave, mostly a photoreceptor response, is impaired when

Figure 14.1 (*Facing page*) Fundus photograph, visual field and multifocal ERG of a 53-year-old woman who had complete amaurosis fugax of the right eye lasting 5 min followed by almost complete recovery except for a persistent inferior area of blurred vision. Visual acuity was 20/20 in each eye and fundus appearance was normal. Visual field showed a consistent inferior defect. Multifocal ERG revealed impaired responses (*circled*) corresponding to the inferior visual field defect due to ischemic retinal damage. Further work-up with echocardiogram revealed patent foramen ovale and pulmonary hypertension as the cause of her embolic events.

choroidal circulation is compromised but is relatively spared if the retinal circulation is reduced.

Ophthalmic Artery Occlusion

Disruption of blood flow of the ophthalmic artery may occur due to atherosclerosis, thrombosis, or embolism. In addition, the ophthalmic artery is a branch of the internal carotid artery, and any significant impediment of carotid artery blood flow may produce hypoperfusion of the ophthalmic artery. Ophthalmic artery hypoperfusion, in turn, results in hypoperfusion of not only the central retinal artery supplying the inner retinal layers but also the ciliary arteries providing circulation to the choroid and the outer retinal layers. The extent of ERG findings in ophthalmic artery occlusion correlates with the degree of retinal ischemia. All components of the full-field ERG including scotopic and photopic a- and b-waves are impaired in ophthalmic artery occlusion (1). In contrast to central retinal artery or vein occlusion, a selective decrease in b-wave amplitude due to ischemia of the inner retinal layers does not typically occur in ophthalmic artery occlusion. The EOG light-peak to dark-trough ratios are usually reduced in ophthalmic artery occlusion because of ischemia to the retinal pigment epithelium and photoreceptor cells (1). The VEP findings parallel ERG responses but may be further impaired due to ischemic optic neuropathy.

Central Retinal Artery Occlusion

Clinical features of central retinal artery occlusion (CRAO) include diffuse retinal edema and the appearance of a "cherry-red spot" at the fovea. Retinal edema does not occur at the fovea where there is no ganglion cell layer and the retina is the thinnest so that the color of the choroidal circulation stands out against the surrounding edematous opaque retina. Fluorescein angiography shows absent or markedly reduced filling of the retinal arteries. Thrombosis or embolus of the central retinal artery at the laminar cribosa is often the cause of CRAO. Risk factors for CRAO include atherosclerosis, embolism from carotid intravascular plaques, diseased cardiac valves, or intracardiac deposits, and vasculitic disorders such as giant cell arteritis. With time, the central retinal artery opens or recanalizes and flow is at least partially restored, but the ischemic damage is irreversible. Visual prognosis is unfavorable with final visual acuity of 20/200 or worse in most patients. Hayreh et al. found irreversible damage to the retina of rhesus monkeys after 107 min of complete mechanical clamping of the central retinal artery but the retina recovered well after 97 min (2). Treatments include reduction of intraocular pressure to increase ocular blood perfusion by ocular massage and aqueous removal with anterior chamber paracentesis. Other treatments include inhalation of supplemental oxygen or carbogen (a mixture of increased concentration of carbon dioxide and oxygen), hyperbaric oxygen treatment, and intravenous thrombolytic medications.

The diagnosis of CRAO is by retinal appearance with fluorescein angiography support if needed. However, in a patient with a remote history of CRAO, retinal appearance may be nearly normal, and ERG is helpful in detecting retinal dysfunction. In addition, ERG can differentiate a CRAO from an ophthalmic artery occlusion. Disruption of the retinal arterial circulation from CRAO produces ischemia of the inner retinal layers whereas ophthalmic artery occlusion results in hypoperfusion of the entire retina.

Standard full-field ERG in CRAO typically reveals a selective reduction of b-wave amplitude due to ischemia of the inner retinal layers (Fig. 14.2) (3–6). The a-wave, which receives contribution from photoreceptor activity, is relatively spared in CRAO but some impairment may occur. Of interest, the photopic negative response (PhNR) of the full-field ERG is severely reduced in CRAO (7). The PhNR is a negative response occurring after the b-wave and is a measure of retinal ganglion cell function. The reduction of PhNR in CRAO implicates that the damage also involves the retinal ganglion cells and their axons in the optic nerve.

In general, patients with CRAO have the following on standard full-field ERG: (1) scotopic rod flash response—marked reduced and prolonged b-wave, (2) scotopic combined rod–cone bright flash response—normal or reduced a-wave

Central Retinal Artery Occlusion

77-Year-Old Woman

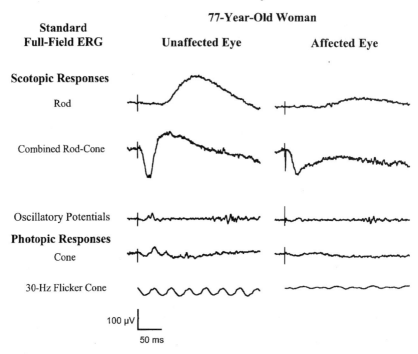

Figure 14.2 Full-field ERG responses of a 77-year-old patient with CRAO of the right eye. All responses are impaired in the affected eye with a relative selective reduction of b-wave such that the b- to a-wave amplitude ratio is less than 1 for the scotopic combined rod–cone response ("negative ERG pattern").

with normal or prolonged implicit time and a marked selective decrease in b-wave amplitude with prolonged implicit time, producing a reduced b-wave/a-wave amplitude ratio of less than 1 (negative ERG pattern), (3) oscillatory potentials—severely reduced, (4) photopic cone flash response—normal or reduced a-wave with normal or prolonged implicit time and a decrease in b-wave amplitude with prolonged implicit time, producing a reduced b-wave/a-wave amplitude ratio, and (5) photopic 30-Hz cone flicker response—reduced and prolonged b-wave.

Yotsukara and Adachi-Usami (6) documented full-field ERG improvement with scotopic combined rod–cone bright-flash response in 8 of 15 CRAO patients treated with ocular massage, intravenous urokinase, and hyperbaric oxygen. Delayed b-wave implicit times and reduced b-wave/a-wave amplitude ratios were noted in the affected eyes as compared with the unaffected eyes. Improvements of the ERG parameters correlated with visual improvement.

Branch Retinal Artery Occlusion

Branch retinal artery occlusion (BRAO) caused by embolus or thrombosis results in regional retinal edema. Intravascular embolic plaque may be visible, and fluorescein angiography typically shows reduced perfusion in the distribution of the retinal artery. Risk factors for BRAO include atherosclerosis, hematologic disorders, vasculitis, and embolism from carotid artery or diseased cardiac valves. With time, the retinal arteriole opens or recanalizes with at least partial restoration of the blood flow, but the ischemic damage is irreversible. Visual prognosis is related to macular involvement and the size of the involved retina. The diagnosis of BRAO is by retinal appearance with support from fluorescein angiography if needed. The effect of BRAO on full-field ERG is related to the size of the involved retina, and the full-field ERG may be normal or mildly impaired with a selective decrease in b-wave amplitude similar to CRAO. Multifocal ERG is more likely than full-field ERG to detect regional retinal dysfunction from BRAO and may be potentially useful in patients with a remote history of branch retinal vein occlusion (BRVO) when retinal signs are minimal (Fig. 14.3). Of interest, Hasagawa et al. (8) found that the second-order multifocal ERG response was more impaired than the first-order responses in the retinal region affected by BRAO in five patients. The authors concluded that the reduction in first- and second-order multifocal ERG responses was due to inner retinal dysfunction.

Central Retinal Vein Occlusion

Clinical features of central retinal vein occlusion (CRVO) include dilated tortuous retinal veins, scattered intraretinal

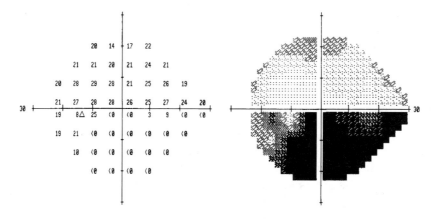

Branch Retinal Artery Occlusion

69-Year-Old Woman - Left Eye

24-2 Threshold Humphrey Visual Field

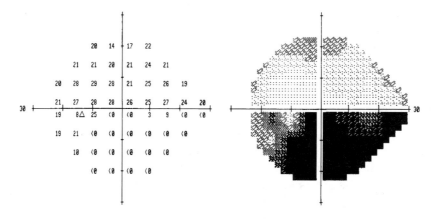

Multifocal ERG

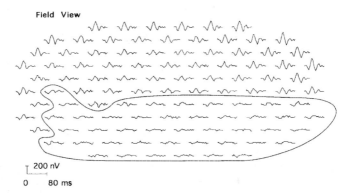

Figure 14.3 Visual field and multifocal ERG of a 69-year-old woman with a superior BRAO producing an inferior visual field defect. The area of markedly impaired multifocal ERG responses (*circled*) corresponds well to the visual field defect.

and nerve fiber layer hemorrhages, retinal edema, and optic disc edema. Physiologic mechanism of CRVO is likely related to atherosclerosis of the central retinal artery, which impinges on the adjacent central retinal vein and results in reduced venous flow with or without thrombosis. Risk factors for CRVO include hypertension, diabetes mellitus, and glaucoma.

Two types of CRVO are recognized, non-ischemic, and ischemic. Non-ischemic CRVO, also called as venous stasis retinopathy, is less severe and characterized by mild dilation and tortuosity of retinal veins with scattered retinal hemorrhages. Fluorescein angiography shows prolonged retinal venous filling with minimal areas of non-perfusion. Development of neovascularization of the anterior segment as a reaction to retinal ischemia is rare. Visual prognosis is generally favorable in non-ischemic CRVO, but some patients diagnosed initially with non-ischemic CRVO may progress to ischemic CRVO.

In contrast to non-ischemic CRVO, ischemic CRVO also called as hemorrhagic retinopathy is associated with marked retinal venous dilation and tortuosity, hemorrhages, edema, nerve fiber infarcts (cotton–wool spots) and prominent areas of capillary non-perfusion on fluorescein angiography. The risk for development of neovascularization of the anterior segment (iris and/or angle) and neovascular glaucoma is highest during the first four months after CRVO.

Neovascularization is treated with panretinal laser photocoagulation or, in severe cases, with cryotherapy or laser destruction to the ciliary body. In the past, macular edema was treated with grid laser photocoagulation but results from the Central Vein Occlusion Study (9), a multicenter randomized clinical trial, do not support this treatment. Visual prognosis is poor in ischemic CRVO.

The diagnosis of CRVO is primarily by retinal appearance with support from fluorescein angiography if needed. However, in a patient with a remote history of CRVO, the retinal signs may be minimal, consisting of only mild venous tortuosity, and ERG is helpful in diagnosing retinal ischemia.

The extent of ERG findings in CRVO correlates with the degree of retinal ischemia, and the full-field ERG may be minimally to severely impaired. In those with mild non-ischemic CRVO, the ERG responses may show amplitude loss or prolonged implicit time or both (Fig. 14.4) (10). In ischemic CRVO, both amplitude and timing are affected, and a relative selective reduction of b-wave amplitude occurs due to ischemia of the inner retinal layers (Fig. 14.5) (5). The selectively impaired b-wave is most apparent on the scotopic combined rod–cone bright flash response, and the b- to a-wave amplitude ratio may be reduced to less than 1.0 producing the so-called "negative" ERG pattern.

Predicting which CRVO patients will develop neovascularization is helpful so that panretinal laser photocoagulation is given promptly after neovascularization is detected. Prophylactic panretinal photocoagulation to all CRVO patients does not totally prevent neovascularization in some patients and is not recommended by the Central Vein Occlusion Study (11). In the same study, initial visual acuity, amount of non-perfused retina from fluorescein angiography, and the extent of retinal hemorrhage are predictors of neovascularization (12). Because none of the predictors reached

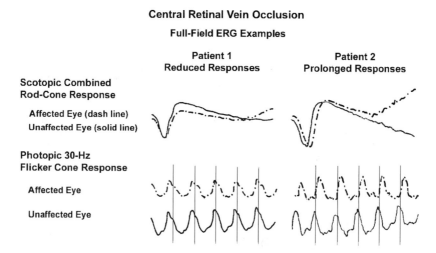

Figure 14.4 Examples of full-field ERG responses in CRVO. The degree of ERG impairment is related to the extent of retinal ischemia and ranges from minimal to severe. The responses may show amplitude loss or prolonged implicit time or both. (From Ref. 10, with permission from the American Medical Association.)

Central Retinal Vein Occlusion
Examples of Initial Full-Field ERG

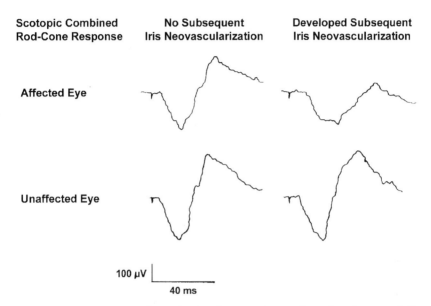

Figure 14.5 Examples of initial scotopic combined rod–cone full-field ERG responses in CRVO in patients with and without subsequent iris neovascularization. Note the greater impairment of the ERG response and the relatively selective impairment of the b-wave in the patient with subsequent iris neovascularization. Several ERG parameters have been demonstrated as predictors of iris neovascularization, including b-wave amplitude, b-wave implicit time, and b- to a-wave amplitude ratio of the scotopic combined rod–cone response as well as b-wave implicit time of the photopic 30-Hz flicker cone response. (From Ref. 22) with permission from the American Medical Association.)

100% sensitivity and specificity, the Central Vein Occlusion Study (13) recommends frequent follow-up examinations in CRVO patients, which theoretically has the potential to detect neovascularization promptly in all patients. However, patient return rate may not be 100%, and less developed health care systems may not have the resources to provide adequate number of follow-up examinations to all CRVO patients.

Other predictors of neovascularization in CRVO include the relative afferent pupillary defect and the ERG (14). Hayreh et al. (15) reported that a relative afferent pupillary defect of ≥ 0.7 log units has a sensitivity of 88% and a specificity of 90% in differentiating ischemic from non-ischemic CRVO, and scotopic or photopic bright-flash b-wave amplitudes had a sensitivity of 80–90% with a specificity of 70–80%. Larsson et al. (16) in a study of 32 CRVO patients found that iris neovascularization was predicted by fluorescein angiography in 82% of the patients and with ERG scotopic 30-Hz flicker implicit time in 94% of the patients. In addition, Matsui et al. (17) found a significant correlation between b-wave/a-wave amplitude ratio and capillary dropout on fluorescein angiography.

Full-field ERG parameters proposed for predicting neovascularization include b-wave/a-wave amplitude ratio, b-wave amplitude, b-wave implicit time, and 30-Hz photopic flicker b-wave implicit time. Additional predictive ERG parameters for neovascularization include $R_{\max}$ and $\log K$, which are derived from the intensity–response function (Naka–Rushton function fit) calculated from the b-wave amplitudes of scotopic responses with increasing stimulus intensity (see Chapter 1). The $R_{\max}$ is the maximal scotopic b-wave amplitude, and $\log K$ is an index of retinal sensitivity defined as the relative log value of the flash intensity that elicits a response of half of $R_{\max}$. Recommendations of ERG parameters for predicting neovascularization vary among studies, and this is due, in part, to the high ERG variability in CRVO as well as differences in ERG methodology among studies. Breton et al. (18) have demonstrated that the predictive power of b-wave implicit time and b-wave/a-wave amplitude ratio for iris neovascularization were influenced by stimulus intensity.

Regarding scotopic full-field ERG studies in predicting neovascularization, Sabates et al. (19) found that the mean b-wave/a-wave amplitude ratios from the scotopic combined rod–cone bright flash response were 1.67 in 27 non-ischemic CRVO patients compared to 0.70 in six ischemic CRVO patients. None of the patients with a b/a-wave ratio of greater than 1 developed neovascularization, and the b/a-wave ratio was useful to categorize "undetermined" CRVO patients into non-ischemic or ischemic CRVO. Likewise, Matsui et al. (20) found a correlation between final visual acuity and initial ERG parameters such as b-wave amplitude and b-wave/a-wave amplitude ratio in a study of 47 CRVO patients. Matsui et al. (21) also reported b-wave/a-wave amplitude ratio improvement in some CRVO patients suggesting that retinal ischemia in CRVO may be reversible in some cases. However, Kaye and Harding (22) found that the prolonged b-wave implicit time was the parameter most significantly associated with neovascularization followed by b-wave/a-wave amplitude ratio and then b-wave amplitude on 26 CRVO patients, seven of whom developed iris neovascularization. In contrast to the studies mentioned, Johnson et al. (10) in a study of 15 CRVO patients noted that all nine eyes with neo-vascularization showed prolonged scotopic a-wave, b-wave, and 30-Hz flicker b-wave responses but only one eye had a reduced b-wave/a-wave amplitude ratio that was close to or less than 1. In a later report from the same investigators, ERG retinal sensitivity ($\log K$) was found to have a sensitivity of 90% and a specificity of 91% in predicting neovascularization (23). Similarly, Moschos et al. (24) found a-wave and b-wave implicit times to be better than b-wave/a-wave amplitude ratio in predicting neovascularization. The use of scotopic 30-Hz flicker implicit time was further supported by studies by Larsson et al. (25,26). These investigators suggest that the optimal time to perform the scotopic 30-Hz flicker response to predict neovascularization may be three weeks after the onset of CRVO as there may be considerable change in ERG during the first three weeks.

Taken together, the results of these scotopic full-field ERG studies suggest that prolonged scotopic bright-flash b-wave implicit time and 30-Hz flicker b-wave implicit time may be better predictors of neovascularization than the scotopic bright-flash b-wave/a-wave amplitude ratio. Both scotopic and photopic 30-Hz bright-flash flicker elicit cone-generated responses, and the full-field ERG international standard includes a 30-Hz flicker stimulus under photopic condition.

Larsson and Andréasson (27) compared scotopic and photopic 30-Hz flicker responses as predictor for iris neovascularization in 44 CRVO patients and both 30-Hz flicker responses had high predictive value.

With respect to other full-field ERG studies with scotopic and photopic stimuli, Breton et al. (28) studied 21 CRVO patients during initial clinical visit and found that R_{max} and the scotopic bright-flash b-wave/a-wave amplitude ratio were better in predicting iris neovascularization than the retinal sensitivity ($\log K$) and 30-Hz flicker implicit time obtained after only 2–3 min of light adaptation. A later report from Breton et al. (29) on 39 CRVO patients reached similar conclusions. Roy et al. (30) noted that ERG responses to photopic red flash are also a predictor of neovascularization. Barber et al. (31) performed ERG with undilated pupils and found the photopic cone flash responses to have prolonged a-wave implicit time and reduced b-wave amplitude in 15 CRVO patients. Taken together, the results of these studies, which included photopic stimuli, suggest that photopic ERG parameters such as the photopic 30-Hz flicker are also predictors of neovascularization.

As evident by the studies mentioned, ERG impairments are common in CRVO. However, some studies have noted that a significant percentage of CRVO patients have supernormal response in the affected as well as the fellow eye (32). The reason for this finding is unclear. Sakaue et al. (33) found that 36% of the unaffected fellow eyes of 50 patients with unilateral CRVO had full-field scotopic bright flash ERG responses above the normal range with 30% having increased b-wave amplitudes and 6% with increased a-wave amplitudes. In the same study, of the 50 affected eyes with CRVO, 42% were normal, 34% had increased b-wave amplitudes and 10% had increased a-wave amplitudes. In contrast to other studies, only 14% of affected eyes had reduced ERG amplitudes. In addition, Gouras and MacKay (34) showed that eyes with CRVO had slower but larger, supernormal full-field ERG responses to long-wavelength stimulus when compared to the unaffected eye. The authors concluded that the long-wavelength cones are less able to reduce their responsiveness to light with increasing levels of light adaptation in a retina affected by CRVO.

In a preliminary study, the P1 amplitudes and latencies of the first-order multifocal ERG response correlated significantly with the full-field 30-Hz cone flicker amplitudes and latencies (35). The authors concluded that wide-field multifocal ERG is a sensitive indicator of disease in CRVO and may potentially have a role in the clinical setting.

Electro-oculogram generally parallels ERG response in CRVO although patients with reduced EOG light-peak/dark-trough amplitude ratio and normal full-field ERG have been reported (36,37). Ohn et al. (37) performed EOG and full-field ERG on 24 CRVO patients, 13 of whom had ischemic CRVO. The mean EOG ratio for patients with ischemic and non-ischemic CRVO were 1.38 ± 0.38 (standard deviation) and 1.92 ± 0.43, respectively (normal ≥ 1.85), and this difference was statistically significant. However, the sensitivity and specificity for differentiating ischemic from non-ischemic CRVO based on EOG was only 92% and 55%, respectively. Papakostopoulos et al. (38) in a study of 28 CRVO patients noted that EOG light-peak amplitude in the affected eyes was 48% or less than that of the unaffected eye in the eight patients who developed iris neovascularization. Pattern ERG is a measure of ganglion cell function and is reduced in CRVO (14). The VEP in CRVO parallels ERG function.

Branch Retinal Vein Occlusion

Branch retinal vein occlusion usually occurs at an arteriovenous intersection. Signs of the vein occlusion such as scattered retinal hemorrhages, edema, and venous tortuosity are visible in the region distal to the site of the occlusion. Risk factors for BRVO are similar to CRVO and include hypertension and diabetes mellitus. In contrast to CRVO, neovascularization of the retina or optic nerve head may occur but iris neovascularization is rare. Visual prognosis is dependent on the extent of retinal ischemia and macular involvement. The diagnosis of BRVO is by retinal appearance with support from fluorescein angiography if needed.

Multifocal ERG is more likely than full-field ERG to detect regional retinal dysfunction from BRVO and may be potentially useful in patients with a remote history of BRVO when retinal signs are minimal. In contrast, the effect of BRVO on full-field ERG is related to the size of the involved retina, and the full-field ERG in BRVO may be normal or mildly impaired with a selective decrease in b-wave amplitude similar to CRVO. Of interest, Hara and Miura (39) noted full-field ERG oscillatory potentials to be reduced in the affected eyes of 34 unilateral BRVO patients presumably due to inner retinal ischemia. In the same study, the EOG light-peak to dark-trough amplitude ratios and the light-peak amplitudes were significantly reduced in the affected eye compared to the unaffected eye. The investigators hypothesized that the EOG impairment was due to inner retina dysfunction that hampered the EOG amplitude rise to light. Lastly, Gündüz et al. (40) found pattern ERG and VEP to be impaired in BRVO patients without systemic disease and attributed these findings to retinal dysfunction.

OTHER PROLIFERATIVE NEOVASCULAR DISORDERS

Retinopathy of Prematurity

Retinopathy of prematurity (ROP) is a retinal vascular proliferative disease of premature and low-birth-weight infants. Fetal retinal vascularization occurs from the optic nerve head toward the peripheral retina and is completed at approximately 36 and 40 weeks of gestation in the nasal and temporal retinal regions, respectively. The severity of ROP is categorized into five stages: stage 1—demarcation line between vascularized and non-vascularized retina, stage 2—raised demarcation line forming a ridge, stage 3—extraretinal fibrovascular proliferation of the ridge, stage 4—subtotal retinal detachment, and stage 5—total funnel-shaped retinal detachment. The diagnosis of ROP is by retinal appearance. Treatments include laser or cryotherapy to the non-vascularized retina. Flash VEP may be helpful as objective evidence of

visual function in infants with stage 5 ROP. Clarkson et al.
(41) advocated bright-flash VEP and ocular ultrasound to
evaluate stage 5 ROP infants before and after retinal reattachment surgery. Eyes with regressed ROP are more likely
to develop delayed retinal detachment, cataract, glaucoma,
strabismus, anisometropia, amblyopia, and myopia.

Using a-wave amplitudes of scotopic full-field ERG
responses from increasing stimulus intensity to estimate the
saturated maximal rod response amplitude (R_{mp3}) (see
Chapter 1), Fulton and Hansen (42) reported mild photoreceptor dysfunction in five infants and children with complete
regression of previous mild ROP. The same investigators also
noted reduced oscillatory potentials in nine infants and
children with previous stage 1, 2, or 3 ROP.

Diabetes Retinopathy

Diabetic retinopathy is one of the leading causes of visual
impairment and blindness worldwide. Two forms of diabetes
are recognized. Type 1 diabetes, also called juvenile-onset or
insulin-dependent diabetes, is characterized by pancreatic
beta-cell destruction leading to absolute insulin deficiency.
Type 2 diabetes, also called adult-onset or non-insulin-
dependent diabetes, is characterized by insulin resistance
with insulin secretory defect and relative insulin deficiency.
Type 2 diabetes is more common and makes up approximately
90% of diabetic patients. However, patients with type 1 diabetes are more likely to develop severe diabetic retinopathy.
The risk of developing diabetic retinopathy is related to duration of the disease, and nearly all patients with diabetes for
more than 20 years will have some degree of retinopathy. Diabetic retinopathy is categorized into non-proliferative or proliferative stages. In the mild to moderate non-proliferative
stage, previously called background retinopathy, retinal
findings include small intraretinal hemorrhages and
microaneurysms. In the severe non-proliferative stage,
previously called preproliferative retinopathy, signs of
increasing ischemia such as severe intraretinal hemorrhages,
microaneurysms, venous abnormalities, and intraretinal

microvascular abnormalities occur. In proliferative diabetic retinopathy, retinal neovascularization in response to ischemia takes place, which if left untreated may progress to vitreous hemorrhage, fibrovascular formation, and retinal detachment. Diabetic macular edema due to microvascular disease is also a major cause of visual impairment and may occur with non-proliferative or proliferative retinopathy.

Clinical electrophysiologic testing of patients with diabetic retinopathy is not commonly performed because of the reliance by most clinicians on retinal appearance. However, ERG abnormalities occur early in the disease even in the absence of any visible retinopathy, indicating that the ERG is a sensitive indicator of mild disturbance of retinal circulation. Reduced and delayed oscillatory potentials without any impairment of the a-wave and b-wave amplitudes may occur in diabetic patients with early or no retinopathy, with the most consistent finding being an increase in the implicit time of the first oscillatory potential wavelet (OP_1) presumably due to early, mild ischemia of the inner retinal layers (44–47). Aside from impaired oscillatory potentials, other less consistent full-field ERG abnormalities found in diabetic patients without visible retinopathy include prolonged b-wave implicit times and reduced scotopic b-wave amplitude, with the latter observed in type 1 diabetic children (46,48). Likewise, multifocal ERG of diabetic patients without visible retinopathy showed prolonged oscillatory potentials and delayed first-order responses (49,50). Amplitude reduction of the second-order multifocal ERG components was also noted (51).

Clinical ERG testing in diabetic patients to assess the risk of progression to proliferative retinopathy is seldom performed because of the reliance on retinal appearance and fluorescein angiographic examinations. However, Bresnick et al. (52–54) examined the predictive value of full-field ERG findings for progression to proliferative diabetic retinopathy in 85 patients in the Early Treatment Diabetic Retinopathy Study. The investigators showed that the summed amplitudes of the oscillatory potentials, the overall severity of retinopathy, and the severity of fluorescein angiographic leakage were independent predictors of progression to severe proliferative retinopathy. Similarly, in another longitudinal study, Simonsen (55) found that low oscillatory potential amplitudes were a predictive factor in the development of proliferative diabetic retinopathy.

With progression of diabetic retinopathy, all ERG parameters including scotopic and photopic a-wave and b-wave responses become impaired due to retinal ischemia, vitreous hemorrhage, and retinal detachment (51,56). In patients with mild to moderate non-proliferative retinopathy, scotopic and photopic b-waves are impaired in addition to impaired oscillatory potentials (57). In proliferative diabetic retinopathy, the ERG reductions are variable and dependent on the degree of microvascular damage and the presence of complications such as vitreous hemorrhage and retinal detachment.

Several studies have examined the effect of panretinal photocoagulation on ERG. Lawwill and O'Connor (58) performed ERG and EOG on diabetic patients before and after photocoagulation and noted a 10% decrease in a- and b-wave amplitudes when approximately 20% of the retina was photocoagulated. However, Ogden et al. (59) found that a decrease of ERG amplitude varied from 10% to 95% after photocoagulation. These conflicting results were clarified by Wepman et al. (60) who found a correlation between b-wave amplitude reduction and area of photocoagulated retina, but this relationship was evident only after the magnitude of the ERG response prior to treatment was taken into account. Patients with larger pretreatment amplitudes showed a greater amplitude reduction than patients with small pretreatment signals even though they had equivalent amounts of retina destroyed, because laser destruction of functionally active retina would result in a greater net reduction of ERG after treatment.

Diabetic macular edema may produce focal ERG impairment but by itself is unlikely to reduce full-field ERG responses significantly. Greenstein et al. (61,62) evaluated 11 patients with multifocal ERG before and after laser treatment for clinically significant diabetic macular edema. Their findings suggest that local ERG timing delays were not good predictors of visual field deficits and that focal laser treatment produced increases in implicit time and decreases in amplitude of local ERG responses which were not restricted to the treated macular area.

In terms of other electrophysiologic testing, pattern ERG studies in diabetic patients without apparent retinopathy have mixed results due in part to differences in technique among studies (46). In patients with non-proliferative diabetic retinopathy, most pattern ERG studies have reported decrease in amplitude and delay in implicit time (46). Lastly, VEP may be helpful to predict final visual acuity in diabetic eyes with vitreous hemorrhage when retinal appearance is obscured (63).

Sickle Cell Retinopathy

Hereditary hemoglobulinopathies occur when mutant hemoglobins (Hgb) S and C are inherited rather than normal hemoglobin A, resulting in sickle trait (Hgb AS), sickle cell disease (Hgb SS), and hemoglobin SC disease. Intravascular sickling of red blood cells, hemolysis, and thrombosis can produce preretinal, intraretinal and subretinal hemorrhages and peripheral retinal neovascularization leading to retinal detachment. Sickle cell disease is most common in blacks. The diagnosis of sickle cell retinopathy is by retinal appearance and hemoglobulin electrophoresis if not yet performed.

Peachey et al. (64) noted normal full-field ERG responses in sickle cell disease patients without retinal neovascularization. Patients with neovascularization were found to have generalized reduced ERG components including a-wave, b-wave, and oscillatory amplitudes, presumably due to ischemia. In a later study of 44 patients with sickle cell retinopathy from the same research group, a correlation between ERG amplitude measures and capillary non-perfusion determined by fluorescein angiography was documented (65). In the same study, the maximal scotopic b-wave amplitude, R_{max}, derived from the intensity–response function (Naka–Rushton function fit) (see Chapter 1), was also reduced but the retinal sensitivity, $\log K$, defined as the flash intensity that elicits a response of half of R_{max}, was unaffected in sickle cell disease patients. The findings of EOG and VEP in sickle cell disease are rarely reported. The EOG is likely to parallel ERG responses, and VEP is likely to parallel macular function.

OTHER OCULAR VASCULAR DISORDERS

Hypertensive Retinopathy

Chronic systemic arterial hypertension produces atherosclerosis and increased vascular permeability and is a major cause of coronary arterial disease, cerebral arterial occlusion, and renal failure. A systolic blood pressure of greater than 130 mm Hg and a diastolic blood pressure of greater than 85 mm Hg on two or more clinical visits are considered elevated. Hypertension is classified as stage 1 (140–159/90–99, systolic/diastolic), stage 2 (160–179/100–109), stage 3 (180–209/110–119), and stage 4 ($\geq$210/$\geq$120). In over 90% of patients, the cause is unknown, and the patients are diagnosed with primary or essential hypertension. In the remaining patients, secondary hypertension results from disorders including renal vascular disease, aortic coarctation, Cushing's disease, and pheochromocytoma.

Hypertension may cause retinopathy, choroidopathy, and optic neuropathy. Retinal signs of hypertension include arteriolar narrowing, arteriovenous crossing changes (arteriovenous nicking), arteriolar sclerosis, arteriolar tortuosity, hemorrhages, exudates, inner retinal infarcts (cotton–wool spots), and retinal edema. Hypertensive retinopathy may be categorized by Scheie's classification. Grade I retinopathy has visible arteriolar narrowing; grade II retinopathy has arteriolar narrowing plus focal arteriolar abnormalities and arteriolar sclerosis; grade III has grade II findings plus retinal hemorrhages and exudates; and Grade IV has grade III findings plus optic disc edema. Findings of hypertensive choroidopathy include retinal pigment epithelium and choroidal infarcts (Elschnig spots), subretinal exudates, serous retinal detachments, and choroidal sclerosis. Optic disc edema may be associated with hypertensive retinopathy or occur due to anterior ischemic optic neuropathy. The diagnosis of hypertensive retinopathy and choroidopathy is based on clinical examination, blood pressure measurement, and a history of hypertension. Treatment is control of the hypertension.

Clinical electrophysiologic testing of patients with hypertensive retinopathy is seldom performed because of the reliance by most clinicians on retinal appearance. However, similar to diabetic retinopathy, reduced and delayed oscillatory potentials without any impairment of the a-wave and b-wave amplitudes on full-field ERG may occur in hypertensive patients with early or no retinopathy, indicating that the ERG is a sensitive indicator of mild disturbance of retinal circulation. Eichler et al. (66) found prolonged and reduced oscillatory potential wavelets in patients with mild hypertension and grade I hypertensive retinopathy. Likewise, Müller et al. (67) noted reduced oscillatory potential wavelets O_2 and O_4 in 24 patients with hypertension of more than 10 years with grade I or grade II hypertensive retinopathy. Further, Rivalico et al. (68) performed full-field ERG performed initially and repeated after a mean period of eight months after treatment in 24 patients with untreated stage 1 hypertension and early or no hypertensive retinopathy. Increased systolic blood pressure correlated with reduced sum of the amplitudes of oscillatory potential wavelets O_1, O_2, and O_3. After instituting medical antihypertensive therapy, oscillatory potential amplitudes did not improve significantly except in patients treated with angiotensin-converting enzyme inhibitors, presumably because of the vasodilation effects of the medications that may have increased retinal blood flow (69). Of note, Henkes and van der Kam (70) reported generalized supernormal full-field ERG responses in hypertensive patients without retinopathy, but this finding is not well studied by others.

With progression of hypertensive retinopathy, other ERG parameters including scotopic and photopic a-wave and b-wave responses become impaired due to retinal and choroidal ischemia. Talks et al. (71) performed full-field ERG and pattern VEP in 34 patients with grade III or grade IV hypertensive retinopathy. Analysis of the ERG a-wave was not reported, but the b-wave was significantly reduced and prolonged in all patients and the impairment persisted in the 12 patients who had 2–4 years of follow up. In the same study, pattern VEP was significantly reduced and prolonged due to the retinopathy and anterior ischemic optic neuropathy if present. EOG light-peak to dark-trough amplitude ratio is reduced in some patients with hypertensive retinopathy, and EOG impairment is likely to parallel the degree of retinal and choroidal ischemia (72).

Idiopathic Polypoidal Choroidal Vasculopathy

Idiopathic polypoidal choroidal vasculopathy is a rare disorder characterized by polypoidal-shaped choroidal vascular lesions (73). The recognition of these particular lesions is enhanced by fluorescein or indocyanine green angiography. The orange subretinal lesions are variable in size and appear to be polypoidal dilations arising from a choroidal vascular network. Peripapillary lesions are common but macular lesions have also been described (74). Serosanguineous detachment of the retinal pigment epithelium may occur over the choroidal lesion. Other names for the disorder include posterior uveal bleeding syndrome and multiple recurrent serosanguineous retinal pigment epithelial detachment syndrome. Affected persons have a female to male ratio of about 5:1, and most cases are bilateral. The disease tends to affect pigmented individuals with blacks at the greatest risk in the United States. Decreased vision is the most common symptom.

Reports of electrophysiologic findings in idiopathic polypoidal choroidal vasculopathy are extremely scarce. In theory, multifocal ERG is more likely to detect localized areas of retinal dysfunction (than full-field ERG), and the VEP is likely to parallel ERG and macular function.

REFERENCES

1. Ulrich WD, Ulrich CH, Kästner R, Reimann J. ERG and EOG in carotid artery occlusion disease. Doc Ophthal Proc Ser 1980; 23:49–55.

2. Hayreh SS, Kolder HE, Weingeist TA. Central retinal artery occlusion and retinal tolerance time. Ophthalmology 1980; 87: 75–78.

3. Flower RW, Speros P, Kenyon KR. Electroretinographic changes and choroidal defects in a case of central retinal artery occlusion. Am J Ophthalmol 1977; 83:451–459.

4. Henkes HE. Electroretinography in circulatory disturbances of the retina: electroretinogram in cases of occlusion of the central retinal artery. Arch Ophthalmol 1954; 51:42–53.

5. Karpe G, Uchermann A. The clinical electroretinogram, VII: the electroretinogram in circulatory disturbances of the retina. Acta Ophthalmol 1955; 33:492–516.

6. Yotsukara J, Adachi-Usami E. Correlation of electroretinographic changes with visual prognosis in central retinal artery occlusion. Ophthalmologica 1993; 207:13–18.

7. Machida S, Gotoh Y, Tanaka M, Tazawa Y. Predominant loss of the photopic negative response in central retinal artery occlusion. Am J Ophthalmol 2004; 137:938–940.

8. Hasagawa S, Ohshima A, Hayakawa Y, Takagi M, Abe H. Multifocal electroretinograms in patients with branch retinal artery occlusion. Invest Ophthalmol Vision Sci 2001; 42: 298–304.

9. The Central Vein Occlusion Study Group. Evaluation of grid pattern photocoagulation for macular edema in central vein occlusion. The Central Vein Occlusion Study Group M Report. Ophthalmology 1996; 102:1425–1433.

10. Johnson MA, Marcus S, Elman MJ, McPhee TJ. Neovascularization in central retinal vein occlusion: electroretinographic findings. Arch Ophthalmol 1988; 106:348–352.

11. The Central Vein Occlusion Study Group. A randomized clinical trial of early panretinal photocoagulation for ischemic central vein occlusion. The Central Vein Occlusion Study Group N report. Ophthalmology 1995; 102:1434–1444.

12. The Central Vein Occlusion Study Group. Natural history and clinical management of central retinal vein occlusion. The Central Vein Occlusion Study Group. Arch Ophthalmol 1997; 115:486–491.

13. The Central Vein Occlusion Study Group. Baseline and early natural history report. The Central Vein Occlusion Study. Arch Ophthalmol 1993; 111:1087–1095.

14. Morrell AJ, Thompson DA, Gibson JM, Kritzinger EE, Drasdo N. Electroretinography as a prognostic indicator for neovascularisation in CRVO. Eye 1991; 5:362–368.

15. Hayreh SS, Klugman MR, Podhajsky P, Kolder HE. Electroretinography in central retinal vein occlusion. Correlation of electroretinographic changes with pupillary abnormalities. Graefes Arch Clin Exp Ophthalmol 1989; 227:549–561.

16. Larsson J, Bauer B, Cavalin-Sjöberg U, Andréasson S. Fluorescein angiography versus ERG for predicting the prognosis in central retinal vein occlusion. Acta Ophthalmol 1998; 76:456–460.

17. Matsui Y, Katsumi O, Mehta M, Hirose T. Correlation of electroretinographic and fluorescein angiographic findings in unilateral central retinal vein obstruction. Graefes Arch Clin Exp Ophthalmol 1994; 232:449–457.

18. Breton ME, Schueller AW, Montzka DP. Electroretinogram b-wave implicit time and b/a wave ratio as a function of intensity in central retinal vein occlusion. Ophthalmology 1991; 98:1845–1853.

19. Sabates R, Hirose T, McMeel JW. Electroretinography in the prognosis and classification of central retinal vein occlusion. Arch Ophthalmol 1983; 101:232–235.

20. Matsui Y, Katsumi O, McMeel JW, Hirose T. Prognostic value of initial electroretinogram in central retinal vein obstruction. Graefes Arch Clin Exp Ophthalmol 1994; 232:75–81.

21. Matsui Y, Katsumi O, Hiroshi S, Hirose T. Electroretinogram b/a wave ratio improvement in central retinal vein obstruction. Br J Ophthalmol 1994; 78:191–198.

22. Kaye SB, Harding PS. Electroretinography in unilateral central retinal vein occlusion as a predictor of rubeosis iridis. Arch Ophthalmol 1988; 106:353–356.

23. Johnson MA, McPhee TJ. Electroretinographic findings in iris neovascularization due to acute central retinal vein occlusion. Arch Ophthalmol 1993; 111:806–814.

24. Moschos M, Brouzas D, Moschou M, Theodossiadis G. The a- and b-wave latencies as a prognostic indicator of neovascularization in central retinal vein occlusion. Doc Ophthalmol 1999; 99:123–133.

25. Larsson J, Andreasson S, Bauer B. Cone b-wave implicit time as an early predictor of rubeosis in central retinal vein occlusion. Am J Ophthalmol 1998; 125:247–249.

26. Larsson J, Bauer B, Andréasson S. The 30-Hz flicker cone ERG for monitoring the early course of central retinal vein occlusion. Acta Ophthalmol 2000; 78:187–190.

27. Larsson J, Andréasson S. Photopic 30 Hz flicker ERG as a predictor for rubeosis in central retinal vein occlusion. Br J Ophthalmol 2001; 85:683–685.

28. Breton ME, Quinn GE, Keene SS, Dahmen JC, Brucker AJ. Electroretinogram parameters at presentation as predictors of rubeosis in central retinal vein occlusion patients. Ophthalmology 1989; 96:1343–1352.

29. Breton ME, Montzka DP, Brucker AJ, Quinn GE. Electroretinogram interpretation in central retinal vein occlusion. Ophthalmology 1991; 98:1837–1844.

30. Roy MS, Mackay CJ, Gouras P. Cone ERG subnormality to red flash in central retinal vein occlusion: a predictor of ocular neovascularization. Eye 1997; 11:335–341.

31. Barber C, Galloway N, Reacher M, Salem H. The role of electroretinogram in the management of central retinal vein occlusion. Doc Ophthalmol Proc Ser 1984; 40:348–352.

32. Henkes HE. Electroretinogram in circulatory disturbances of the retina, I: electroretinogram in cases of occlusion of the central retinal vein or one of its branches. Arch Ophthalmol 1953; 49:190–201.

33. Sakaue H, Katsumi O, Hirose T. Electroretinographic findings in fellow eyes of patients with central retinal vein occlusion. Arch Ophthalmol 1989; 107:1459–1462.

34. Gouras P, MacKay CJ. Supernormal cone electroretinograms in central retinal vein occlusion. Invest Ophthalmol Vision Sci 1992; 33:508–515.

35. Dolan FM, Parks S, Keating D, Dutton GN, Evans AL. Multi-focal electroretinographic features of central retinal vein occlusion. Invest Ophthalmol Vision Sci 2003; 44:4954–4959.

36. Carr RE, Siegel IM. Electrophysiologic aspects of several retinal diseases. Am J Ophthalmol 1964; 58:95–107.

37. Ohn Y-H, Katsumi O, Kruger-Leite E, Larson EW, Hirose T. Electrooculogram in central retinal vein obstruction. Ophthalmologica 1991; 203:189–195.

38. Papakostopoulos D, Bloom PA, Grey RHB, Hart JDH. The electro-oculogram in central retinal vein occlusion. Br J Ophthalmol 1992; 76:515–519.

39. Hara A, Miura M. Decreased inner retinal activity in branch retinal vein occlusion. Doc Ophthalmol 1994; 88:39–47.

40. Gündüz K, Zengin N, Okuda S, Okka M, Özbayrak N. Pattern-reversal electroretinograms and visual evoked potentials in branch retinal vein occlusion. Doc Ophthalmol 1996; 91:155–164.

41. Clarkson JG, Jacobson SG, Frazier-Byrne S, Flynn JT. Evaluation of eyes with stage-5 retinopathy of prematurity. Graefes Arch Clin Exp Ophthalmol 1989; 227:332–334.

42. Fulton AB, Hansen RM. Photoreceptor function in infants and children with a history of mild retinopathy of prematurity. J Opt Soc Am 1996; 13:566–571.

43. Fulton AB, Hansen RM. Electroretinogram responses and refractive errors in patients with a history of retinopathy of prematurity. Doc Ophthalmol 1995; 91:87–100.

44. Bresnick GH, Palta M. Temporal aspects of the electroretinogram in diabetic retinopathy. Arch Ophthalmol 1987; 105:660–664.

45. Shirao Y, Okumura T, Ohta T, Kawasaki K. Clinical importance of electroretinographic oscillatory potentials in early detection and objective evaluation for diabetic retinopathy. Clin Vision Sci 1991; 6:445–450.

46. Tzekov E, Arden GB. The electroretinogram in diabetic retinopathy. Surv Ophthalmol 1999; 44:53–60.

47. Yonemura D, Kawasaki K, Okumua T. Early deterioration in the temporal aspect of the human electroretinogram in diabetes mellitus. Folia Ophthalmol Jpn 1977; 28:379–388.

48. Chung NH, Kim SH, Kwak MS. The electroretinogram sensivity in patients with diabetes. Korean J Ophthalmol 1993; 7: 43–47.

49. Fortune B, Schneck ME, Adams AJ. Multifocal electroretinogram delays reveal local retinal dysfunction in early diabetic retinopathy. Invest Ophthalmol Vision Sci 1999; 40:2638–2651.

50. Kurtenbach A, Langrova H, Zrenner E. Multifocal oscillatory potentials in type 1 diabetes without retinopathy. Invest Ophthalmol Vision Sci 2000; 41:3234–3241.

51. Palmowski AM, Sutter EE, Bearse MA, Fung W. Mapping of retinal function in diabetic retinopathy using the multifocal electroretinogram. Invest Ophthalmol Vision Sci 1997; 38:2586–2596.

52. Bresnick GH, Korth K, Groo A, Palta M. Electroretinographic oscillatory potentials predict progression of diabetic retinopathy: preliminary report. Arch Ophthalmol 1984; 102:1307–1311.

53. Bresnick GH, Palta M. Oscillatory potential amplitudes relation to severity of diabetic retinopathy. Arch Ophthalmol 1987; 105:929–933.

54. Bresnick GH, Palta M. Predicting progression to severe proliferative diabetic retinopathy. Arch Ophthalmol 1987; 105:810–814.

55. Simonsen SE. The value of oscillatory potential in selecting juvenile diabetics at risk of developing proliferative retinopathy. Acta Ophthalmol 1980; 58:403.

56. Kim S-H, Lee S-H, Bae J-Y, Cho J-H, Kang Y-S. Electroretinographic evaluation in adult diabetes. Doc Ophthalmol 1998; 94:201–213.

57. Holopigian K, Seiple W, Lorenzo M, Carr R. A comparison of photopic and scotopic electroretinographic changes in early diabetic retinopathy. Invest Ophthalmol Vision Sci 1992; 33:2773–2780.

58. Lawwill T, O'Connor PR. ERG and EOG in diabetes pre- and post- photocoagulation. Doc Ophthal Proc Ser 1972; 2:17–23.

59. Ogden TE, Callahan F, Riekhof FT. The electroretinogram after peripheral retinal ablation in diabetic retinopathy. Am J Ophthalmol 1976; 81:397–402.

60. Wepman B, Sokol S, Price J. The effects of photocoagulation on the electroretinogram and dark adaptation in diabetic retinopathy. Doc Ophthal Proc Ser 1977; 13:139–147.

61. Greenstein VC, Chen H, Hood DC, Holopigian K, Seiple W, Carr RE. Retinal function in diabetic macular edema after focal laser photocoagulation. Invest Ophthalmol Vision Sci 2000; 41:3655–3664.

62. Greenstein VC, Holopigian K, Hood DC, Seiple W, Carr RE. The nature and extent of retinal dysfunction associated with diabetic macular edema. Invest Ophthalmol Vision Sci 2000; 41:3643–3654.

63. Vadrevu VL, Cavender S, Odom JV. Use of 10-Hz flash visual evoked potentials in prediction of final visual acuity in diabetic eyes with vitreous hemorrhage. Doc Ophthalmol 1992; 79: 371–382.

64. Peachey NS, Charles HC, Lee CM, Fishman GA, Cunba-Vaz JG, Smith RT. Electroretinographic findings in sickle cell retinopathy. Arch Ophthalmol 1987; 105:934–938.

65. Peachey NS, Gagliano DA, Jacobson MS, Derlacki DJ, Fishman GA, Cohen SB. Correlation of electroretinographic findings and peripheral retinal nonperfusion in patients with sickle cell retinopathy. Arch Ophthalmol 1990; 108:1106–1109.

66. Eichler J, Stave J, Bohm J. Oscillatory potentials in hypertensive retinopathy. Doc Ophthal Proc Ser 1984; 40:161–165.

67. Müller W, Gaub J, Spittel U, Dück K-H. Oscillatory potentials in cases of systemic hypertension. Doc Ophthal Proc Ser 1984; 40:167–171.

68. Ravalico G, Rinoldi G, Solimano N, Bellini G, Cosenzi A, Sacerdote A, Bocin E. Oscillatory potentials in subjects with treated hypertension. Ophthalmologica 1995; 209:187–189.

69. Ravalico G, Rinoldi G, Solimano N, Bellini G, Cosenzi A, Bocin E. Oscillatory potentials of the electroretinogram in hypertensive patients with different antihypertensive treatment. Doc Ophthalmol 1998; 94:321–326.

70. Henkes HE, van der Kam JP. Electroretinographic studies in general hypertension and in arteriosclerosis. Angiology 1954; 5:49–58.

71. Talks SJ, Good P, Clough CG, Beevers DG, Dodson PM. The acute and long-term ocular effects of accelerated hypertension: a clinical and electrophysiological study. Eye 1996; 10:321–327.

72. Ashworth B. The electro-oculogram in disorders of the retinal circulation. Am J Ophthalmol 1966; 61:505–508.

73. Yannuzzi LA, Ciardella A, Spaide RF, Rabb M, Freund B, Orlock DA. The expanding clinical spectrum of idiopathic polypoidal choroidal vasculopathy. Arch Ophthalmol 1997; 115:478–485.

74. Moorthy RS, Lyon AT, Rabb MF, Spaide RF, Yannuzzi LA, Jampol LM. Idiopathic polypoidal choroidal vasculopathy of the macula. Ophthalmology 1998; 105:1380–1385.

15

Nutritional, Toxic, and Pharmacologic Effects

The retina and the optic nerve are susceptible to numerous nutritional deficiencies, toxicities, and pharmacologic effects. The electrophysiologic findings of the more commonly encountered conditions in this group of disorders are discussed in this chapter, and electrophysiologic testing is of value in some of these conditions. The topics covered are:

- Vitamin A deficiency
- Nutritional optic neuropathy
- Metallic intraocular foreign bodies—ocular siderosis
- Methanol poisoning
- Synthetic retinoids—isotretinoin (Accutane®)
- Chloroquine/hydroxychloroquine
- Thioridazine (Mellaril®), chlorpromazine, and other phenothiazines
- Quinine
- Deferoxamine (Desferrioxamine®)
- Vigabatrin
- Sildenafil (Viagra®)

- Gentamicin
- Ethambutol
- Cisplatin
- Indomethacin

VITAMIN A DEFICIENCY

Vitamin A is a fat-soluble vitamin that is absorbed by the small intestine and transported to the liver where it is stored as vitamin A ester. Vitamin A is delivered to the target tissues by retinol binding protein, a transport protein produced by the liver, as vitamin A alcohol (retinol). In the retina, retinol is stored in the retinal pigment epithelium and enters the outer segments of the photoreceptors as 11-cis retinol where it is transformed to 11-cis retinaldehyde (retinal) and combined with the protein opsin to form the light sensitive rhodopsin. Therefore, vitamin A deficiency may arise from inadequate nutritional intake, poor intestinal absorption, impaired liver storage, ineffective retinol binding protein transport, or impaired conversion of retinol to retinaldehyde.

Children are especially susceptible to vitamin A deficiency from malnutrition, and the major cause of blindness in children worldwide is xerophthalmia due to vitamin A deficiency (1). Night vision impairment from retinal dysfunction in affected individuals is common. The reason why certain persons are affected in impoverished communities while the majority is spared remains unclear, and the condition is often accompanied by generalized malnutrition with multiple dietary deficiencies.

In developed countries, vitamin A deficiency from malnutrition is extremely rare, and the condition occurs most commonly from poor intestinal absorption (e.g., congenital or post-surgical short bowel syndrome and Crohn's disease) and liver dysfunction (e.g., alcoholism, liver failure). In some cases, treatment with oral vitamin A supplements may be ineffective and intravenous treatment is necessary.

In the 1950s, Dhanda (2) using early ERG techniques in India found reduced and non-detectable ERG responses in

patients with xerophthalmia and night blindness due to vitamin A deficiency. After oral vitamin A, the night blindness
resolved rapidly with ERG responses returning to normal at
a slower rate. The xerosis patches, on the other hand, were
more refractive to treatment. Children younger than age 15
are particularly prone to develop night blindness from vitamin A deficiency. Multiple scattered retinal gray-white spots
may occur with prolonged vitamin A deficiency, but at the
onset of night blindness, the retina usually appears normal.
The dark adaptation threshold curves in vitamin A deficiency
are prolonged and show delayed initial cone dark adaptation
followed by a marked prolongation of early rod adaptation
("rod plateaux") but normal final rod threshold is eventually
reached (3).

Studies in developed countries where vitamin A
deficiency occurs in the setting of liver dysfunction (4,5),
intestinal bypass (6,7), Crohn disease (8), cystic fibrosis (9),
and abetalipoproteinemia (10) have shown reduced ERG
responses as well as abnormal dark adaptometry. Rod ERG
responses are more reduced than cone ERG responses in vitamin A deficiency, but both can be substantially reduced
depending on the stage of the disease (Fig. 15.1). Implicit
times are less prolonged than those in rod–cone dystrophy
(retinits pigmentosa), and the shape of the dark-adapted
bright-flash combined rod–cone response may have some
similarity to the light-adapted cone response (7). Dark adaptometry reveals elevated rod and cone thresholds (8). With
vitamin A supplementation, ERG responses and dark
adapting thresholds improve. In the central retina, the cone
function recovers more quickly than rod function, while in
the retinal periphery the opposite occurs perhaps because of
regional differences in rod–cone density and rod–cone
competition for available vitamin A during visual pigment
regeneration (8).

In general, ERG and dark adaptometry are useful in supporting the diagnosis of vitamin A deficiency and in following
patients who are refractive to treatment. Serum vitamin A
level remains the first ancillary test of choice when the condition is suspected. Nevertheless, ERG and dark adaptometry

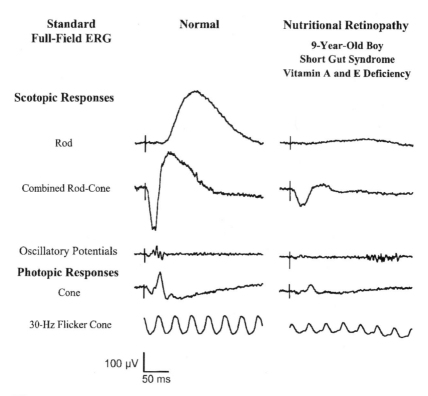

Figure 15.1 Full-field ERG responses of an 8-year-old boy with nutritional retinopathy due to malabsorption from short gut syndrome. The patient had vitamin A and vitamin E deficiency. The scotopic rod and combined rod–cone responses were more impaired than the photopic cone responses. The oscillatory potentials were also reduced.

are beneficial especially in cases where xerophthalmia is not obvious or when long-term follow-up is necessary because the deficiency is the result of chronic intestinal or liver disorders.

NUTRITIONAL OPTIC NEUROPATHY

Optic neuropathy related to deficiency of nutrient to the optic nerve is called nutritional optic neuropathy. Other names for the disorder include nutritional amblyopia and tobacco–alcohol amblyopia. The condition may be caused by malnutrition and in some cases, is associated with tobacco and alcohol use. Rapid onset of bilateral loss of central vision with cecocentral scotomas is followed by the development of optic nerve head pallor. A deficiency of B complex vitamins appears to be the underlying cause in some causes, but causative factors may be multiple. Prognosis is generally favorable, if malnutrition is rectified and use of alcohol and tobacco are discontinued in the early stage of the disease. Reversible VEP abnormalities in patients with nutritional optic neuropathy have been reported (11–13). Impairments of VEP are more likely to occur with lower contrast pattern stimulus, and P1 latency may not necessary increase in some patients (14).

METALLIC INTRAOCULAR FOREIGN BODIES—OCULAR SIDEROSIS

Metallic intraocular foreign bodies may produce progressive visual loss by continued release of dissolving toxic material. The extent and rapidity of the induced ocular toxicity depend on the type of metal, size, and location. For instance, copper-containing foreign bodies usually produce severe ocular toxicity (ocular chalcosis) with rapid loss of vision and diminishing ERG responses but aluminum foreign bodies typically are associated with mild ocular toxicity. Ocular toxicity from iron-containing foreign bodies may result in ocular siderosis (siderosis bulbi) with clinical features such as tonic pupil, iris heterochromia, cataract, and progressive pigmentary retinopathy. Symptoms of ocular siderosis include decreased central and peripheral vision and impaired night vision.

When the risks of surgical removal of the metallic intraocular foreign body appear to outweigh the likelihood of ocular toxicity, periodic examinations and serial ERGs are recommended. If progressive loss of visual function due to ocular toxicity is detected, prompt removal of the foreign body is indicated (15,16). Full-field ERG in early ocular siderosis is normal or may demonstrate a transient supernormal

Toxic Retinopathy from Retained Metallic Foreign Body
44-Year-Old Man with Progressive Visual Loss of Left Eye
Foreign Body Lodged in Peripheral Temporal Retina for 10 Years

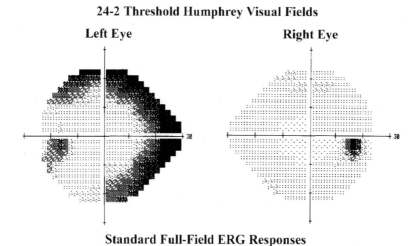

Figure 15.2 (*Caption on facing page*)

response (17,18). Damage from the impact of the foreign body such as retinal edema or retinal detachment may also result in transient as well as permanent reduced ERG responses and should be considered in ERG interpretation. Over time, full-field ERG responses become reduced and prolonged, often with more scotopic than photopic impairment (Fig. 15.2). A greater selective decrease in b-wave amplitude as compared to a-wave occurs and is most notable on the scotopic combined rod–cone bright flash response (19). The oscillatory potentials also decrease correspondingly indicating more dysfunction of the inner retina. With further progression, a negative ERG pattern with b-wave to a-wave amplitude ratio of less than 1 may occur and the ERG eventually becomes non-detectable.

In early ocular siderosis, visual function and ERG responses improve after foreign body removal. In more advance cases, improvements are variable but visual acuity and ERG responses are likely to stabilize with removal of the foreign body (18). Of interest, in patients with ocular siderosis and cataract, reduced or non-detectable full-field ERG responses do not preclude a visual acuity of 20/25 or better after cataract extraction and foreign body removal despite persisting visual field defects (16,20). Impairment of EOG also occurs with ocular siderosis but has not been extensively studied.

Figure 15.2 (*Facing page*) Visual fields and full-field ERG responses of a 44-year-old man with a retained metallic foreign body in the left eye for 10 years. Visual acuity was 20/20 right eye and 20/60 left eye. Visual fields showed nasal constriction in the left eye. Ophthalmoscopy revealed normal appearance of the maculas and the optic nerve heads. Full-field ERG responses were markedly asymmetric indicating toxic retinopathy of the left eye. The scotopic rod and combined rod–cone responses of the left eye were more impaired than the photopic cone responses. The scotopic combined rod–cone response demonstrated a relatively selective reduction in b-wave such that the b- to a-wave amplitude ratio is less than 1 ("negative ERG"). The oscillatory potentials were essentially absent. Prompt removal of the metallic foreign body was recommended.

METHANOL POISONING

Methanol (methyl alcohol) is a toxic chemical used as an industrial solvent and is also found in automotive antifreeze fluid. Methanol may be found in home-brewed alcohol or used unethically as a cheap substitute for ethanol in alcoholic drinks. Absorption of methanol can occur through the skin, lung, and gastrointestinal tract. Methanol poisoning can result in permanent blindness and death, and absorption of as little as 10 ml of methanol can cause blindness. Methanol is primarily oxidized to formaldehyde by hepatic alcohol dehydrogenase, and formaldehyde is then rapidly converted by aldehyde dehydrogenase to formic acid, which is subsequently oxidized to carbon dioxide by a hepatic folate dependent pathway. The accumulation of formic acid not only produces severe metabolic acidosis but also inhibits mitochondrial cytochrome oxidase, which results in dysfunction of the photoreceptors, Müller cells, and axoplasmic flow of the retrolaminar optic nerve (21–24).

Patients with methanol toxicity usually report a history of recent alcohol ingestion and have headache, nausea, vomiting, and weakness. Visual symptoms typically occur 12–48 hr after methanol ingestion and is variable ranging from mild blurred vision to complete blindness (25). The degree of impaired pupillary light reaction is an important prognostic indicator of visual outcome and death (25). Ocular findings include hyperemia of the optic nerve, followed by peripapillary retinal edema which subsequently spreads radially as greyish streaks throughout the retina accompanied commonly by retinal vein engorgement. Over weeks, some visual recovery may occur, and the optic nerve head becomes atrophic and occasionally develops glaucomatous-like cupping (25,26). Treatment strategies of methanol toxicity have principally been directed at inhibiting alcohol dehydrogenase.

In general, visual electrophysiologic tests may help in detecting retinal and optic nerve dysfunction due to methanol toxicity. The findings of ERG and VEP are variable and dependent on degree of toxicity and stage of recovery (27–29). Virtually all components of the standard full-field ERG, both scotopically and photopically, are likely to be impaired during the acute stage of methanol toxicity. Because photoreceptors as well as Müller cells are sensitive to damage from formic acid, both a- and b-wave are impaired (27,28,30). However, a relatively selective impairment of b-wave has been reported and a negative pattern ERG may occur with a b-wave to a-wave amplitude ratio of less than 1 on scotopic combined rod–cone response (31). Further, an increased a-wave and a reduced b-wave in the acute stage of methanol poisoning have been documented in humans as well as primates during acute toxicity (32,33). With visual recovery, the full-field ERG improves (27). In methanol toxicity, VEP responses are likely to be impaired in part from retinal dysfunction, but reports of VEP in methanol toxicity are sparse. Responses of VEP ranging from normal to transient reduction of pattern VEP with normal latency have been noted (27,29).

SYNTHETIC RETINOIDS—ISOTRETINOIN (ACCUTANE®)

Analogues of vitamin A such as isotretinoin (Accutane®), a synthetic retinoid, are used in the treatment of acne and other dermatologic diseases. Impaired night vision, abnormal dark adaptation, and reduced scotopic ERG responses have been reported with isotretinoin use and are reversed with cessation of the medication (34,35). The pathogenesis is likely related to the synthetic retinoid competing for normal vitamin A binding sites on the retinol binding protein or on the target cell surface. In light of the number of persons on synthetic retinoids, the frequency of significant retinal toxicity is relatively low, and mass screening is impractical and unnecessary. However, detailed clinical work-up is warranted in those with visual symptoms.

CHLOROQUINE/HYDROXYCHLOROQUINE

Chloroquine and its derivative hydroxychloroquine (Plaquenil®) are medications used in the treatment of malaria, rheumatoid arthritis, systemic lupus erythematosus, and Sjögren's syndrome. The clinical features of toxic retino- pathy from chloroquine and hydroxychloroquine include reduced visual acuity, peripheral visual loss, pigmentary macular atrophy often acquiring a bull's eye appearance, per- ipheral retinal changes, and eventual optic nerve atrophy. Binding of chloroquine and hydroxychloroquine to melanin granules in the ciliary body, retina, and choroid has been implicated as a cause of the toxicity but the exact mechanism is unclear (36). Toxic retinopathy is more frequent with the use of chloroquine than with hydroxychloroquine. In general, the incidence of hydroxychloroquine retinal toxicity from more recent studies ranges from less than 1% to up to 6% (37–40). The risk of toxicity increases with higher daily dosages and is likely to be related to the amount of total cumulative dosage. Patients with normal retinal function placed on hydroxychloroquine at a maximal daily dosage of 6.5 mg/kg are safe from retinal toxicity for the first six years of treatment (40). In general, visual loss from toxic retinopa- thy may be reversible with discontinued use of these medica- tions if toxicity is detected early, but in some cases, visual loss is irreversible and continues to progress even after drug cessation (41,42).

In most cases, serial periodic automated static perimetry of the central 10-degree visual field and multifocal ERG test- ing at the start of the treatment and periodically thereafter as indicated is the preferred method of detecting maculopathy from chloroquine or hydroxychloroquine. In additional

Figure 15.3 (*Facing page.*) Multifocal ERG of a 55-year-old woman treated with hydroxychloroquine, 200 mg twice daily for 5 years. The patient was asymptomatic and had 20/20 vision in each eye. Ophthalmoscopy was normal. Multifocal ERG showed impaired responses centrally. Notable decreases in response density of the center and perifoveal concentric rings are apparent. Clinically asymptomatic patients on hydroxychloroquine may have decreases in multifocal ERG responses possibly indicating a preclinical stage of drug-related toxicity.

Impaired Multifocal ERG Responses from Hydroxychloroquine

55-Year-Old Visually Asymptomatic Woman

Trace Array from 103-Hexagonal Stimulus

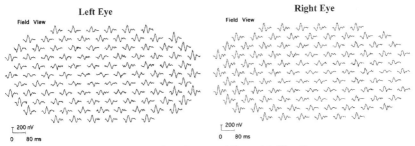

Response Density from Center and Concentric Ring Groups
(Patient tracing - black, Normal tracing - grey)

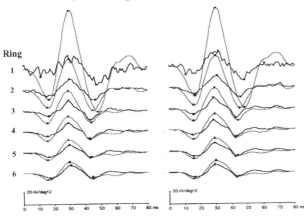

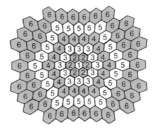

Figure 15.3 (*Caption on facing page*)

fluorescein angiography may facilitate the visualization of early subtle bull's-eye maculopathy. Areas of localized decreased multifocal ERG responses are found bilaterally in patients with hydroxychloroquine maculopathy, and clinically asymptomatic patients may have decreases in multifocal ERG responses (Fig. 15.3) possibly indicating a preclinical stage of drug-related toxicity or pharmacologic actions of the drug (43–46).

Because of the localized nature of toxic retinopathy from chloroquine or hydroxychloroquine especially in the early stages, neither full-field ERG or EOG are diagnostically useful although both tests will demonstrate abnormalities in advance cases (47). Full-field ERG is usually normal or only mildly reduced in chloroquine or hydroxychloroquine maculopathy. With progression to diffuse retinal involvement, full-field ERG abnormalities become evident. In general, full-field ERG cone response is more likely to be affected than rod response. However, with advance cases, all components of the full-field ERG are affected, and both full-field ERG and EOG become non-detectable or minimally recordable (41). For instance, Weiner et al. (48) documented marked impairment of virtually all components of the full-field ERG, both scotopically and photopically, in two patients with advanced hydroxychloroquine retinopathy and cumulative doses of about 1800 and 2900 g. Of interest, the autoimmune disease that is being treated by these agents may itself produce mild ERG and EOG impairment. Sassaman et al. (49) found smaller foveal ERG responses in patients with untreated systemic lupus erythematosus compared to normals. In the same report, the authors also noted mild full-field ERG alterations in systemic lupus erythematosus patients treated with hydroxychloroquine with no apparent retinopathy compared to untreated patients; this finding may imply that treated patients had more severe systemic lupus erythematosus which produced the full-field ERG alterations than untreated patients or that altered ERG responses from retinal dysfunction occur before any visible retinopathy. With regard to EOG, several authors found reduced EOG light-peak to dark-trough amplitude ratios in untreated patients with autoimmune disease and in patients treated with chloroquine or hydroxychloroquine (47,50). In the latter study, Pinckers and Broekhuyse (47) studied 918 rheumatoid arthritis patients and found EOG abnormality rates of 20%, 23%, and 37% in the untreated, hydroxychloroquine-treated, and chloroquine retinopathy groups, respectively. The authors concluded that EOG is not a method of choice in detecting early toxic retinopathy in these patients, because impaired EOG is found in untreated patients and was not sensitive enough to determine.

THIORIDAZINE (MELLARIL®), CHLORPROMAZINE, AND OTHER PHENOTHIAZINES

Thioridazine (Mellaril®) is a phenothiazine derivative used in the treatment of psychiatric disorders. Symptoms of thioridazine-induced toxic retinopathy include decreased visual acuity, visual field loss, and night blindness. In the early stage, the macula and sometimes other regions of the retina acquire a granular appearance. With time, these changes evolve into patchy areas of pigmentary disturbance that may be hypopigmented or hyperpigmented. Binding of phenothiazines to melanin granules is implicated as the etiology of the toxic retinopathy. If toxicity is detected early, visual loss may be reversed with drug cessation, but in advance cases, visual loss is irreversible and may continue to progress even after discontinuation of the medication (51–53). The risk of developing thioridazine retinopathy is related to daily and cumulative dosage. The risk of toxic retinopathy is generally low for dosages below the recommended maximal total daily dose of 800 mg but retinal toxicity may still rarely occur (54). Pigmentary deposits of the skin, cornea and lens are also common with 800 mg thioridazine daily for over 44 months (55).

The diagnosis of thioridazine-induced toxic retinopathy as well as other phenothiazine-induced retinopathy is arrived on the basis of visual symptoms, visual field defects, retinal appearance, and ERG findings. Serial periodic assessment is helpful in patients suspected of thioridazine-induced toxic retinopathy.

In thioridazine-induced toxic retinopathy, virtually all scotopic and photopic components of the full-field ERG are affected to a various degree correlating to the extent of pigmentary retinopathy. However, in some cases, Marmor (51) has shown that visual function parameters including the full-field ERG may improve despite visible progression of the pigmentary retinopathy. With continued progression, full-field ERG eventually becomes non-detectable and EOG light-peak absent. Filip and Balik (56) demonstrated acute thioridazine-induced full-field ERG changes and found an impaired a-wave and b-wave in 10 normal volunteers 90 min after ingestion of 50 mg of thioridazine as compared to baseline, but the ERG was performed only after 5 min of dark adaptation and 5 min of light adaptation, respectively, Miyata et al. (57) reported reduced amplitudes of the O_2, O_3, and O_4 wavelets of the oscillatory potentials and delayed peak time of the O_2 wavelet in 28 patients treated with thioridazine, one of whom had visible pigmentary retinopathy. However, the authors reported results only from the combined rod–cone full-field ERG response obtained only after 15 min of dark adaptation. Godel et al. (58) examined the effect of thioridazine cessation on the full-field ERG and found improved ERG amplitudes in two patients and no improvement in one patient. In general, EOG tends to parallel ERG responses and the extent of thioridazine-induced pigmentary retinopathy. Also VEP is likely to parallel ERG findings and macular function. However, Saletu et al. (59) reported prolonged and reduced flash VEP responses in 21 hyperkinetic children who were treated only with up to 80 mg thioridazine daily for 8 weeks. Since such brief regimen is unlikely to produce retinal toxicity, these results suggest that thioridazine may have a physiologic effect on the VEP.

Chlorpromazine is a phenothiazine derivative used for psychiatric disorders and has far less ocular toxic effect than thioridazine (60). The risk of pigmentary retinopathy increases significantly with prolonged treatment of over

800 mg chlorpromazine daily (55). Pigmentary deposits of the skin, conjunctiva, cornea, and lens can also occur with chlorpromazine therapy. Siddall (55) found pigmentary retinopathy in 13 (26%) of 50 patients treated with chlorpromazine alone as compared with 13 (46%) of 28 patients treated with a combination of chlorpromazine and other phenothiazine derivatives including thioridazine. Of the 13 patients with chlorpromazine-induced pigmentary retinopathy, nine had retinal granularity and four had fine pigmentary clumping which was reversed with reduced chlorpromazine dosage. Visual loss as well as the corresponding pigmentary retinopathy were less severe in the chlorpromazine only group.

Of note, despite the binding of phenothiazines to melanin granules and the occurrence of associated pigmentary retinopathy, EOG is not of value in the early detection of phenothiazine-induced retinopathy. In a study of 203 eyes of patients less than age 46 treated with phenothiazines including perazine, thioridazine, levo-mepromazine, and promethazine, Henkes (61) found that of the 92 eyes with "just visible" retinal pigmentary changes, 20 eyes had reduced EOG light-peak to dark-trough amplitude ratios, and of 18 eyes with "clearly visible" pigmentary retinopathy, only 12 had reduced EOG ratios. Based on these data, Henkes (61) concluded that EOG was not sensitive enough to detect early phenothiazine retinopathy. Likewise, in a study of 99 female patients, less than age 45, initially treated with phenothiazine derivatives, Alkemade (62) found 15 (15%) patients with pigmentary retinopathy, and of these, only nine of the 13 patients who had EOG testing had reduced EOG.

QUININE

Quinine, an alkaloid originally derived from the bark of the South American cinchoma tree, is used in the treatment of malaria and nocturnal muscle cramps. Quinine toxicity occurs with overdose from over-medication, attempted suicide, attempted abortion, or exposure to quinine filler in illegal narcotics. Symptoms of acute quinine poisoning include nausea, vomiting, tinnitus, deafness, blindness, and confusion. These symptoms usually occur with an ingestion of greater than 4 g of quinine with the mean fatal dose being in the range of 8 g. However, rare idiosyncratic sensitivity to quinine at lower dosages may occur. Treatment is aimed at reducing quinine serum levels.

With non-lethal acute quinine toxicity, severe visual loss occurs within hours after ingestion followed often by partial central visual improvement over days to weeks and marked persistent loss of peripheral vision. Ocular findings include large non-reactive pupils, retinal arteriolar narrowing, retinal edema, and the development of optic nerve head pallor. If needed, visual electrophysiologic tests may help in assessing visual function particularly in those who test unreliably subjectively with visual acuity and fields. The mechanism of visual dysfunction from quinine toxicity is not completely understood. Retinal dysfunction with abnormal ERG response is evident in humans as well as animals (63). The development of optic nerve head pallor has led to the speculation of retinal ganglion cell dysfunction.

Clinical and visual electrophysiologic findings in quinine toxicity are variable depending on the severity of toxicity and degree of recovery. In addition, studies of electrophysiologic findings in quinine toxicity consist mostly of case reports with differences in methodology. In general, during the early stage of acute quinine toxicity when severe acute visual loss occurs, the full-field ERG may be normal or demonstrate both rod and cone response impairment with absent oscillatory potentials. Over the next few days, some visual improvement usually occur, and impaired full-field ERG becomes more apparent with a greater selective reduction in b-wave so that a negative ERG pattern with b-wave to a-wave amplitude ratio of less than 1 is common (Fig. 15.4). The cone ERG response is generally more impaired than the rod response, and absent oscillatory potentials persist. Subsequently over weeks and months as the vision stabilizes, the ERG may improve or may demonstrate delayed slow progression of impairment. With regard to EOG and VEP, reduced EOG light-peak to dark-trough amplitude ratio and increased VEP latency occur

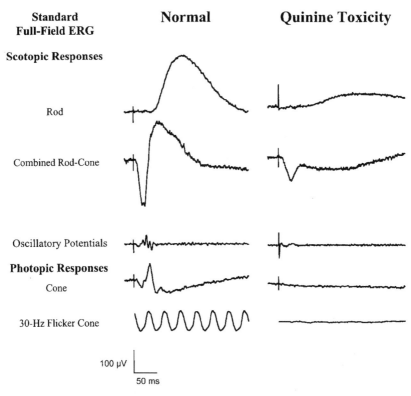

Figure 15.4 Full-field responses of a patient with persistent visual impairment from quinine toxicity. The cone responses are more impaired than the rod responses. The scotopic combined rod–cone response demonstrates a relatively selective reduction in b-wave such that the b- to a-wave amplitude ratio is less than one ("negative ERG"). The oscillatory potentials are essentially absent.

in the early stage of quinine toxicity and may show some subsequent improvement.

Several studies have documented electrophysiologic findings during the early phase of quinine toxicity. Brinton et al. (64) found slowed but increased a-wave, reduced and delayed b-wave, and absent oscillatory potentials for the scotopic combined rod–cone full-field ERG response in a patient with no light perception 18 h after ingestion of about 4 g of quinine, but the ERG was performed only after 15 min of dark adaptation. The next day, the patient's central vision improved, and the ERG a-wave and b-wave returned to normal in a few days, but a late progressive decrease in b-wave amplitude was noted within 6 months of follow-up. Visual acuity recovered to 20/15 in each eye but visual fields remained severely constricted with peripheral vision consisting of temporal islands only. The EOG amplitude ratio was initially 1.3 in each eye but improved to 1.6 by day nine. The pattern VEP showed persistent increased latency. In contrast, Yospaiboon et al. (65) reported small a-wave, non-detectable b-wave, and non-detectable oscillatory potentials for the scotopic combined rod–cone full-field ERG response and non-detectable VEP in a patient with no light perception after ingesting 12.6 g of quinine over 1 week for the treatment of malaria, but the ERG was performed after only 15 min of dark adaptation. After 21 weeks of follow-up, gradual partial a-wave and b-wave recovery and near complete VEP recovery were observed concomitantly with a visual acuity recovery to 20/30. Further, Canning and Hague (66) noted normal full-field ERG amplitude to presumably scotopic blue, red, and white stimuli, reduced ERG oscillatory potentials, markedly reduced pattern ERG, non-detectable pattern VEP to grading stimuli, and small but not delayed flash VEP in a patient with visual acuity of 6/18 right eye and 6/24 left eye with markedly constricted visual fields one day after ingesting 9 g of quinine. After 66 days, the full-field ERG amplitudes became reduced, the reduced pattern ERG persisted, and the pattern VEP became detectable with increased latency.

Several other studies have further provided electrophysiologic responses after the acute phase of quinine toxicity. Moloney et al. (67) documented improved scotopic variable-intensity stimuli response function of the full-field ERG from day 10 to 24 months in a patient with light perception vision after ingesting 6 g of quinine. However, despite an eventual visual acuity of 20/30 in each eye, reduced full-field ERG cone response and reduced oscillatory potentials persisted with rod response improving after 12 months. The EOG at day 10 had no light peak but eventually improved to a light-peak to dark-trough amplitude ratio of 1.8 at 24 months. Flash VEP response was absent at day 10 but improved to near normal after 60 days. In another case report, Bacon et al. (68) found increased a-wave and absent b-wave for the scotopic combined rod–cone full-field ERG response, reduced EOG light-peak and dark-trough amplitude ratio of 1.3, and delayed pattern VEP with P_2 component at 125–145 ms in a patient 4 weeks after ingestion of 10 g of quinine. When these tests were repeated 10 weeks after quinine toxicity, only a modest improvement was found with a small detectable full-field ERG b-wave and slightly improved VEP latency. Of interest, François et al. (69) found a relatively selective b-wave impairment with a negative pattern full-field ERG, greater photopic than scotopic impaired full-field ERG response, absent ERG oscillatory potentials, and reduced EOG in three patients examined at 15 months, 36 years and 37 years, respectively, after quinine toxicity. Similar findings were also noted by Behrman and Mushin (70) in a 10-month follow-up of a patient ingested 24 g of quinine but this patient was also on central nervous system medications for schizophrenia.

DEFEROXAMINE (DESFERRIOXAMINE)

Deferoxamine, also called desferrioxamine, is an iron chelator used for the treatment of iron overload. Patients with hematologic conditions such as beta-thalassemia major requiring frequent transfusions may develop hemosiderosis or iron overload that if left untreated may produce diabetes, cardiac disease, and hepatic dysfunction. Deferoxamine treatment in these patients dramatically increases urinary iron excretion. Other indications of deferoxamine have included acute iron intoxication, removal of iron deposits in synovial membranes in rheumatoid arthritis, and as a challenge test to diagnose aluminum overload in chronic renal failure. Deferoxamine is generally tolerated and is administered subcutaneously, intramuscularly, or intravenously (71). However, adverse toxic effects of deferoxamine therapy may involve visual, auditory, cutaneous, cardiovascular, respiratory, gastrointestinal, and nervous systems. Ocular signs of deferoxamine toxicity include cataract, pigmentary retinopathy, and optic neuropathy. The mechanism of deferoxamine toxicity is not completely understood. The fact that deferoxamine also chelates other metals such as copper, zinc, cobalt, and nickel has been implicated as a potential cause of toxicity (72). Patients with preexisting blood–retinal barrier breakdown associated with diabetes, rheumatoid arthritis, metabolic encephalopathy, and renal failure are at increased risk of developing deferoxamine-induced retinopathy (73). Ocular histopathology of deferoxamine toxicity reveals degenerative retinal pigment epithelial cells and thickened Bruch's membrane (74). The relationship between deferoxamine dosage and the development of induced toxic retinopathy is highly variable. In a recent study of 16 patients with deferoxamine-induced retinal toxicity, the duration of deferoxamine therapy before presentation of 13 of the patients was known and varied from 4 weeks to 10 years, and the total dosage of deferoxamine was calculable in six patients and ranged from 243 to 10,950 g with a mean of 2785 g (73). Moreover, irreversible and reversible visual loss from optic nerve hyperemia, cystoid macular edema, and pigmentary retinopathy have been reported with a single small dose of deferoxamine (40 mg/kg) used as an aluminum overload challenge test in patients with chronic renal failure and on dialysis (75,76).

Visual symptoms of deferoxamine toxicity include decreased vision, impaired color vision, and night blindness. Ocular findings include cataract, pigmentary retinopathy, and optic neuropathy. Concomitant deferoxamine-induced deafness may occur. The earliest sign of deferoxamine retinopathy is often a subtle opacification or loss of transparency of the outer retina and retinal pigment epithelium followed by development of retinal pigment epithelium pigment mottling (73). With time, macular or peripheral retinal pigmentary alterations occur (77,78). Late hyperfluorescence of the affected region of the retina on fluorescein angiography is a reliable sign of active toxic retinopathy (73). Following deferoxamine cessation, visual improvement may or may not improve, and retinal pigmentary changes may progress or develop despite improvement in visual function (78,79). Isolated optic neuropathy associated with deferoxamine use is likely to be less frequent than deferoxamine-induced retinopathy. In a series of eight patients with deferoxamine ocular toxicity reported by Lakhampal et al. (78), five of six patients with "presumed" retrobulbar optic neuropathy also had macular pigmentary degeneration.

The diagnosis of deferoxamine-induced ocular toxicity is arrived on the basis of visual symptoms, visual field defects, ophthalmoscopy, and fluorescein angiography. Visual electrophysiologic tests including full-field ERG, focal ERG, EOG, pattern ERG, and VEP are also of diagnostic value to determine earlier or more widespread injury than is suggested by ophthalmoscopic examination alone (73).

Visual electrophysiologic findings in deferoxamine toxicity are variable and are generally related to the severity of toxicity (77). Full-field ERG ranges from normal in mild cases to marked reduced and prolonged rod and cone responses in severe cases (73,78). Likewise, EOG may be normal or demonstrate a substantial impaired light rise with marked reduced light-peak to dark-trough amplitude ratio (73,78). Impaired VEP may reflect toxic retinopathy, optic neuropathy or both. In a study of 120 beta-thalassemia patients undergoing long-term deferoxamine treatment, Triantafyllou et al. (80) found impaired pattern VEP in 27% of the patients, which was mostly reversible with modification of deferoxamine treatment. Similarly, Taylor et al. (81) noted prolonged pattern VEP in 21% of 77 patients on chronic deferoxamine therapy and without clinical apparent retinopathy. Further, in a study of 43 patients with beta-thalassemia undergoing long-term deferoxamine treatment, Arden et al. found no or only mild abnormal retina appearance but pattern ERG abnormalities were much more pronounced than full-field or EOG findings. Of interest, siderosis or iron overload itself may also produce electrophysiologic alterations. For example, Gelmi et al. (82) found that thalassemia major patients treated with transfusions, who have no visual symptoms and had never received high doses of deferoxamine, may exhibit ERG and VEP findings that resemble early siderosis bulbi.

VIGABATRIN

Vigabatrin is an antiepileptic medication used for complex partial, secondarily generalized seizures, and infantile spasm. Vigabatrin increases concentration of γ-aminobutyric acid (GABA), an inhibitory neurotransmitter in the central nervous system, by interfering with the production of the enzyme γ-aminobutyric transaminase which inactivates GABA. However, GABA is also an important inhibitory neurotransmitter in the retina, and GABA receptors are found on photoreceptor terminals and horizontal, bipolar, and amacrine cells of the inner retina. Bilateral visual field constriction, often concentric or binasal, from toxic retinopathy occurs in about one-third of patients on vigabatrin therapy; however, only about 10% of vigabatrin patients have visual symptoms such as reduced peripheral vision, blurred vision, and impaired color vision (83–86). Vigabatrin produces accumulation of GABA in the retina but precise mechanisms of vigabatrin-induced retinopathy are not well understood. Three subtypes of GABA receptors, type A, B, and C are known, and subtypes of GABA-ergic rod bipolar, cone bipolar, and amacrine cells have been identified. However, subtypes of GABA receptors are not necessarily evenly distributed. For instance, bipolar cells express both $GABA_A$ and $GABA_C$ receptors but the ratio of $GABA_C$ to $GABA_A$ receptors is greater in rod bipolar cells than cone bipolar cells. Activation of $GABA_C$ receptors increases ERG b-wave, and activation of $GABA_A$ receptors decreases ERG b-wave, but vigabatrin also produces GABA accumulation in Müller cells which are involved in generating the ERG b-wave (87–89).

The retinal appearance is usually normal in vigabatrin-induced retinopathy. Rarely, the retina may show narrow retinal arterioles, surface wrinkling retinopathy, and abnormal macular reflexes (85). The diagnosis of vigabatrin-induced retinopathy is typically made on the basis of visual symptoms, bilateral concentric or binasal visual field constriction, and progressive deterioration of full-field ERG responses. Visual impairment may persist even after cessation of vigabatrin therapy (90,91).

While impaired full-field ERG responses are commonly found in vigabatrin-treated patients, the impaired ERG responses may be the result of not only the toxic effect of vigabatrin but also the non-toxic pharmacological effect of vigabatrin (92). Therefore, in vigabatrin-treated patients who are visually asymptomatic with stable visual fields and abnormal ERG responses, the abnormal ERG responses could be due to physiologic effect of vigabatrin or early toxic effect of vigabatrin or both (93,94). Only careful follow-up with serial visual fields and full-field ERG will determine whether further progression occurs supporting a toxic effect (Fig. 15.5).

Several authors have reported a greater cone than rod full-field ERG impairment in vigabatrin-treated patients with the b-wave amplitude of the photopic cone flicker response being the strongest correlate of the degree of visual field constriction (85,89,95,96). For instance, in most children treated with vigabatrin, the cone flicker amplitude declines between 6 months and 1 year of treatment (97). Although photopic b-wave reduction is the most frequent full-field ERG finding in vigabatrin-treated patients, reduced scotopic b-wave amplitudes and impaired oscillatory potentials can also occur (87,98,99). Taken together, these findings indicate a more selective dysfunction of the inner retina.

Focal and multifocal ERG may be reduced centrally as well as peripherally in vigabatrin-treated patients (86,100–102). Reduced light-peak to dark-trough EOG amplitude ratio is noted often in vigabatrin-treated patients (103). However, EOG abnormality is not significantly associated with the degree of vigabatrin-induced visual field loss (95,104).

Impairment of conventional VEP is common in vigabatrin-treated patients and does not necessarily correlate with severity of ERG changes (89). A specialized VEP called "special VEP H-Stimulus" has been developed by Harding et al. (105,106) to assess the effect of vigabatrin. The technique elicits pattern VEP response from the central 5° radius and from

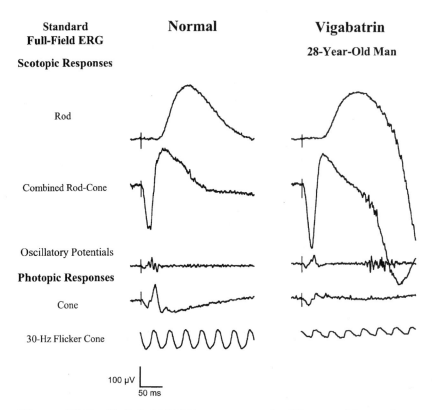

Figure 15.5. Full-field ERG responses of a 28-year-old man treated with vigabatrin for seizure disorder for 1 year. Note the reduced cone single-flash and 30-Hz responses as well as the impaired oscillatory potentials. Despite the ERG impairment, the patient has been visually asymptomatic with stable visual fields and ERG responses after 4 years of follow-up. Therefore, the non-progressive impaired ERG responses in this patient are likely related to the non-toxic pharmacological effect of vigabatrin.

a peripheral outer rim between 30° and 60° radius. The technique has a sensitivity of 75% and a specificity of 87.5% in identifying visual field defect and may be used in young children older than 3 years, who are unable to perform reliable visual fields.

   With discontinuation of vigabatrin, visual field defects and electrophysiologic abnormalities may persist (91,101,107). In patients with minimal or no visual field loss, visual impairment as well as ERG amplitude loss are more likely to be reversible (91). In patients with vigabatrin-associated visual field constrictions, the ERG and the EOG may demonstrate recovery after discontinuation of the medication without corresponding improvement of visual field (108).

SILDENAFIL (VIAGRA®)

Sildenafil (Viagra®) is a medication for penile erectile dysfunction and acts by potentiating the vascular dilation effect of sexual stimulation on the corpus cavernosum of the penis. Cyclic guanosine monophsophate (cGMP) is a potent vascular smooth muscle relaxant of the corpus cavernosum and is inactivated by phosphodiesterase 5. Sildenafil limits the inactivation of cGMP by directly inhibiting phosphodiesterase 5. However, sildenafil also has about a 10% cross inhibitory effect on phosphodiesterase 6 which is involved in the process of phototransduction in retinal photoreceptor cells.

Incidence of visual symptoms is dose-related ranging from about 3% after ingesting sildenafil 50 mg to near 50% after ingesting 200 mg (109). Visual disturbance is likely to occur 1 hr after ingesting sildenafil and resolves over 3–4 hr. The transient visual symptoms from sildenafil include bluish vision, increased light sensitivity, and diminished color perception. Transient mild visual field and ERG alterations may occur (109,110). Vobig et al. (111) found reduced a-wave and b-wave of the scotopic combined rod–cone full-field ERG response to 63% and 77% of baseline, respectively, 1 hr after ingesting sildenafil 100 mg in five healthy subjects. Other parameters of the full-field ERG showed only small insignificant reductions, and the implicit times remained unaffected. The ERG changes correlated well with peak sildenafil plasma concentration and resolved 6 hr after ingestion. In contrast, Gabrieli et al. (112) noted higher full-field ERG scotopic rod response and greater rod sensitivity as determined by variable-intensity stimuli in a patient with visual halos 2 hr after sildenafil administration. This result was confirmed by the same research group in a subsequent study of 12 subjects (113).

In a study with both full-field and multifocal ERG, Luu et al. (114) found slightly depressed cone function in the macula and the peripheral retina for at least 5 hr after dildenafil 200 mg in 14 healthy persons, but the ERG parameters still remained within normal limits. In the same study, the authors also noted a slightly increased scotopic combined rod–cone full-field ERG response; similar to the findings of Gabrieli but unlike those of Vobig. In a randomized, double-blind, placebo-controlled clinical trial of 20 men, Jagle et al. (115) performed full-field ERG responses 65 min after ingestion of 100 mg of sidenafil or placebo and found significant prolongations in the implicit times of scotopic a-wave (combined rod–cone response) and photopic b-wave (cone single-flash and flicker responses) after sidenafil ingestion. The ERG responses returned to normal after 24 hr.

Although the visual symptoms and ERG alterations of sildenafil appear to be transient, the effect of chronic sildenafil use in affected persons and asymptomatic carriers of retinal dystrophy is unknown. Because of this, caution regarding sildenafil use in affected persons and known carriers of retinal dystrophy has been advocated by some investigators. In a study of mice, heterozygous for a recessive mutation causing absence of γ subunit of rod phosphodiesterase 6, Behn and Potter (116) reported a significant reversible dose-dependent decrease in ERG a-wave and b-wave after intraperitoneal injection of sildenafil in these heterozygous carriers as compared to normal mice. However, whether sildenafil is likely to produce a greater transient ERG effect in asymptomatic human carriers of retinal dystrophy is unknown and whether these transient retinal effects would cause permanent dysfunction has not been demonstrated.

GENTAMICIN

Retinal toxicity from intravitreal or subconjunctival gentamicin, an aminoglycoside antibiotic, is well recognized. D'Amico et al. (117,118) using a rabbit model found that gentamicin was the most toxic aminoglycoside compared to netilmicin, tobramycin, amikacin, and kanamycin, and an intravitreal dose of 200 μg or greater of gentamicin resulted in electron microscopic damage to the photoreceptors and retinal pigment epithelium as well as reduced ERG. The risk of toxicity decreased markedly with a gentamicin dosage of 100 μg or less (119–121). Further, subconjunctival gentamicin injection adjacent to thinned sclera may lead to localized retinal toxicity (122). Moreover, inadvertent intraocular injection during subconjunctival injection of gentamicin produces retinal whitening with a macular cherry-like spot, diffuse retinal necrosis, and a rapid extinction of ERG (123). Clinically, this may mimic a central retinal artery occlusion or a combined central retinal artery and vein occlusion. In such cases, full-field ERG is helpful, because in retinal vascular occlusions, the ERG is usually not completely extinguished but demonstrates detectable a-waves.

ETHAMBUTOL

Ethambutol is a medication used in the treatment of tuberculosis and may produce optic nerve toxicity resulting in impaired visual acuity and visual field defects such as central scotoma, arcuate scotoma, and enlarged blind spot. Visual impairment is generally, at least partially, reversible if the drug is discontinued promptly but may be irreversible in some cases. The severity of the optic neuropathy does not necessarily correlate with the total cumulative intake of ethambutol. Several studies have documented reduced and prolonged VEP in ethambutol optic neuropathy (124–126). In addition, impaired VEP may occur in asymptomatic patients indicating subclinical optic neuropathy. With prompt drug cessation, visual acuity improves over months but recovery may not be complete, and in about one-third of the patients, prolonged VEP persists (127,128). Full-field ERG and EOG responses are usually normal although one study reported reduced EOG light-peak to dark-trough amplitude ratio in 26% of eyes with ethambutol optic neuropathy (129).

CISPLATIN

Cisplatin is an antineoplastic agent used in the treatment of several types of carcinoma. Visual impairment is reported rarely as a consequence of cisplatin neurotoxicity that may produce cortical blindness, optic neuritis, and retinopathy. Wilding et al. (130) examined 13 cisplatin-treated patients with ocular symptoms of blurred vision or altered color vision and found reduced cone full-field ERG response and considerably less affected rod ERG responses in 11 patients who underwent ERG testing. Loss of color discrimination and saturation, particularly on the blue–yellow axis, was common, and the retinal appearance was usually normal with irregular macular pigmentation in six (46%) of the patients. Hilliard et al. (131) reported two children, aged 4 and 7, treated with high-dose cisplatin and etoposide, who suffered visual loss to 20/600 with granular pigmentary retinopathy, optic nerve head pallor, and non-detectable full-field ERG. The authors proposed that the retinal toxicity was related to decreased renal clearance of cisplatin due to previous nephrotoxic drugs and perhaps also to cisplatin-induced nephrotoxicity. Of interest, Marmor (132) studied a 68-year-old woman with decreased vision after inadvertent overdosage with cisplatin. Both scotopic and photopic full-field ERG responses were marked reduced with a relative selective decrease in b-wave amplitude that was large enough to produce a negative ERG pattern with b-wave to a-wave amplitude ratios of less than 1 on scotopic bright-flash combined rod–cone response and photopic cone flash response. Oscillatory potentials were also notably decreased, and long-duration flash ERG demonstrated marked reduced photopic on-responses with near normal off-responses. Katz et al. reported a 55-year-old man who received four times the intended dose of intravenous cisplatin as part of therapy for non-Hodgkin lymphoma. Vision decreased to 20/300 in each eye immediately and never improved. Full-field ERG was non-detectable except for scotopic bright-flash rod–cone response where a reduced a-wave was visible with no b-wave. At autopsy 8 months later, photoreceptors appeared normal, and splitting of the outer plexiform layer of the retina was present (133). Because cisplatin may also produce optic neuritis, and cortical blindness, impaired VEP responses may also occur and may be more likely in those receiving intra-arterial cisplatin (134).

INDOMETHACIN

Indomethacin is a frequently used non-steroidal antiinflammatory analgesic medication that very rarely produces a pigmentary retinopathy associated with reduced visual acuity, visual field defects, impaired scotopic full-field ERG responses, and reduced EOG light-peak to dark-trough amplitude ratio (135,136). Improvement of visual function usually occurs with discontinuation of the medication. Burns (136) reported ocular findings of 34 patients treated with indomethacin, most of the whom had rheumatoid arthritis and were seen for ocular symptoms. Six (18%) of the 34 patients were found to have indomethacin-induced corneal deposits and 10 (29%) had macular pigmentary disturbance. Abnormal full-field ERG responses were also noted in some of the patients. Henkes et al. (135) documented reduced EOG light-peak to dark-trough amplitude ratio and impaired scotopic full-field ERG responses, obtained after 15 min of dark adaptation, with no impairment of photopic responses in a 58-year-old man with rheumatoid arthritis and treated with indomethacin. After discontinuation of indomethacin, visual function, EOG, and ERG improved after several months.

REFERENCES

1. Mclaren DS. Vitamin A deficiency disorders. J Indian Med Assoc 1999; 97:320–323.

2. Dhanda RP. Electroretinography in night blindness and other vitamin A deficiencies. Arch Ophthalmol 1955; 54:841–849.

3. Cideciyan AV, Pugh EN, Lamb TD, Huang Y, Jacobson SG. Rod plateaux during dark adaptation in Sorsby's fundus

dystrophy and vitamin A deficiency. Invest Ophthalmol
Vision Sci 1997; 38:1786–1794.

4. Newman NJ, Capone A, Leeper HF, O'Day DG, Mandell B,
Lambert SR, Thaft RA. Clinical and subclinical ophthalmic
findings with retinol deficiency. Ophthalmology 1994;
101:1077–1083.

5. Sandberg MA, Rosen JB, Berson EL. Cone and rod function in
vitamin A deficiency with chroinic alcoholism and in retinitis
pigmentosa. Am J Ophthalmol 1977; 84:658–665.

6. Brown GC, Felton SM, Benson WE. Reversible night blindness associated with intestinal bypass surgery. Am J
Ophthalmol 1980; 89:776–779.

7. Perlman I, Barzilai D, Haim T, Schramek A. Night vision in a
case of vitamin A deficiency due to malabsorption. Br J
Ophthalmol 1983; 67:37–42.

8. Kemp CM, Jacobson SG, Faulkner DJ, Walt RW. Visual
function and rhodopsin levels in humans with vitamin A
deficiency. Exp Eye Res 1988; 46:185–197.

9. Neugebauer MA, Vernon SA, Brimlow G, Tyrrell JC, Hiller
EJ, Marenah C. Nyctalopia and conjunctival xerosis indicating vitamin A deficiency in cystic fibrosis. Eye 1989; 3:
360–364.

10. Sperling MA, Hiles DA, Kennerdell JS. Electroretinographic
responses following vitamin A therapy in abetalipoproteinemia. Am J Ophthalmol 1972; 73:342–351.

11. Krumholz A, Weiss HD, Goldstein PJ, Harris KC. Evoked
responses in vitamin B_{12} deficiency. Ann Neurol 1980;
9:407–409.

12. Troncoso J, Mancall EL, Schatz NJ. Visual evoked responses
in pernicious anemia. Arch Neurol 1979; 36:168–169.

13. Kriss A, Carroll WM, Blumhardt LD, Halliday AM. Pattern-
and flash-evoked potential changes in toxic (nutritional) optic
neuropathy. Adv Neurol 1982; 32:11–19.

14. Kupersmith MJ, Weiss PA, Carr RE. The visual-evoked
potential in tobacco-alcohol and nutritional amblyopia. Am
J Ophthalmol 1983; 95:307–314.

15. Neumann R, Belkin M, Loewenthal E, Gorodtsky R. A long-term follow-up of metallic intraocular foreign bodies, employing diagnostic X-ray spectrometry. Arch Ophthalmol 1992; 110:1269–1272.

16. Sneed SR, Weingeist TA. Management of siderosis bulbi due to a retained iron-containing intraoxular foreign body. Ophthalmology 1990; 97:375–379.

17. Hope-Ross M, Mahon GJ, Johnston PB. Ocular siderosis. Eye 1993; 7:419–425.

18. Knave B. Electroretinography in eyes with retained intraocular metallic foreign bodies. Acta Ophthalmol 1969; 100 (suppl):3–63.

19. Schechner R, Miller B, Merksamer E, Perlman I. A long term follow up of ocular siderosis: quantitative assessment of the electroretinogram. Doc Ophthalmol 1991; 76:231–240.

20. Ghoraba H, Al-Nahrawy O, Mohamed OAZ, Sabagh H. Non-recordable electroretinogram in siderosis bulbi might not indicate poor visual outcome. Retina 2001; 21:277–279.

21. Baumbach GL, Cancilla PA, Martin-Amat G, Tephly TR, McMartin KE, Makar AB, Hayreh MS, Hayreh SS. Methyl alcohol poisoning, IV: alternations of the morphological findings of the retina and optic nerve. Arch Ophthalmol 1977; 95:1859–1865.

22. Garner CD, Lee EW, Louis-Ferdinand RT. Muller cell involvement in methanol-induced retinal toxicity. Toxicol Appl Pharmacol 1995; 130:101–107.

23. Hayreh MS, Hayreh SS, Baumbach GL, Cancilla P, Martin-Amat G, Tephly TR, McMartin KE, Makar AB. Methyl alcohol poisoning, III: ocular toxicity. Arch Ophthalmol 1977; 95:1851–1858.

24. Seme MT, Summerfelt P, Neitz J, Eells JT, Henry MM. Differential recovery of retinal function after mitochondrial inhibition by methanol intoxication. Invest Ophthalmol Vision Sci 2001; 42:834–841.

25. Benton CD, Calhoun FP. The ocular effects of methyl alcohol poisoning. Trans Am Acad Ophthalmol Otolaryngol 1952; 56:875–883.

26. Stelmach MZ, O'Day J. Partly reversible visual failure with methanol toxicity. Aust NZ J Ophthalmol 1992; 20:57–64.

27. McKellar MJ, Hidajat RR, Elder MJ. Acute ocular methanol toxicity. Aust NZ J Ophthalmol 1997; 25:225–230.

28. Ruedemann AD. The electroretinogram in chronic methyl alcohol poisoning in human beings. Am J Ophthalmol 1962; 54:34–53.

29. Ingemansson SO. Clinical observations on ten cases of methanol poisoning with particular reference to ocular manifestations. Acta Ophthalmol 1984; 62:15–24.

30. Murray TG, Burton TC, Rajani C, Lewandowski MF, Burke JM, Eells JT. Methanol poisoning: a rodent model with structural and functional evidence for retinal involvement. Arch Ophthalmol 1991; 109:1012–1016.

31. Fishman GA, Birch DG, Holder GE, Brigell MG. Methanol. Electrophysiologic Testing in Disorders of the Retina, Optic Nerve, and Visual Pathway. San Francisco: The Foundation of the American Academy of Ophthalmology, 2001:95–96.

32. Karpe G. The basis of clinical electroretinography. Acta Ophthalmol 1945: 24 (suppl):1–118.

33. Potts AM, Proglin J, Farkas I, Orbison L, Chickering D. Studies on the visual toxicity of methanol. Am J Ophthalmol 1955; 40:76–83.

34. Brown RD, Grattan CEH. Visual toxicity of synthetic retinoids. Br J Ophthalmol 1989; 73:286–288.

35. Weleber RG, Denman ST, Hanifin JM, Cunningham WJ. Abnormal retinal function associated with isotretinoin therapy for acne. Arch Ophthalmol 1986; 104:831–837.

36. Bernstein HN. Chloroquine ocular toxicity. Surv Ophthalmol 1967; 12:415–447.

37. Finbloom DS, Silver K, Newsome DA, Gunkel RD. Comparison of hydroxychloroquine and chloroquine use and the development of retinal toxicity. J Rheumatol 1985; 12:692–694.

38. Morsman CD, Liversey SJ, Richards JM, Jessop JD, Mills PV. Screening for hydroxychloroquine retinal toxicity: is it necessary? Eye 1990; 4:572–576.

39. Rynes RI. Ophthalmologic safety of long-term hydroxychloroquine sulfate treatment. Am J Med 1983; 75:35–39.

40. Mavrikakis I, Sfikakis PP, Rougas K, Nikolaou A, Kostopoulos C, Mavrikakis M. The incidence of irreversible retinal toxicity in patients treated with hydroxychloroquine: a reappraisal. Ophthalmology 2003; 110:1321–1326.

41. Krill AE, Potts AM, Johanson CE. Chloroquine retinopathy: investigation of discrepancy between dark adaptation and electroretinographic findings in advanced stages. Am J Ophthalmol 1971; 71:530–534.

42. Mavrikakis M, Papazoglou S, Sfikakis PP, Vaiopoulos G, Rougas K. Retinal toxicity in long term hydroxychloroquine treatment. Ann Rheum Dis 1996; 55:187–189.

43. Penrose PJ, Tzekov RT, Sutter EE, Fu AD, Allen AW, Fung WE, Oxford KW. Multifocal electroretinography evaluation for early detection of retinal dysfunction in patients taking hydroxychloroquine. Retina 2003; 23:503–512.

44. So SC, Hedges TR, Schuman JS, Quireza ML. Evaluation of hydroxychloroquine retinopathy with multifocal electroretinography. Ophthalmic Surg Lasers Imaging 2003; 34:251–258.

45. Moschos MN, Moschos MM, Apostolopoulos M, Mallias JA, Bouros C, Theodossiadis GP. Assessing hydroxychloroquine toxicity by the multifocal ERG. Doc Ophthalmol 2004; 108:47–53.

46. Tzekov RT, Serrato A, Marmor MF. ERG findings in patients using hydroxychloroquine. Doc Ophthalmol 2004; 108:87–97.

47. Pinckers A, Broekhuyse RM. The EOG in rheumatoid arthritis. Acta Ophthalmol 1983; 61:831–837.

48. Weiner A, Sandberg MA, Gaudio AR, Kini MM, Berson EL. Hydroxychloroquine retinopathy. Am J Ophthalmol 1991; 112:528–534.

49. Sassaman FW, Cassidy JT, Alpern M. Electroretinography in patients with connective tissue diseases treated with hydroxychloroquine. Am J Ophthalmol 1970; 77:515–523.

50. Percival SP. The ocular toxicity of chloroquine. Trans Ophthalmol Soc UK 1967; 87:355–357.

51. Marmor MF. Is thioridazine retinopathy progressive? Relationship of pigmentary changes to visual function. Br J Ophthalmol 1990; 74:739–742.

52. Meredith TA, Aaberg TM, Willerson WD. Progressive chorioretinopathy after receiving thioridazine. Arch Ophthalmol 1978; 96:1172–1176.

53. Davidorf FH. Thioridazine pigmentary retinopathy. Arch Ophthalmol 1973; 90:251–255.

54. Appelbaum A. An ophthalmoscopic study of patients under treatment with thioridazine. Arch Ophthalmol 1963; 69:578–580.

55. Siddall JR. Ocular toxic changes associated with chlorpromazine and thioridazine. Can J Ophthalmol 1966; 1:190–198.

56. Filip V, Balik J. Possible indication of dopaminergic blockade in man by electroretinography. Int Pharmacopsychiatry 1978; 13:151–156.

57. Miyata M, Imai H, Ishikawa S, Nakajima S. Change in human electroretinography associated with thioridazine administration. Ophthalmologica 1980; 181:175–180.

58. Godel V, Loewenstein A, Lazar M. Spectral electroretinography in thioridazine toxicity. Ann Ophthalmol 1990; 22: 293–296.

59. Saletu B, Saletu M, Simeon J, Viamontes G, Itil TM. Comparative symptomatological and evoked potential studies with d-amphetamine, thioridazine, and placebo in hyperkinetic children. Biol Psychiatry 1975; 10:253–275.

60. Boet D. Toxic effects of phenothiazines on the eye. Doc Ophthalmol 1970; 28:16–69.

61. Henkes HE. Electro-oculography as a diagnostic aid in phenothiazin retinopathy. Trans Ophthalmol Soc UK 1967; 87:285–287.

62. Alkemade PP. Phenothiazine-retinopathy. Ophthalmologica 1968; 155:70–76.

63. Cibis BW, Burian HM, Blodi FC. Electroretinogram changes in acute quinine poisoning. Arch Ophthalmol 1973; 90: 307–309.

64. Brinton GS, Norton EWD, Zahn JR, Knighton RW. Ocular quinine toxicity. Am J Ophthalmol 1980; 90:403–410.

65. Yospaiboon Y, Lawtiantong T, Chotibutr S. Clinical observations of ocular quinine intoxication. Jpn J Ophthalmol 1984; 28:409–415.

66. Canning CR, Hague S. Ocular quinine toxicity. Br J Ophthalmol 1988; 72:23–26.

67. Moloney JB, Hillery M, Fenton M. Two year electrophysiology follow-up in quinine amblyopia: a case report. Arch Ophthalmol 1987; 65:731–734.

68. Bacon P, Spalton DJ, Smith SE. Blindness from quinine toxicity. Br J Ophthalmol 1988; 72:219–214.

69. François J, de Rouck A, Cambie E. Retinal and optic evaluation in quinine poisoning. Ann Ophthalmol 1972; 4:177–185.

70. Behrman J, Mushin A. Electrodiagnostic findings in quinine amblyopia. Br J Ophthalmol 1968; 52:925–928.

71. Cohen A, Martin M, Mizanin J, Kankle DF, Schwartz E. Vision and hearing during deferoxamine therapy. J Pediatr 1990; 117:326–330.

72. De Virgiliis S, Congia M, Turco MP, Trau F, Dessi C, Argiolu F, Sorcinelli R, Sitzia A, Cao A. Depletion of trace elements and acute ocular toxicity induced by desferrioxamine in patients with thalassaemia. Arch Dis Child 1988; 63:250–255.

73. Haimovici R, D'Amico DJ, Gragoudas ES, Sokol S. The expanded clinical spectrum of deferoxamine retinopathy. Ophthalmology 2002; 109:164–171.

74. Rahi AH, Hungerford JL, Ahmed AI. Ocular toxicity of desferrioxamine: light microscopic histochemical and ultrastructural findings. Br J Ophthalmol 1986; 70:373–381.

75. Bene C, Manzler A, Bene D, Kranias G. Irreversible ocular toxicity from single "challange" dose of deferoxamine. Clin Nephrol 1987; 31:45–48.

76. Ravelli M, Scaroni P, Mombelloni S, Movilli E, Feller P, Apostoli P, De Maria G, Valotti C, Sciuto G, Maiorca R. Acute visual disorders in patients on regular dialysis given

desferrioxamine as a test. Nephrol Dial Transplant 1990; 5:945–949.

77. Davies SC, Marcus RE, Hungerford JL, Miller MH, Arden GB, Huehns ER. Ocular toxicity of high-dose intravenous desferrioxamine. Lancet 1983; 2:181–184.

78. Lakhampal V, Schocket SS, Jiji R. Deferoxamine (desferal)-induced toxic retinal pigmentary degeneration and presumed optic neuropathy. Ophthalmology 1984; 91:443–451.

79. Orton RB, de Veber LL, Sulh HM. Ocular and auditory toxicity of long-term, high-dose subcutaneous deferoxamine therapy. Can J Ophthalmol 1985; 20:153–156.

80. Triantafyllou N, Fisfis M, Sideris G, Triantafyllou D, Rombos A, Vrettou H, Mantouvalos V, Politi C, Malliara S, Papageorgiou C. Neurophysiological and neuro-otological study of homozygous beta-thalassemia under long-term desferrioxamine (DFO) treatment. Acta Neurol Scand 1991; 83:306–308.

81. Taylor MJ, Keenan NK, Gallant T, Skarf B, Freedman MH, Logan WJ. Subclinical VEP abnormalities in patients on chronic deferoxamine therapy. Longitudinal studies. Electroencephalogr Clin Neurophysiol 1987; 68:81–87.

82. Gelmi C, Borgna-Pignatti C, Franchin S, Tacchini M, Trimarchi F. Electroretinographic and visual-evoked potential abnormalities in patients with beta-thalassemia major. Ophthalmologica 1988; 196:29–34.

83. Daneshvar H, Racette L, Coupland SG, Kertes PJ, Guberman A, Zackon D. Symptomatic and asymptomatic visual loss in patients taking vigabatrin. Ophthalmology 1999; 106: 1792–1798.

84. Käfviäinen R, Nousiainen I, Mäntyjävi M, Nikoskelainen E, Partanen J, Partanen K, Riekkinen P. Vigabatrin, a gabaergic antiepileptic drug, causes concentric visual field defects. Neurology 1999; 53:922–926.

85. Krauss GL, Johnson MA, Miller NR. Vigabatrin-associated retinal cone system dysfunction: electroretinogram and ophthalmologic findings. Neurology 1998; 50:614–618.

86. Lawden MC, Eke T, Degg C, Harding GF, Wild JM. Visual field defects associated with vigabatrin therapy. J Neurol Neurosurg Psychiatry 1999; 67:716–722.

87. Coupland SG, Zackon DH, Leonard BC, Ross TM. Vigabatrin effect on inner retinal function. Ophthalmology 2001; 108:1493–1496.

88. Dong C-J, Hare WA. GABAc feedback pathway modulates the amplitude and kinetics of ERG b-wave in a mammalian retina in vivo. Vision Res 2002; 42:1081–1087.

89. Miller NR, Johnson MA, Paul SR, Girkin CA, Perry JD, Endres M, Krauss GL. Visual dysfunction in patients receiving vigabatrin: clinical and electrophysiologic findings. Neurology 1999; 53:2082–2087.

90. Eke T, Talbot JF, Lawden MC. Severe persistent visual field constriction associated with vigabatrin. Br Med J 1997; 314:180–181.

91. Johnson MA, Krauss GL, Miller NR, Medura M, Paul SR. Visual function loss from vigabatrin: effect of stopping the drug. Neurology 2000; 55:40–45.

92. Weatall CA, Nobile R, Morong S, Buncic JR, Logan WJ, Panton CM. Changes in the electroretinogram resulting from discontinuation of vigabatrin in children. Doc Ophthalmol 2003; 107:299–309.

93. Jensen H, Sjö O, Udall P, Gram L. Vigabatrin and retinal changes. Doc Ophthalmol 2002; 104:171–180.

94. van der Torren K, Graniewski-Wijnands HS, Polak BCP. Visual field and electrophysiological abnormalities due to vigabatrin. Doc Ophthalmol 2002; 104:181–188.

95. Harding GF, Wild JM, Robertson KA, Rietbrock S, Martinez C. Separating the retinal electrophysiologic effects of vigabatrin: treatment versus field loss. Neurology 2000; 55:347–352.

96. Ponjavic V, Andreasson S. Multifocal ERG and full-field ERG in patients on long-term vigabatrin medication. Doc Ophthalmol 2001; 102:63–72.

97. Westall CA, Logan WJ, Smith K, Buncic JR, Panton CM, Abdolell M. The hospital for sick children, Toronto, longitudi-

nal ERG study of children on vigabatrin. Doc Ophthalmol 2002; 104:133–149.

98. Besch D, Kurtenbach A, Apfelstedt-Sylla E, Sadowski B, Dennig D, Asenbauer C, Zrenner E, Schieter U. Visual field constriction and electrophysiological changes associated with vigabatrin. Doc Ophthalmol 2002; 104:151–170.

99. Morong S, Weatall CA, Nobile R, Buncic JR, Logan WJ, Panton CM, Abdolell M. Longitudinal changes in photopic OPs occurring with vigabatrin treatment. Doc Ophthalmol 2003; 107:289–297.

100. Ruether K, Pung T, Kellner U, Schmitz B, Hartmann C, Seeliger M. Electrophysiologic evaluation of a patient with peripheral visual field contraction associated with vigabatrin. Arch Ophthalmol 1998; 116:817–819.

101. Harding GF, Wild JM, Robertson KA, Lawden MC, Betts TA, Barber C, Barnes PM. Electro-oculography, electroretinography, visual evoked potentials, and multifocal electroretinography in patients with vigabatrin-attributed visual field constriction. Epilepsia 2000; 41:1420–1431.

102. Banin E, Shalev RS, Obolnesky A, Neis R, Chowers I, Gross-Tsur V. Retinal function abnormalities in patients treated with vigabatrin. Arch Ophthalmol 2003; 121:811–816.

103. Arndt CF, Derambure P, Defoort-Dhellemmes S, Hache JC. Outer retinal dysfunction in patients treated with vigabatrin. Neurology 1999; 52:1201–1205.

104. Hardus P, Verduin WM, Berendschot TT, Kamermans M, Postma G, Stilma JS, van Veelen CW. The value of electrophysiology results in patients with epilepsy and vigabatrin associated visual field loss. Acta Ophthalmol Scand 2001; 79:169–174.

105. Harding GFA, Robertson K, Spencer EL, Holliday I. Vigabatrin: its effect on the electrophysiology of vision. Doc Ophthalmol 2002; 104:213–229.

106. Spencer EL, Harding GFA. Examining visual field defects in the paediatric population exposed to vigabatrin. Doc Ophthalmol 2003; 107:289–297.

107. Comaish IF, Gorman C, Brinlow GM, Barber C, Orr GM, Galloway NR. The effects of vigabatrin on electrophysiology and visual fields in epileptics: a controlled study with a discussion of possible mechanisms. Doc Ophthalmol 2002; 104:195–212.

108. Graniewski-Wijnands HS, van der Torren K. Electro-ophthalmological recovery after withdrawal from vigabatrin. Doc Ophthalmol 2002; 104:189–194.

109. Marmor MF, Kessler R. Sildenafil (viagra) and ophthalmology. Surv Ophthalmol 1999; 44:153–162.

110. McCulley TJ, Lam BL, Marmor MF, Hoffman KB, Luu JK, Feuer WJ. Acute effects of sildenafil on blue-on-yellow and white-on-white Humphrey perimetry. J Neuro-Ophthalmol 2000; 20:227–228.

111. Vobig MA, Klotz T, Staak M, Bartz-Schmidt KU, Engelmann U, Walter P. Retinal side-effects of sildenafil. Lancet 1999; 353:375.

112. Gabrieli CB, Regine F, Vingolo EM, Rispoli E, Fabbri A, Isodori A. Subjective visual halos after sildenafil (viagra) administration: electroretinographic evaluation. Ophthalmology 2001; 108:877–881.

113. Gabrieli CB, Regine F, Vingolo EM, Rispoli E, Isidori A. Acute electroretinographic changes during sildenafil (viagra) treatment for erectile dysfunction. Doc Ophthalmol 2003; 107:111–114.

114. Luu JK, Chappelow AV, McCulley TJ, Marmor MF. Acute effects of sildenafil on the electroretinogram and multifocal electroretinogram. Am J Ophthalmol 2001; 132:388–394.

115. Jagle H, Jagle C, Serey L, Yu A, Rilk A, Sadowski B, Besch D, Zrenner E, Sharpe LT. Visual short-term effects of viagra: double blind study in healthy young subjects. Am J Ophthalmol 2004; 137:842–849.

116. Behn D, Potter MJ. Sildenafil-mediated reduction in retinal function in heterozygous mice lacking the gamma-subunit of phosphodiesterase. Invest Ophthalmol Vision Sci 2001; 42:523–527.

117. D'Amico DJ, Caspers-Velu L, Libert J, Shanks E, Schrooyen M, Hanninen LA, Kenyon KR. Comparative toxicity of intravitreal aminoglycoside antibiotics. Am J Ophthalmol 1985; 100:264–275.

118. D'Amico DJ, Libert J, Kenyon KR, Hanninen LA, Caspers-Velu L. Retinal toxicity of intravitreal gentamicin. An electron microscopic study.. Invest Ophthalmol Vision Sci 1984; 25:564–572.

119. Kawasaki K, Ohnogi J. Nontoxic concentration of kanamycin and gentamicin for intravitreal use—evaluated by in vitro ERG. Doc Ophthalmol 1988; 70:301–308.

120. Kawasaki K, Mochizuki K, Torisaki M, Yamashita Y, Shirao Y, Wakabayashi K, Tanabe J. Electroretinographical changes due to antimicrobials. Lens Eye Toxic Res 1990; 7:693–704.

121. Palimeris G, Moschos M, Chimonidou E, Panagakis E, Andreanos D, Smirnof T. Retinal toxicity of antibiotics: evaluation by electroretinogram. Doc Ophthal Proc Ser 1978; 15:45–52.

122. Loewenstein A, Zemel E, Vered Y, Lazar M, Perlman I. Retinal toxicity of gentamicin after subconjunctival injection performed adjacent to thinned sclera. Ophthalmology 2001; 108:759–764.

123. Brown GC, Eagle RC, Shakin EP, Gruber M, Arbizio VV. Retinal toxicity of intravitreal gentamicin. Arch Ophthalmol 1990; 108:1740–1744.

124. Yiannikas C, Walsh JC, McLeod JG. Visual evoked potentials in the detection of subclinical optic toxic effects secondary to ethambutol. Arch Neurol 1983; 40:645–648.

125. Kakisu Y, Adachi-Usami E, Mizota A. Pattern electroretinogram and visual evoked cortical potential in ethambutol optic neuropathy. Doc Ophthalmol 1987; 67:327–334.

126. Nasemann J, Zrenner E, Riedel KG. Recovery after severe ethambutol intoxication—psychophysical and electrophysiological correlations. Doc Ophthalmol 1989; 71:279–292.

127. Kumar A, Sandramouli S, Verma L, Tewari HK, Khosla PK. Ocular ethambutol toxicity: is it reversible? J Ocul Pharmacol Ther 1995; 11:411–419.

128. Woung LC, Jou JR, Liaw SL. Visual function in recovered ethambutol optic neuropathy. J Ocul Pharmacol Ther 1995; 11:411–419.

129. Yen MY, Wang AG, Chiang SC, Liu JH. Ethambutol retinal toxicity: an electrophysiologic study. J Formos Med Assoc 2000; 99:630–634.

130. Wilding G, Caruso RC, Lawrence TS, Ostchega Y, Ballintine EJ, Young RC, Ozols RF. Retinal toxicity after high-dose cisplatin therapy. J Clin Oncol 1985; 3:1683–1689.

131. Hilliard LM, Berkow RL, Watterson J, Ballard EA, Balzer GK, Moertel CL. Retinal toxicity associated with cisplatin and etoposide in pediatric patients. Med Pediatr Oncol 1997; 28:310–313.

132. Marmor MF. Negative-type electroretinogram from cisplatin toxicity. Doc Ophthalmol 1993; 84:237–246.

133. Katz BJ, Ward JH, Digre KB, Creel DJ, Mamalis N. Persistent severe visual and electroretinographic abnormalities after intravenous cisplatin therapy. J Neuro-Ophthalmol 2003; 23:132–135.

134. Maiese K, Walker RW, Gargan R, Victor JD. Intra-arterial cisplatin-associated optic and otic toxicity. Arch Neurol 1992; 49:83–86.

135. Henkes HE, van Lith GH, Canta LR. Indomethacin retinopathy. Am J Ophthalmol 1972; 73:846–856.

136. Burns CA. Indomethacin, reduced retinal sensitivity, and corneal deposits. Am J Ophthalmol 1968; 66:825–835.

16

Non-Organic Visual Loss and Other Ocular and Systemic Disorders

This chapter provides electrophysiological information on non-organic visual loss as well as other ocular and systemic conditions not covered by other chapters. Awareness of the potential effects of common ocular conditions such as refractive error and cataract is important in the interpretation of electrophysiological tests. In addition, some systemic disorders such as muscular dystrophy and liver dysfunction do not typically cause significant visual symptoms but may nevertheless be associated with abnormal electrophysiological responses. The outline of the chapter is as follows:

Non-organic visual loss (functional visual loss):
    Ocular disorders:
        • Hyperopia, myopia, and myopic retinal degeneration
        • Cataract and media opacities
        • Retinal detachment
        • Pigment dispersion syndrome
    Systemic disorders:
        Human immunodeficiency virus (HIV) infection

- Thyroid dysfunction
- Adrenocortical hyperactivity and corticosteroid
- Liver dysfunction
- Duchenne and Becker muscular dystrophies
- Myotonic dystrophy
- Albinism

NON-ORGANIC VISUAL LOSS

Non-organic or functional visual loss occurs when the nature or the amount of visual impairment is incompatible with objective clinical findings. Non-organic visual loss has been classified into two categories. In the "malingering" type, will-ful pretension or exaggeration of symptoms is consciously made for personal gains. In the so-called "hysteria" type, non-organic symptoms are the result of subconscious process. Because differentiation between the two types depends on knowing the psychological origin of the symptoms, determin-ing whether the non-organic visual loss is strictly due to "malingering" or "hysteria" is not always possible. Thompson (1) further categorized patients with non-organic visual loss into four groups. The "deliberate malingerer" pur-posely feigns visual loss. The "worried imposter" willingly exaggerates visual loss but worries that there may be serious disease. The "impressionable exaggerator" believes disease is present and is determined not to hide his disease. The "sug-gestible innocent" is convinced the symptoms are real but remains inappropriately complacent. The diagnosis of non-organic visual loss is made on the basis of excluding organic diseases, which requires thorough clinical examination and appropriate work-up. Therefore, patients with occult or early organic disease may be erroneously diagnosed as having non-organic visual loss. Further, non-organic visual loss may occur in the presence of concurrent unrelated organic ocular disease as well as in visually asymptomatic patients who have non-physiological test results such as tunneling of visual fields. On the other hand, patients with mild vague com-plaints and normal clinical examinations may not necessarily be given a diagnosis of non-organic visual loss. The prognosis of non-organic visual loss is variable and unpredictable (2,3).

Many techniques and maneuvers are available to elicit non-physiological subjective visual acuity and field results in patients suspected of non-organic visual loss (4,5). However, with minimal coaching, some normal persons can easily imitate reproducible quadrantic, hemianopic, and altitudinal visual fields with automated or manual perimetry (6). In cases of equivocal non-organic visual loss, electrophysiological tests are helpful to exclude organic diseases. Diffuse retinal dysfunction can be determined by full-field ERG. Focal retinal dysfunction may be detected by focal and multifocal ERG, but the patient should be monitored for intentional or unintentional poor fixation that may produce falsely impaired results. Suppressed multifocal ERG responses have been reported in patients with non-organic visual loss as well as healthy volunteers who attempted suppression with inattention, poor fixation, and by adjusting the focus to the greatest blur (7).

The use of pattern and flash VEP in diagnosing non-organic visual loss has been advocated by several investigators (8–12). Steele et al. (10) found that objective estimate of visual acuity based on pattern VEP is useful in diagnosing non-organic visual loss. Subsequently, Xu et al. (12) reached the same conclusion in a study of 72 patients. In addition, Towle et al. (11) found that the P300 component of the VEP, whose amplitude is not influenced by stimulus pattern size, can also be helpful in determining non-organic visual loss.

Voluntary suppression of the VEP response is possible in some normal persons so an abnormal result in patients suspected of non-organic visual loss should not be attributed automatically to organic disease. Pattern onset/offset and flash VEP are less susceptible to this effect than pattern reversal VEP. Uren et al. (13) found that both the amplitude and the latency of the VEP response may be impaired in normal persons by deliberate poor fixation and defocusing. Therefore, direct observation of the patient during VEP is essential to reduce poor fixation. Bumgartner and Epstein (14) noted that of the 15 normal subjects they studied, one-third was capable of altering or obliterating the pattern reversal VEP responses by maneuvers such as meditation, daydreaming, and convergence. Likewise, Morgan et al. (15) found approximately 20% of their 42 normal subjects were able to consciously extinguish or alter the pattern reversal VEP, but only about 10% could extinguish the flash VEP. In the same study, no significant change in pattern reversal VEP implicit time and no change in flash VEP amplitude were found in the normal subjects who tried but failed to extinguish their VEP.

Taken together, a diagnosis of non-organic visual loss is well supported when unequivocal normal responses are obtained from a combination of retinal and cortical electrophysiological tests that may include the full-field ERG, multifocal ERG, pattern ERG, pattern VEP, and flash VEP. For instance, Röver and Bach (9) pointed out that in the presence of an impaired VEP in suspected non-organic visual loss patients, a normal pattern ERG is helpful to confirm the diagnosis. Similarly, the diagnosis of non-organic visual loss is reasonably founded when the full-field ERG, multifocal ERG, and pattern VEP are all well within normal limits. On the other hand, impaired results in tests that require good fixation or attention or both such as the multifocal ERG and pattern VEP, may be due to voluntary maneuvers and may not necessarily be signs of organic disease.

OCULAR DISORDERS

Hyperopia, Myopia, and Myopic Retinal Degeneration

The ERG responses are impaired in moderate and high myopia even in the absence of myopic retinal degeneration. The reduction in both scotopic and photopic ERG amplitudes correlates directly with increased axial eye length rather than directly with refractive error (16–19). The ERG amplitude reductions generally are more likely to reach clinical significance for myopia of more than -5 diopters. Compared to ERG amplitudes, the b-wave to a-wave amplitude ratios, implicit times, and retinal sensitivity, as measured by increased stimulus intensity ERG responses, are less likely to be affected (17–19). Reduced and delayed multifocal ERG is also found in myopia and is primarily the result of cone function loss (20). In addition, EOG reductions are associated with myopia but a clear correlation between axial eye length and EOG light-peak to dark-trough amplitude ratios was not found (16,21).

Myopic retinal degeneration refers to progressive retinal thinning and chorioretinal atrophy that occur in some highly myopic persons. In contrast to myopia without retinal degeneration, myopic retinal degeneration causes notable reduction in EOG that is somewhat related to the extent of the chorioretinal atrophy (21,22). Scotopic and photopic full-field ERG responses are generally moderate to severe impaired with the b-wave being more likely to be affected than the a-wave (Fig. 16.1) (22).

Electrophysiological responses in hyperopia are less well studied. In a study of 31 patients with refractive errors of greater than +5 diopters, Perlman et al. (17) noted no consistent full-field ERG abnormalities nor a correlation between ERG responses and axial eye length.

Cataract and Media Opacities

Cataract and other media opacities affect electrophysiological responses by absorbing, reflecting, and scattering the incoming light stimulus. Dense opacities such as brunescent cataract and dense vitreous hemorrhage that absorb light are likely to result in reduced and prolonged full-field ERG responses, but even an extremely dense media opacity is unlikely to completely extinguish standard full-field ERG responses in an otherwise normal eye. Opacities such as mature white cataract that scatters light are unlikely to diminish the full-field ERG responses. On the contrary, a unilateral dense white mature cataract produces a modest increase in the pupil–light reaction indicating greater visual afferent input (23).

When the view to the retina and the optic nerve head is obscured by a dense media opacity, the integrity of the visual

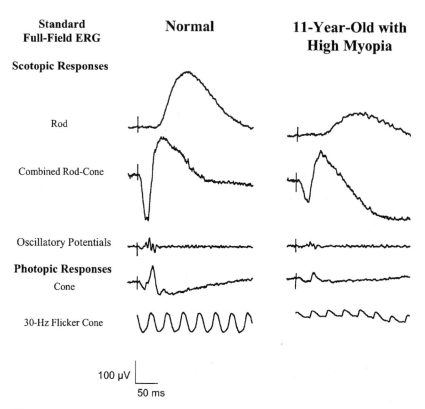

Standard Full-Field ERG | Normal | 11-Year-Old with High Myopia

Scotopic Responses

Rod

Combined Rod-Cone

Oscillatory Potentials

Photopic Responses
Cone

30-Hz Flicker Cone

100 μV
50 ms

Figure 16.1 Full-field ERG responses of an 11-year-old boy with high myopia (–14 diopters) and myopic retinal degeneration. Visual acuity was 20/200. Note the reduced and prolonged cone and rod responses.

pathway can still be assessed by a combination of diagnostic tests such as afferent pupillary defect testing, ultrasound, full-field ERG, and flash VEP. A visual pathway defect should be suspected if an afferent pupillary defect is seen in an eye with a cataract, even a very dense one (23). Ultrasound is helpful to detect anatomical alterations behind the media opacity. Several investigators have demonstrated better visual outcome after cataract extraction in patients with dense cataracts and normal or near normal preoperative full-field ERG or VEP, or both (24–28). Because full-field ERG is a measure of retinal function and VEP tests the entire visual system, VEP testing is helpful to determine whether optic neuropathy or more posterior visual pathway defect is present. In patients with unilateral media opacity, a comparison of the full-field ERG and VEP responses with those of the fellow eye is important to minimize misinterpretation of test results due to intersubject variability (29,30). Unfortunately, none of the diagnostic tests mentioned can consistently detect amblyopia, which may be confirmed only with an accurate past ocular history (31).

High intensity bright-flash ERG has been advocated to assess visual prognosis in patients with media opacity and preexisting ocular conditions such as diabetic retinopathy (32). Because ERG response may be affected by the media opacity or the retinal condition or both, the results should be interpreted cautiously. For instance, visual improvement may occur after vitrectomy for dense vitreous hemorrhage even when the preoperative ERG responses are non-detectable (33,34).

The effect of cataract on multifocal ERG responses has not been studied in detail. Reductions of central multifocal ERG responses are found in normal persons when light scatter is produced with liquid crustal diffuser or acrylic sheets (35,36). These findings are relatively consistent with findings of a study comparing multifocal ERG responses before and after removal of mild to moderate cataracts (37).

In terms of other cataract-related electrophysiological findings, reduced oscillatory potentials of the full-field ERG are found in patients with aphakic or pseudophakic cystoid macular edema suggesting inner retinal layer dysfunction not only in the macula but also throughout retina (38). Patients treated for unilateral congenital cataract, who have early surgery and contact lens correction and comply with occlusion therapy, show rapid VEP maturation and have a good visual prognosis (39).

Retinal Detachment

A separation between the retinal pigment epithelium and the photoreceptors, often accompanied by accumulation of serous fluid in this potential space, is called retinal detachment. In retinal detachment, the amount of ERG deterioration is related to the size of the detachment and the degree of dysfunction of the detached retina. Both rod and cone responses may be reduced and prolonged with similar effects on the a-wave and b-wave. The ERG is likely to be severely reduced in chronic, large retinal detachment. Interestingly, mild reduced ERG may occur in the contralateral normal eye in patients with unilateral retinal detachment (40). In addition, Sasoh et al. (41) using multifocal ERG technique found impaired ERG in both attached and detached retinal areas before and after successful retinal reattachment surgery and the ERG disturbance was more widespread than the visual field abnormality. The short-wavelength cone (S-cone) system may be more prone to damage in retinal detachment than the long-wavelength and medium-wavelength cone systems (42).

The clinical role of ERG in retinal detachment is limited. Some investigators found the amplitude of the ERG response to be of prognostic value for return of visual function after successful retinal reattachment (43,44). However, this finding is not supported by other studies (45). Regardless, retinal reattachment procedures are usually undertaken without the necessity of a preoperative ERG although postoperatively ERG may be helpful to assess retinal function when expected visual improvement fails to occur. The EOG is diminished in retinal detachment, because to maintain a retinal resting potential, the integrity of the retinal pigment epithelium as well as its contact with the photoreceptors must be intact.

Injection of silicone oil or 20% sulfur hexafluoride (SF_6) gas into the vitreous chamber as intraocular tamponade is an integral part of a number of retinal reattachment procedures. Frumar et al. (46) found similar impaired ERG responses in patients treated with silicone oil or SF_6 gas. A progressive recovery of the ERG was observed over a 6-month follow-up period with accelerated ERG recovery following either the removal of the silicone oil or absorption of the intraocular SF_6 gas bubble. The authors proposed that the insulation effect of the tamponade agents produced the impaired ERG responses. Similar ERG recovery following silicone oil removal was also reported by Foerster et al. (47) and Thaler et al. (48). Further, Foerster found that the EOG also recovered after silicone oil removal but the EOG recovery was not as consistent as the ERG and may reflect the continued effect on the EOG from previous detachment. In contrast, Thaler found EOG fast and slow oscillations non-detectable preoperatively or postoperatively before or after silicone oil removal. Of interest, an ERG model for determining the volume conductor effect of silicone oil on the ERG was developed by Doslek (49). Based on the model, a small reduction in the ERG was not produced until at least 50% of the vitreous was replaced with silicone oil, and the ERG diminished non-linearly as the percentage of silicone oil increased further. Despite the observed ERG impairment due to silicone oil in humans, Meredith et al. (50) did not find any ERG reduction in rabbits following vitrectomy and silicone oil injection.

Pigment Dispersion Syndrome

Pigment dispersion syndrome is characterized by dispersed pigment in the anterior chamber caused by disruption of the iris pigment epithelium from friction with lens zonules during physiological changes in pupil size. The condition is associated with glaucoma, lattice degeneration, and retinal detachment. Abnormal function of the retinal pigment epithelium is suspected. In support of this hypothesis, Scuderi et al. (51) found reduced EOG light-peak to dark-trough amplitude ratios in patients with pigment dispersion syndrome compared with patients with chronic open-angle glaucoma and normal subjects. Likewise, Greenstein et al. (52) noted significantly reduced EOG amplitude ratios in patients with pigment dispersion syndrome (2.00 ± 0.33, mean $\pm$ variance, 14 subjects) and patients with pigmentary glaucoma (1.78 ± 0.29, 11 subjects) as compared to the control group (2.68 ± 0.52).

SYSTEMIC DISORDERS

Human Immunodeficiency Virus (HIV) Infection

Human immunodeficiency virus (HIV) infection often results in acquired immunodeficiency syndrome (AIDS). Ocular findings include cotton wool spots, retinal hemorrhages, and cytomegalovirus retinitis. Significantly impairment of virtually all parameters of the full-field ERG are found in patients with cytomegalovirus retinitis (53). In addition, subclinical retinopathy and visual pathway dysfunction in HIV patients with normal retinal appearance may occur and can be detected by mild to moderate impairment of color vision, contrast sensitivity, ERG, or VEP (53–57). In general, full-field ERG responses of HIV patients are more likely to have impaired amplitude rather than prolonged implicit time when compared to those of control subjects (53). Transient pattern ERG responses are more affected than steady-state responses in HIV patients (55). Impaired VEP responses may also occur in neurologically asymptomatic HIV patients (58,59).

Thyroid Dysfunction

Full-field ERG, pattern ERG, and VEP are generally reduced in hypothyroidism and improve with thyroid hormone replacement therapy (60–63). Tamburini et al. (62) noted a significant correlation between increased VEP P100 latency and decreased thyroxine (T4) levels. In a study of pattern ERG and pattern VEP, Holder and Condon concluded that pattern VEP delay in hypothyroidism is at least in part due to reversible central retinal dysfunction. Of interest, infants with congenital hypothyroidism demonstrate delayed visual maturation which becomes normal even without treatment (64).

Increased or supernormal full-field ERG responses have been reported in hyperthyroidism (61,65). However, Mitchell et al. (66) found no significant change in pattern VEP responses in hyperthyroid patients. The electrophysiological findings of compressive optic neuropathy from thyroid-associated ophthalmopathy are discussed in Chapter 17.

Adrenocortical Hyperactivity and Corticosteroid

Increased or supernormal full-field ERG responses have been reported in patients with hyperadrenocorticism as well as patients receiving corticosteroid therapy (67). Increases in both the scotopic and photopic a- and b-waves are found and are particularly notable in eyes of normal subjects during the early period of corticosteroid therapy (68). However, the effects of chronic corticosteroid therapy on the ERG have not been studied in detail.

Liver Dysfunction

Patients with hepatic failure are at risk for developing hepatic encephalopathy. Eckstein et al. (69) showed that both the scotopic and photopic a- and b-waves of the full-field ERG are decreased and delayed in patients with more advanced stages of hepatic encephalopathy. The oscillatory potentials were delayed even in patients with minimal encephalopathy and were significantly decreased in patients with more severe encephalopathy. Despite these ERG alterations, the patients were asymptomatic and were found to have only very mild pigmentary retinal changes that are not definitively attributable to the liver disease. Studies of VEP as a diagnostic tool for encephalopathy are limited and show mixed results (70,71).

Duchenne and Becker Muscular Dystrophies

Mutations of the gene encoding dystrophin, located on the X chromosome (Xp12), are associated with X-linked recessive muscular dystrophies ranging from the severe Duchenne type to the milder Becker type. Dystrophin, a cytoskeletal protein, is not only expressed in muscle but also in numerous tissues including heart, brain, and retina. Patients with Duchenne muscular dystrophy have early-onset progressive proximal muscular dystrophy with pseudohypertrophy of the calves. Death from cardiac and respiratory deficiency occurs in the second or third decade of life.

Patients with muscular dystrophy are visually asymptomatic with normal retinal appearance. However, full-field ERG demonstrates negative responses such that a selective impairment of the b-wave occurs in the scotopic bright-flash combined rod–cone response and results in a b-wave to a-wave amplitude ratio of less than one (72–75). Other ERG features include impaired rod response and decreased oscillatory potentials. Taken together, these ERG characteristics of muscular dystrophy resemble those of congenital stationary night blindness (CSNB), but in contrast to CSNB, the cone flash response is well preserved in muscular dystrophy and the decrease in oscillatory potentials is more selective to the OP_2 component especially under photopic conditions (74,76). In addition, patients with muscular dystrophy have no night blindness and have normal dark adaptation measurements despite reduced rod ERG response (77,78). Nevertheless, long duration stimulus full-field ERG to separate ON- and OFF-bipolar cell activity in muscular dystrophy shows abnormal transmission of signals of the ON-response (73). Some correlations of phenotype by ERG in patients with dystrophin mutations have been demonstrated (79,80). The most important determinant of the ERG b-wave phenotype is the mutation position rather than disease severity (79). Female muscular dystrophy carriers may also have abnormal ERG responses but these are much milder than affected males (81). Lastly, a combination of muscular dystrophy, glycerol kinase deficiency, and congenital adrenal hypoplasia is found in association with a deletion at Xp21 (82). These rare patients also demonstrate negative scotopic responses and some may have features of ocular albinism.

Myotonic Dystrophy

Myotonic dystrophy is an autosomal dominant disorder resulting from an expansion of a variable trinucleotide (CTG) repeat in the untranslated 3′-terminus region of the gene encoding dystrophia myotonica protein kinase on chromosome 19 (DM1) or, less commonly, the disorder is associated with a genetic locus on chromosome 3q (DM2). Systemic manifestations include facial weakness, distal weakness with difficulty releasing hand grip, frontal baldness, and dysarthria. The diagnosis is usually evident by family history and clinical features.

The most consistent ocular findings in myotonic dystrophy are cataract and low intraocular pressure. Up to 50% of affected persons may have retinal pigmentary disturbance at the macula, which may be reticular or butterfly-shaped in appearance (83). Peripheral retinal atrophic pigmentary changes may also occur alone or concurrently with the macular disturbance. The retinal changes may slowly progress but rarely do they produce severe visual impairment.

In general, ERG in myotonic dystrophy shows impaired scotopic responses with a relatively selective impairment of the b-wave with reduced b-wave amplitude and prolonged b-wave implicit time for rod response and the combined rod–cone response. Photopic cone b-wave response amplitude may also be reduced. The ERG abnormalities may occur in the absence of any apparent clinical retinal changes, and correlation between clinical and ERG findings is variable (84). In an early report, Burian and Burns (85) performed scotopic ERG on 24 patients with myotonic dystrophy and found the responses to be reduced primarily due to a selective reduction of the b-wave. Dark adaptation thresholds were found to be slightly elevated than normal, but the patients reported no nyctalopia. Subsequently, Stanescu and Michiels (86) performed ERG on 11 patients with myotonic dystrophy and reported decrease of scotopic as well as photopic b-wave amplitude with delayed scotopic implicit time (86). These ERG findings are supported by other reports (87,88). Correlations between VEP P100 latency and ERG b-wave amplitude and those between VEP P100 amplitude and ERG b-wave amplitude have been demonstrated (89).

Albinism

Albinism refers to a group of genetically diverse disorders characterized by hypopigmentation of the skin, hair, and eyes. Albinism may be divided into oculocutaneous or ocular albinism. In both oculocutaneous and ocular albinism, iris transillumination defects, hypopigmentation of the retinal pigment epithelium, and foveal hypoplasia are apparent, but in ocular albinism, the skin and hair appear normal (Fig. 16.2). Oculocutaneous albinism is usually autosomal recessive or dominant while ocular albinism is typically autosomal or X-linked recessive. Other ocular manifestations of albinism include nystagmus, photoaversion, and reduced visual acuity. In female carriers of X-linked ocular albinism, the retinal appearance may be normal or demonstrate classic

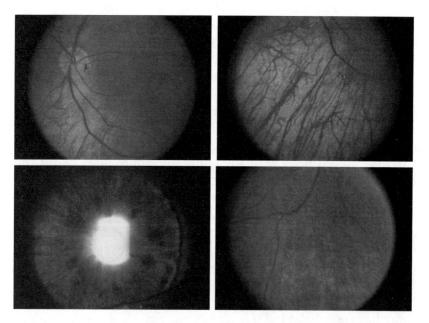

Figure 16.2 X-linked ocular albinism (previous unpublished photographs of pedigree reported in Ref. 92). *Top left and top right:* Fundus of the left eye of a 25-year-old affected man with 20/60 vision showing indistinct fovea and retinal depigmentation. *Bottom left:* Iris illumination defects in the 76-year-old affected maternal cousin. *Bottom right:* "Mud-splattered" retinal appearance of the 55-year-old mother who is an obligatory carrier. The full-field ERG responses of the affected males in this family were normal. (Refer to the color insert.)

"mud-splattered" appearance of the peripheral retina or focal or diffuse hypopigmentation (Fig. 16.2).

Full-field ERG responses in albinism are generally normal. In an early report, Krill and Lee (90) found normal EOG and supranormal scotopic ERG responses. The authors hypothesized that increased intraocular reflection of light due to lack of light-absorbing pigment was the cause of the increased ERG responses. However, subsequent studies showed that full-field ERG responses in albinism are generally similar rather than increased in comparison to normal subjects (91–95).

In albinism, abnormal crossing of retinal ganglion cell fibers occurs at the optic chiasm and can be demonstrated by VEP testing (96,97). Normal persons have hemidecussation of ganglion cell fibers at the chiasm with fibers from the nasal retina crossing to the contralateral side. For patients with albinism, majority of the fibers from the temporal retina also cross and an excessive amount of fibers from the eye is projected to the contralateral cerebral hemisphere. This misrouting of the visual pathway can be detected as asymmetry in the VEP responses from the occipital cortex with monocular light stimulation. For example, when the right eye is stimulated in an albino, VEP activity is greater over the left occipital cortex, and the reverse occurs when the left eye is stimulated. This phenomenon can be demonstrated by several different VEP methodologies but is best seen with a bipolar electrode setup that compares the differences in responses between the left and right occipital hemispheres during monocular stimulation (98,99). If misrouting is present, the bipolar VEP recording is inverted when the response from stimulation of one eye is compared to the stimulation of the other eye. If significant nystagmus is present, pattern-reversal VEP may not be feasible due to poor fixation, and flash VEP or pattern onset/offset VEP is employed. The extent of misrouting of the visual pathway is somewhat variable among albinos (100). In addition, this phenomenon should not be considered as pathognomonic for albinism since crossed VEP asymmetry has also been observed in patients with incomplete congenital stationary night blindness (101).

REFERENCES

1. Thompson HS. Functional visual loss. Am J Ophthalmol 1985; 100:209–213.

2. Barris MC, Kaufman DI, Barberio D. Visual impairment in hysteria. Doc Ophthalmol 1992; 82:369–382.

3. Kathol RG, Cox TA, Corbett JJ, Thompson HS. Functional visual loss. Follow-up of 42 cases. Arch Ophthalmol 1983; 101:729–735.

4. Bose S, Kupersmith MJ. Neuro-ophthalmologic presentations of functional visual disorders [review]. Neurol Clin 1995; 13:321–339.

5. Kramer KK, La Piana FG, Appleton B. Ocular malingering and hysteria: diagnosis and management. Surv Ophthalmol 1979; 24:89–96.

6. Thompson JC, Kosmorsky GS, Ellis BD. Fields of dreamers and dreamed-up fields. Ophthalmology 1996; 103:117–125.

7. Vrabec TR, Affel EL, Gaughan JP, Foroozan R, Tennant MTS, Klancnik JMJ, Jordan CS, Savino PJ. Voluntary suppression of the multifocal electroretinogram. Ophthalmology 2004; 111:169–176.

8. Bobak P, Khanna P, Goodwin J, Brigell M. Pattern visual evoked potentials in cases of ambiguous acuity loss. Doc Ophthalmol 1993; 85:185–192.

9. Röver J, Bach M. Pattern electroretinogram plus visual-evoked potential: a decisive test in patients suspected of malingering. Doc Ophthalmol 1987; 66:245–251.

10. Steele M, Seiple WH, Carr RE, Klug R. The clinical utility of visual-evoked potential acuity testing. Am J Ophthalmol 1989; 108:572–577.

11. Towle VL, Sutcliffe E, Sokol S. Diagnosing functional visual defects with the P300 component of the visual evoked potential. Arch Ophthalmol 1985; 103:47–50.

12. Xu S, Meyer D, Yoser S, Mathews D, Elfervig JL. Pattern visual evoked potential in the diagnosis of functional visual loss. Ophthalmology 2001; 108:76–80.

13. Uren SM, Stewart P, Crosby PA. Subject cooperation and the visual evoked response. Invest Ophthalmol Vis Sci 1979; 18:648–652.

14. Bumgartner J, Epstein CM. Voluntary alteration of visual evoked potentials. Ann Neurol 1982; 12:475–478.

15. Morgan RK, Niugent B, Harrison JM, O'Connor PS. Voluntary alteration of pattern visual evoked responses. Ophthalmology 1985; 92:1356–1363.

16. Pallin O. The influence of the axial length of the eye on the size of the recorded b-potential in the clinical single-flash electroretinogram. Acta Ophthalmol 1969; 101 (suppl): 1–57.

17. Perlman I, Meyer E, Haim T, Zonis S. Retinal function in high refractive error assessed electroretinographically. Br J Ophthalmol 1984; 68:79–84.

18. Westall CA, Dhaliwal HS, Panton CM, Sigesmun D, Levin AV, Nischal KK, Heon E. Values of electroretinogram responses according to axial length. Doc Ophthalmol 2001; 102:115–130.

19. Chen JF, Eisner AE, Burns SA, Hansen RM, Lou PL, Kwong KK, Fulton AB. The effect of eye shape on retinal responses. Clin Vision Sci 1992; 7:521–530.

20. Kawabata H, Adachi-Usami E. Multifocal electroretinogram in myopia. Invest Ophthalmol Vis Sci 1997; 38:2844–2852.

21. Arden GB, Barrada A, Kelsey JH. New clinical test of retinal function based upon the standing potential of the eye. Br J Ophthalmol 1962; 46:449–467.

22. Blach RK, Jay B, Kolb H. Electrical activity of the eye in high myopia. Br J Ophthalmol 1966; 50:629–641.

23. Lam BL, Thompson HS. A unilateral cataract produces a relative afferent pupillary defect in the contralateral eye. Ophthalmology 1990; 97:334–338.

24. Brodie SE. Evaluation of cataractous eyes with opaque media. Int Ophthalmol Clin 1987; 27:153–162.

25. Burian HM, Burns CA. A note on senile cataracts and the electroretinogram. Doc Ophthalmol 1966; 20:141–149.

26. Kennerdell JS. Evaluation of eyes with opaque anterior segments, using both ultrasonography and electroretinography. Am J Ophthalmol 1973; 75:853–860.

27. Knighton RW, Blankenship GW. Electrophysiological evaluation of eyes with opaque media. Int Ophthalmol Clin 1980; 20:1–19.

28. Vrijland HR, van Lith GH. The value of preoperative electro-ophthalmological examination before cataract extraction. Doc Ophthalmol 1983; 55:153–156.

29. Rubin ML, Dawson WW. The transcleral VER: predication of postoperative acuity. Invest Ophthalmol Vis Sci 1978; 17: 71–74.

30. Thompson CRS, Harding GFA. The visual evoked potential in patients with cataracts. Doc Ophthalmol Proc Ser 1978; 15:193–201.

31. Galloway NR. Electrophysiological testing of eyes with opaque media. Eye 1988; 2:615–624.

32. Fuller D. Evaluation of eyes with opaque media by using bright-flash electroretinography. Int Ophthalmol Clin 1978; 18:121–125.

33. Abrams GW, Knighton RW. Falsely extinguished bright-flash electroretinogram: its association with dense vitreous hemorrhage. Arch Ophthalmol 1982; 100:1427–1429.

34. Mandelbaum S, Ober RR, Ogden TE. Nonrecordable electroretinogram in vitreous hemorrhage. Ophthalmology 1982; 89:73–75.

35. Chan HL, Siu AW, Yap MK, Brown B. The effect of light scattering on multifocal electroretinography. Ophthalmol Physiol Opt 2002; 22:482–490.

36. Arai M, Lopes de Faria JM, Hirose T. Effects of stimulus blocking, light scattering and distortion on multifocal electroretinogram. Jpn J Ophthalmol 1999; 43:481–489.

37. Wördehoff UV, Palmowski AM, Heinemann-Vernaleken B, Allgayer R, Ruprecht KW. Influence of cataract on the multifocal ERG recording—a pre- and postoperative comparison. Doc Ophthalmol 2004; 108:67–75.

38. Terasaki H, Miyake K, Miyake Y. Reduced oscillatory potentials of the full-field electroretinogram of eyes with aphakic or pseudophakic cystoid macular edema. Am J Ophthalmol 2003; 135:477–482.

39. McCulloch DL, Skarf B. Pattern reversal visual evoked potentials following early treatment of unilateral, congenital cataract. Arch Ophthalmol 1994; 112:510–518.

40. Karpe G, Rendahl I. Clinical electroretinography in detachment of the retina. Acta Ophthalmol 1969; 47:633–641.

41. Sasoh M, Yoshida S, Kuze M, Uji Y. The multifocal electroretinogram in retinal detachment. Doc Ophthalmol 1998; 94:239–252.

42. Hayashi M, Yamamoto S. Changes of cone electroretinograms to colour flash stimuli after successful retinal detachment surgery. Br J Ophthalmol 2001; 85:410–413.

43. Jacobson JH, Basar D, Carroll J, Stephens G, Safir A. The electroretinogram as a prognostic aid in retinal detachment. Can J Neurol Sci 1958; 59:515–520.

44. Rendahl I. The electroretinogram in detachment of the retina. Arch Ophthalmol 1957; 57:566–576.

45. Schmöger E. The prognostic significance of electroretinograms in conjunction with retinal detachment. Klin Monatsbl Augenheikd 1957; 131:335–343.

46. Frumar KD, Gregor ZJ, Carter RM, Arden GB. Electrophysiological responses after vitrectomy and intraocular tamponade. Trans Ophthalmol Soc UK 1985; 104:129–132.

47. Foerster MH, Esser J, Laqua H. Silicone oil and its influence on electrophysiologic findings. Am J Ophthalmol 1985; 99:201–206.

48. Thaler A, Lessel MR, Gnad H, Heilig P. The influence of intravitreously injected silicone oil on electrophysiological potentials of the eye. Doc Ophthalmol 1986; 62:41–46.

49. Doslak MJ. A theoretical study of the effect of silicone oil on the electroretinogram. Invest Ophthalmol Vis Sci 1988; 29:1881–1884.

50. Meredith TA, Lindsey DT, Edelhauser HF, Goldman AI. Electroretinographic studies following vitrectomy and intraocular silicone oil injection. Br J Ophthalmol 1985; 69:254–260.

51. Scuderi GL, Ricci F, Nucci C, Galasso MJ, Cerulli L. Electrooculography in pigment dispersion syndrome. Ophthalmic Res 1998; 30:23–29.

52. Greenstein VC, Seiple W, Liebmann J, Ritch R. Retinal pigment epithelial dysfunction in patients with pigment dispersion syndrome. Arch Ophthalmol 2001; 119:1291–1295.

53. Latkany PA, Holopigian K, Lorenzo-Latkany M, Seiple W. Electroretinographic and psychophysical findings during early and late stages of human immunodeficiency virus infection and cytomegalovirus retinitis. Ophthalmology 1997; 104:445–453.

54. Gellrich MM, Kade G, Gerling J, Bach M, Hansen LL. Pattern, flicker, and flash electroretinography in human immunodeficiency virus infection: a longitudinal study. Ger J Ophthalmol 1996; 5:16–22.

55. Iragui VJ, Kalmijn J, Plummer DJ, Sample PA, Trick GL, Freeman WR. Pattern electroretinograms and visual evoked potentials in HIV infection: evidence of asymptomatic retinal and postretinal impairment in the absence of infectious retinopathy. Neurology 1996; 47:1452–1456.

56. Malessa R, Agelink MW, Diener HC. Dysfunction of visual pathways in HIV-1 infection. J Neurol Sci 1995; 130: 82–87.

57. Mueller AJ, Berninger TA, Matuschke A, Klauss V, Goebel FD. [Electro-ophthalmologic studies in HIV patients]. Fortschr Ophthalmol 1991; 88:712–715.

58. Jabbari B, Coats M, Salazar A, Martin A, Scherokman B, Laws WA. Longitudinal study of EEG and evoked potentials in neurologically asymptomatic HIV infected subjects. Electroencephalogr Clin Neurophysiol 1993; 86:145–151.

59. Pierelli F, Soldati G, Zambardi P, Garrubba C, Spadaro M, Tilia G, Pauri F, Mororcutti C. Electrophysiological study (VEP, BAEP) in HIV-1 seropositive patients with and without AIDS. Acta Neurol Belg 1993; 93:78–87.

60. Ladenson PW, Stakes JW, Ridgway EC. Reversible alteration of the visual evoked potential in hypothyroidism. Am J Med 1984; 77:1010–1014.

61. Pearlman JT, Burian HM. Electroretinographic findings in thyroid dysfunction. Am J Ophthalmol 1964; 58:216–226.

62. Tamburini G, Tacconi P, Ferrigno P, Cannas A, Massa GM, Mastinu R, Velluzzi F, Loviselli A, Giagheddu M. Visual evoked potentials in hypothyroidism: a long-term evaluation. Electroencephalogr Clin Neurophysiol 1998; 38:201–205.

63. Short MJ, Wilson WP, Gills JP Jr. Thyroid hormone and brain function. IV Effect of triiodothyronine on visual evoked potentials and electroretinogram in man. Electroencephalogr Clin Neurophysiol 1968; 25:123–127.

64. Norcross-Nechay K, Richards GE, Cavallo A. Evoked potentials show early and delayed abnormalities in children with congenital hypothyroidism. Neuropediatrics 1989; 20: 158–163.

65. Wirth A. ERG and endocrine disorders. In: Francois J, ed. Symposium in Ghent. Basel: S Karger AG, 1968:260–266.

66. Mitchell KW, Wood CM, Howe JW. Pattern visual evoked potentials in hyperthyroidism. Br J Ophthalmol 1988; 72:534–537.

67. Wirth A, Tota G. Electroretinogram and adrenal cortical function. In: Schmöger E, ed. Advances in Electrophysiology and Pathology of the Visual System. Proceedings of the 6th ISCERG Symposium. Leipzig: Thieme, 1968:347–350.

68. Zimmerman TJ, Dawson WW, Fitzgerald CR. Electroretinographic changes in normal eyes during administration of prednisone. Ann Ophthalmol 1973; 5:757–765.

69. Eckstein AK, Reichenbach A, Jacobi P, Weber P, Gregor M, Zrenner E. Hepatic retinopathia: changes in retinal function. Vision Res 1997; 37:1699–1706.

70. Johansson U, Andersson T, Persson A, Eriksson LS. Visual evoked potential—a tool in the diagnosis of hepatic encephalopathy? J Hepatol 1989; 9:227–233.

71. Levy LJ, Bolton RP, Losowsky MS. The use of the visual evoked potential (VEP) in delineating a state of subclinical encephalopathy. A comparison with the number connection test (NCT). J Hepatol 1987; 5:211–217.

72. Cibis GW, Fitzgerald KM, Harris DJ, Rothberg PG, Rupani M. The effects of dystrophin gene mutations on the ERG in mice and humans. Invest Ophthalmol Vis Sci 1993; 34:3646–3652.

73. Fitzgerald KM, Cibis BW, Giambrone SA, Harris DJ. Retinal signal transmission in Duchenne muscular dystrophy: evidence for dysfunction in the photoreceptor/depolarizing bipolar cell pathway. J Clin Invest 1994; 93:2425–2430.

74. Pillers DM, Bulman DE, Weleber RG, Sigesmund DA, Musarella MA, Powell BR, Murphey WH, Westall C, Panton C, Becker LE, Worton RG, Tay PN. Dystrophin expression in the human retina is required for normal function as defined by electroretinography. Nat genet 1993; 4:82–86.

75. Sigesmund DA, Weleber RG, Pillers DA, Weatall CA, Panton CM, Powell BR, Heon E, Murphey WH, Musarella MA, Ray PN. Characterization of the ocular phenotype of Duchenne and Becker muscular dystrophy. Ophthalmology 1994; 101:856–865.

76. Tremblay F, De Becker I, Dooley JM, Riddell DC. Duchenne muscular dystrophy: negative scotopic bright-flash electroretinogram but not congenital stationary night blindness. Can J Ophthalmol 1994; 29:274–279.

77. Jensen H, Warburg M, Sjo O, Schwartz M. Duchenne muscular dystrophy: negative electroretinograms and normal dark adaptation: reappraisal of assignment of X linked in complete congenital stationary night blindness. J Med Genet 1995; 32:348–351.

78. Tremblay F, De Becker I, Riddell DC, Dooley JM. Duchenne muscular dystrophy: negative scotopic bright-flash electroretinogram and normal dark adaptation. Can J Ophthalmol 1994; 29:280–283.

79. Pillers DM, Fitzgerald KM, Duncan NM, Rash SM, White RA, Dwinell SJ, Powell BR, Schnur RE, Ray PN, Cibis GW, Weleber RG. Duchenne/Becker muscular dystrophy: correla-

tion of phenotype by electroretinography with sites of dystrophin mutations. Hum Genet 1999; 105:2–9.

80. Ulgenalp A, Oner H, Soylev M, Bora E, Afrashi F, Kose S, Ecal D. Electroretinographic findings in Duchenne/Becker muscular dystrophy and correlations with genotype. Ophthalmic Genet 2002; 23:157–165.

81. Fitzgerald KM, Cibis GW, Gettel AH, Rinaldi R, Harris DJ, White RA. ERG phenotype of a dystrophin mutation in heterozygous female carriers of Duchenne muscular dystrophy. J Med Genet 1999; 36:316–322.

82. Pillers DA, Seltzer WK, Powell BR,Ray PN, Tremblay F, La Roche GR, Lewis RA, McCabe ER, Eriksson AW, Weleber RG. Negative-configuration electroretinogram in Oregon eye disease. Consistent phenotype in Xp21 deletion syndrome. Arch Ophthalmol 1993; 111:1558–1563.

83. Kimizuka Y, Kiyosawa M, Tamai M, Takase S. Retinal changes in myotonic dystrophy: clinical and follow-up evaluation. Retina 1993; 13:129–135.

84. Creel DJ, Crandall AS, Ziter FA. Identification of minimal expression of myotonic dystrophy using electroretinography. Electroencephalogr Clin Neurophysiol 1985; 61: 229–235.

85. Burian HM, Burns CA. Electroretinography and dark adaptation in patients with myotonic dystrophy. Am J Ophthalmol 1966; 61:1044–1054.

86. Stanescu B, Michiels J. Retinal degenerations, electroretinographic aspects in patients with myotonic dystrophy. Doc Ophthalmol Proc Ser 1977; 13:257–262.

87. Cavallacci G, Marconcini C, Perossini M. ERG variations in myotonic dystrophy (Steinert's). Doc Ophthalmol Proc Ser 1980; 23:133–136.

88. Kerty E, Ganes T. Clinical and electrophysiological abnormalities in the visual system in myotonic dystrophy. Ophthalmologica 1989; 198:95–102.

89. Sandrini G, Gelmi C, Rossi V, Bianchi PE, Alfonsi E, Pacchetti C, Verri AP, Nappi G. Electroretinographic and visual

evoked potential abnormalities in myotonic dystrophy. Electroencephalogr Clin Neurophysiol 1986; 64:215–217.

90. Krill AE, Lee GB. The electroretinogram in albinos and carriers of the ocular albino trait. Arch Ophthalmol 1963; 69:32–38.

91. Bergsma DR, Kaiser-Kupfer M. A new form of albinism. Am J Ophthalmol 1974; 77:837–844.

92. Lam BL, Fingert JH, Shutt BC, et al. Clinical and molecular characterization of a family affected with X-linked ocular albinism. Ophthalmic Genet 1997; 18:175–184.

93. Tomei F, Wirth A. The electroretinogram of albinos. Vision Res 1978; 18:1465–1466.

94. Wack MA, Peachey NS, Fishman GA. Electroretinographic findings in human oculocutaneous albinism. Ophthalmology 1989; 96:1778–1785.

95. O'Donnell FE Jr, Hambrick GW Jr, Green WR, Iliff WJ, Stone DL. X-linked ocular albinism: an oculocutaneous macromelanosomal disorder. Arch Ophthalmol 1976; 94: 1883–1892.

96. Creel D, Witkop CJJ, King RA. Asymmetric visually evoked potentials in human albinos: evidence for visual system anomalies. Invest Ophthalmol 1974; 13:430–440.

97. Creel D, O'Donnell FEJ, Witkop CJJ. Visual system anomalies in human ocular albinos. Science 1978; 201:931–933.

98. Apkarian P, Shallo-Hoffmann J. VEP projections in congenital nystagmus, VEP asymmetry in albinism: a comparison study. Invest Ophthalmol Vis Sci 1991; 32:2653–2661.

99. Fitzgerald K, Cibis GW. The value of flash visual evoked potentials in albinism. J Pediatr Ophthalmol Strabismus 1994; 31:18–25.

100. Bouzas EA, Caruso RC, Drews-Bankiewicz MA, Kaiser-Kupfer M. Evoked potential analysis of visual pathways in human albinism. Ophthalmology 1994; 101:309–314.

101. Tremblay F, De Becker I, Cheung C, LaRoche R. Visual evoked potentials with crossed asymmetry in incomplete congenital stationary night blindess. Invest Ophthalmol Vis Sci 1996; 37:1783–1792.

17

Optic Neuropathies and Central Nervous System Disorders

Electrophysiologic tests such as pattern ERG and VEP are affected by optic neuropathies and in some cases may serve as useful objective clinical measures of dysfunction. For instance, residual deficits from recovered mild optic neuritis may be difficult to detect on ophthalmic examination or even with formal visual fields but may be detectable by pattern ERG or pattern VEP. However, these electrophysiologic tests require good fixation and are adjunctive clinical tests that should not be performed in isolation without a comprehensive ophthalmic examination with refraction. Novel electrophysiologic tests such as the multifocal VEP and optic nerve head component of the multifocal ERG are being developed to detect visual pathway dysfunction and their clinical utility requires further investigation. This chapter provides electrophysiologic information on optic neuropathies and central nervous system disorders. Nutritional optic neuropathy is discussed Chapter 15 along with other toxic and nutritional conditions. The outline of this chapter is as follows:

Optic neuropathies:
- Glaucoma
- Optic neuritis/multiple sclerosis
- Ischemic optic neuropathy
- Papilledema
- Compression of optic nerve or chiasm
- Traumatic optic neuropathy
- Optic nerve head drusen
- Hereditary optic neuropathies

Central nervous system disorders:
- Cortical blindness
- Spinocerebellar degeneration, olivopontocerebellar atrophy, and Friedreich ataxia
- Alzheimer disease
- Parkinson disease
- Leukodystrophies

OPTIC NEUROPATHIES

Glaucoma

Glaucoma is a progressive optic neuropathy characterized by loss of retinal ganglion cells associated with increased cupping of the optic nerve head, progressive nerve-fiber-layer visual field defects, and usually, but not always, high intraocular pressure. There are many types of glaucoma with primary open-angle glaucoma being the most common. Glaucoma is one of the leading causes of blindness worldwide, and its prevalence increases with age. Patients with increased intraocular pressure without glaucomatous optic nerve and visual field damage are designated as having "ocular hypertension" and are at risk of developing glaucoma.

Medical and surgical treatments aimed at lowering intraocular pressure have shown to decrease glaucomatous progression and the likelihood of developing glaucoma in ocular hypertension. Early detection of glaucoma and glaucomatous progression is critical so that treatment can be initiated or modified to prevent permanent or future visual loss. Diagnostic tests that are of value in glaucoma must be sensitive enough to detect early glaucoma progression and to identify those ocular hypertensive patients who are at higher risk of developing glaucoma. At the same time, a diagnostic test that is not specific enough will have a high false positive rate rendering the test less useful. Most patients with ocular hypertension do not develop glaucoma, and the rate of conversion to glaucoma is about 1.5% per year (1). Topical antiglaucomatous medication is effective in delaying or preventing the onset of glaucoma in patients with ocular hypertension by reducing this conversion rate to about 0.7% per year (1). Serial examinations with intraocular pressure measurement, visual field testing, and optic nerve head evaluation are recommended for glaucoma and ocular hypertension. However, loss of more than one-third of nerve fibers may occur before a visual field defect becomes detectable.

Despite numerous studies, electrophysiologic testing has yet to gain general acceptance in glaucoma. Long-term prospective studies are needed to determine whether electrophysiologic abnormalities are clinically meaningful in the diagnosis and treatment of glaucoma and ocular hypertension.

The pattern ERG is a measure of retinal ganglion cell function and has been proposed as a diagnostic test in glaucoma (Fig. 17.1). The N95 component of the pattern ERG is generated by retinal ganglion cell function while the P50 component is generated by both retinal ganglion cells and intraretinal cellular elements. For transient pattern ERG responses, earlier studies of P50 in glaucoma yielded variable results (2–4), but subsequent investigations noted more consistent impairment of the N95 in glaucoma and ocular hypertension (5–7). Studies examining correlation between pattern ERG abnormalities and other clinical parameters such as changes in visual field and optic nerve head appearance have yielded inconsistent results (8–12). For instance, one study found that pattern ERG and computerized optic nerve head analysis do not agree in their estimation of glaucomatous risk (8) while a correlation between pattern ERG and nerve fiber layer thickness was reported in another study (13). This lack of consistent correlation is likely due in part to the varied

Impaired Pattern-Reversal VEP and Pattern ERG in Glaucoma

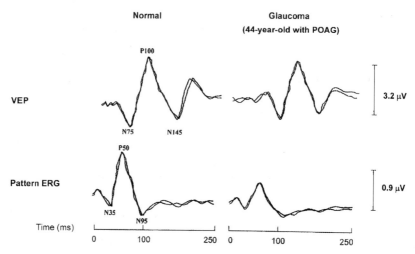

Figure 17.1 Simultaneous recordings of pattern-reversal VEP and pattern ERG. Note the delayed VEP P100 and pattern ERG P50 implicit times and the reduced VEP P100 and pattern P50–N95 amplitudes in the patient with primary open-angle glaucoma (POAG). The recordings were obtained with 15-min check sizes with the stimulus subtending 18 (From Ref. 13 with permission from the American Academy of Ophthalmology.)

effects of glaucoma on multiple physiologic mechanisms. In a cross-sectional study of 203 glaucoma patients, Martus et al. (14) compared optic disc morphometry, automated perimetry, temporal contrast sensitivity, blue-on-yellow VEP, and pattern ERG using confirmatory factor analysis in which the results are not dependent on the preselection of a specific gold standard (14). The investigators found that glaucomatous damage was quantified best by perimetry followed, in order, by neuroretinal rim of the optic disc, temporal contrast sensitivity, pattern ERG, and VEP. However, a combination of short-wavelength automated perimetry (SWAP) and pattern ERG improve the predictive power of progressive defects on standard automated perimetry and could detect glaucomatous optic neuropathy in eyes with normal standard perimetry (13,15,16).

The waveforms of steady-state pattern ERG are dominant by the N95 component, and abnormal steady-state pattern ERG in glaucoma and ocular hypertension have also been noted by several studies (17–20). A comparison of upper hemifield and lower hemifield transient or steady-state pattern ERG responses to detect glaucomatous damage has been demonstrated (21). Reports of correlations between steady-state pattern ERG changes and other clinical parameters are inconsistent (22,23).

In general, pattern ERG abnormalities are found in about 10–40% of patients with ocular hypertension (7,12,17,24,25). This prevalence rate is considerably higher than the approximate 1% per year conversion rate to glaucoma reported in clinical studies. A significant although weak correlation between pattern ERG amplitude and shape of the optic nerve head has been noted (26). Although ocular hypertensives with abnormal pattern ERG are likely to have a greater risk of developing glaucoma when compared to those with normal pattern ERG, the relatively high prevalence of abnormal pattern ERG in ocular hypertensives suggests a false positive rate that is likely too high to be potentially clinically useful in identifying those who would develop glaucoma.

Glaucomatous damage is detectable by multifocal VEP, but further studies are needed to determine whether these changes can be clinically meaningful and better than other clinically measures (Fig. 17.2) (27,28). The second-order response of the multifocal ERG may be reduced in glaucoma but this reduction is variable (29). In one study, multifocal pattern ERG did not reflect localized ganglion cell loss whereas multifocal pattern VEP to a similar stimulus showed the scotoma (30).

The photoreceptors are unaffected in glaucoma and conventional full-field ERG responses are normal (31). The photopic negative response (PhNR), a negative component that immediately follows the full-field ERG b-wave, is related to ganglion cell activity and is reduced in glaucoma (Fig. 17.3) (32). Optimal recording of the PhNR requires specialized techniques and its clinical usefulness requires further study. Mild waveform changes of the first-order multifocal ERG have also

Reduced Multifocal VEP in Glaucoma

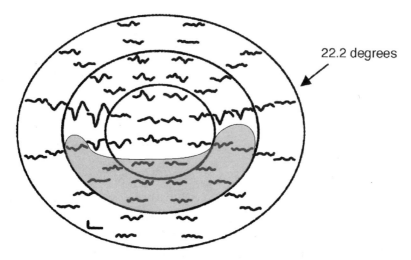

22.2 degrees

Right eye of 50-year-old with glaucoma

Figure 17.2 Multifocal VEP of a patient with glaucoma (right eye). Note the area of decreased VEP responses inferiorly (grey area) related to glaucomatous damage. (From Ref. 141 with permission from the American Medical Association.)

been reported in glaucoma but they are unlikely to be clinically significant (33). However, the optic nerve head component of the multifocal ERG can be extracted and is decreased in glaucoma but its utility requires further investigation (Fig. 17.4).

Optic Neuritis/Multiple Sclerosis

Inflammation of the optic nerve or optic neuritis is associated with a variety of disorders including multiple sclerosis, neuromyelitis optica, sarcoidosis, syphilis, human immunodeficiency virus (HIV) infection, lyme disease, and sinus disease. When the anterior portion of the optic nerve is involved, edema of the optic nerve head is evident. If the involvement is further posterior, the term "retrobulbar" optic neuritis is used, and the optic nerve head appears normal.

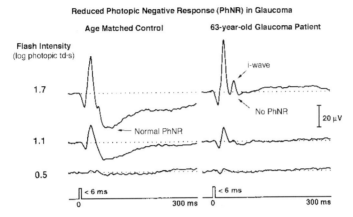

Figure 17.3 Full-field ERG intensity series for a 63-year-old patient with primary open-angle glaucoma demonstrating reduced photopic negative response (PhNR). The recordings were made with a brief (<6 msec) red stimulus on a rod saturating (3.7 log scotopic troland) blue background. (From Ref. 32 with permission of *Investigative Ophthalmology and Visual Science.*)

With time, various degree of optic nerve pallor develops depending on the amount of damage. Symptoms and signs of optic neuritis include decreased vision over days, periocular pain, impaired color perception, visual field defect, and afferent pupillary defect. Severity is highly variable, and visual acuity ranges from 20/20 to no light perception.

The most common type of optic neuritis is acute demyelinating optic neuritis associated with multiple sclerosis, which typically affects young adults of age less than 50. Patients with greater numbers of demyelinating lesions on brain MRI are at higher risk of developing multiple sclerosis. Visual prognosis is generally favorable with most patients recovering to 20/25 or better over 7 weeks or longer. Treatment with intravenous methylprednisolone during the acute phase of optic neuritis hastens visual recovery and delays the development of multiple sclerosis. Chronic use of immunomodulating agents such as beta-interferon 1a (Avonex) helps to reduce future multiple sclerosis attacks.

Optic Nerve Head Component (ONHC) in Glaucoma

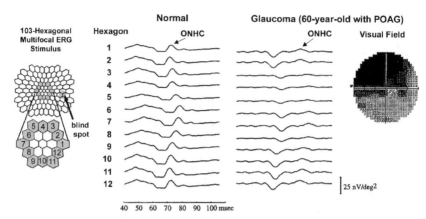

Figure 17.4 The multifocal ERG optic nerve head component (ONHC) of a patient with primary open-angle glaucoma (POAG). The first-order traces of the multifocal ERG are obtained with a sequence of all-black, all-white, and all-black stimulus frames inserted between each of the multifocal stimulus presentations. The traces are then separated into the retinal component (not shown) and the ONHC. The normal ONHC tracings are more delay for hexagons further away from the optic nerve head. Note greater ONHC impairment of the superior hexagons 3, 4, and 5 corresponding to the superior visual field loss. (From Ref. 142 with permission of *Investigative Ophthalmology and Visual Science*.)

The VEP serves as a complementary visual function test in optic neuritis and is particularly useful when visual acuity, visual field, and afferent pupillary defect testing are equivocal (Fig. 17.5). Numerous studies have demonstrated reduced and delayed VEP in optic neuritis (34–37). The VEP elicited with chromatic stimulus is more impaired in optic neuritis than standard VEP (37). Pattern VEP latency and amplitude correlate with other clinical parameters such as visual acuity and field and improve with optic neuritis recovery (38,39). In some cases, VEP may detect subclinical impairment that are not apparent on visual acuity and field testing (38–40). For instance, VEP delays may occur in multiple sclerosis patients

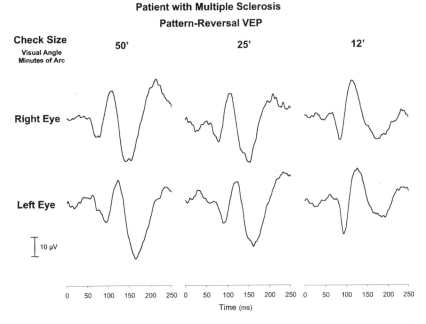

Figure 17.5 Pattern-reversal VEP in a 41-year-old patient with multiple sclerosis. The patient reported abnormal vision of the left eye despite 20/20 visual acuity in each eye along with normal visual fields and normal optic nerve head appearance. The prolonged P100 of the left eye suggests that the patient may have had mild optic neuritis in the left eye.

who never had clinical optic neuritis and are common in the fellow "unaffected" eye of patients with unilateral optic neuritis (37,41). The VEP delays remain in most patients with resolved optic neuritis (42). In general, most studies indicate that delayed VEP is a risk factor for developing clinical definite multiple sclerosis (43–47). Accordingly, the International Panel on the Diagnosis of Multiple Sclerosis recommends that multiple sclerosis be diagnosed on the basis of not only clinical course but also by the use of objective tests such as MRI, cerebrospinal fluid analysis, and VEP (48,49). For example, in patients with insidious neurological progression but no neurologic episodic attacks, the diagnosis of multiple sclerosis may be determined by positive cerebrospinal fluid findings and delayed VEP responses in association with the number of demyelinating MRI lesions (49). Of interest, multifocal VEP is a new tool that can be used to track local optic nerve damage after unilateral optic neuritis (28).

Several studies have documented impaired pattern ERG responses in optic neuritis (34,50,51). The N95 component of the pattern ERG reflects retinal ganglion cell function and is impaired in optic neuritis. The P50 component of the pattern ERG is generated by both retinal ganglion cells and by other intraretinal cellular elements and is relatively preserved in optic neuritis (52). However, P50 may be marked reduced during the acute phase of optic neuritis and recover over weeks (53,54). In a study of 200 eyes with optic neuritis, Holder (54) found abnormal pattern ERG in 40% of the eyes, and of these, 85% had abnormal N95 component without P50 involvement. A subsequent review of 382 eyes by the same investigator showed greater pattern ERG abnormalities in those eyes with attacks of optic neuritis than those eyes with subclinical demyelination (52). In any case, N95 abnormalities may persist after clinical recovery of optic neuritis and may occur in multiple sclerosis patients who never had clinical optic neuritis (53,55). Aside from abnormalities of the transient pattern ERG, steady-state pattern ERG also demonstrates abnormalities in optic neuritis with impairment of the second harmonic component by Fourier analysis (36,37,55,56).

Ischemic Optic Neuropathy

Ischemia of the optic nerve may occur anteriorly at the optic nerve head or posteriorly in the retrobulbar portion of the optic nerve. Anterior ischemia optic neuropathy (AION) is more common and is caused by hypoperfusion of the posterior ciliary arteries. Criteria for the diagnosis of AION include: (1) an acute decrease in vision; (2) nerve fiber layer defect on visual field testing; (3) relative afferent pupillary defect; and (4) optic nerve head edema often with hemorrhage during the acute period with progression to optic pallor over weeks. In contrast, posterior ischemic optic neuropathy (PION) is associated with acute decrease of vision with normal appearance of the optic nerve head followed by the development of optic pallor over weeks. The diagnosis of PION is made on the basis of excluding other disorders and neuroimaging is usually helpful. No established treatment of ischemic optic neuropathy is available, and therapy is aimed at control of risk factors such as hypertension and diabetes. Electrophysiologic testing is not ordinarily performed. Impaired VEP and pattern ERG responses have been documented (27,28,34,57). These impaired responses are non-specific but may serve as complementary tests to determine optic nerve dysfunction especially when other visual function tests or signs of the disease are unreliable or equivocal. In one study, reduction in N95 amplitude of the transient pattern ERG, a measure of retinal ganglion cell response, was found in AION and was suggested as a way to differentiate AION from optic neuritis (58). However, reduced N95 amplitude is also reduced in optic neuritis (51). Clinical multifocal ERG or full-field ERG are unaffected by ischemic optic neuropathy but may help to rule out retinal dysfunction in patients suspected of PION.

Papilledema

Optic nerve head edema due to raised intracranial pressure is typically bilateral and is called papilledema. Intracranial hypertension may be caused by intracranial space-occupying lesion or from idiopathic intracranial hypertension (IIH), traditionally known as pseudotumor cerebri. Prompt neuroimaging is essential in the work-up of papilledema, and if neuroimaging is normal, spinal tap with cerebrospinal fluid pressure measurement is necessary to diagnose IIH. When papilledema is associated with intracranial mass, treatment of the underlying lesion is warranted. In IIH, the papilledema may be treated with medications or if severe, surgically with optic nerve sheath fenestration and ventriculo-peritoneal shunt. Early papilledema produces enlarged blind spot and mild nerve fiber layer field defects, which are reversible with successful therapy. In severe papilledema, hemorrhages and exudates at the optic nerve head are present, and severe visual field defects and decrease in visual acuity loss are encountered. If unchecked, papilledema can lead to permanent loss of nerve fibers and optic nerve pallor. Electrophysiologic testing is not routinely performed. Impaired VEP and pattern ERG responses may occur before disturbances of visual fields and acuity in IIH patients (59,60). However, in a study of 13 patients with IIH, Sorensen et al. (59) found that although the pattern VEP was significantly delayed compared to 20 normal subjects, only four patients had latencies outside the normal range.

Compression of Optic Nerve or Chiasm

Common compressive disorders of the anterior visual pathway include meningioma, thyroid-associated ophthalmopathy, and pituitary adenoma. The diagnosis is made on the basis of impaired visual function and neuroimaging. In general, impaired visual function is evident on clinical examination and established by the results of visual acuity, color, visual field, and afferent pupillary testing. Effective treatments are usually available and include medication, surgery, and radiation. Electrophysiologic tests are not widely performed. Impaired VEP, pattern ERG, and the PhNR on full-field ERG in patients with compressive lesion are common, and these tests may serve as additional diagnostic and monitoring tools especially when other visual tests are equivocal or unreliable (50,51,61–65). For instance, flash and pattern VEP are helpful in monitoring compressive optic neuropathy from thyroid-associated ophthalmopathy (66–69). The results of one study suggest that the delay in VEP responses was smaller and less frequent in patients with compression lesion compared to patients with demyelinating disease (61). In keeping with the general principle that the N95 component of the pattern ERG is a measure of retinal ganglion cell function and the P50 component is relatively spared in optic neuropathy, reduced N95 is common in compressive optic neuropathy (52). For instance, in patients with chiasmal compression from pituitary tumors, prognosis for visual improvement is more favorable when the pre-treatment N95:P50 ratio of the pattern ERG is normal (70). Lastly, the PhNR of the full-field ERG is reduced in patients with optic atrophy induced by compression and show a good correlation with retinal nerve fiber layer thickness on optical coherence tomography (65).

Traumatic Optic Neuropathy

Traumatic injury to the optic nerve may occur from direct penetrating injury caused by objects or, more commonly, from indirect blunt force to the head. The intracanalicular portion of the optic nerve, which is fixed by the bony walls of the optic canal, is most susceptible to traumatic injury. Treatment options include corticosteroid therapy and surgical optic canal decompression but treatment is controversial because evidence is lacking that any treatment is beneficial (71). Prognosis for significant visual improvement is often unfavorable.

In post-trauma patients who are not alert enough for visual function testing and whose pupillary light reflexes are sluggish due to coma or sedation, flash VEP may be helpful in the diagnosis and determining the prognosis of traumatic optic neuropathy (72–75). Attempts have also been made to use flash VEP to determine whether to initiate corticosteroid treatment or to perform surgical decompression, but these treatments remain controversial (76). Pattern ERG responses are also impaired in patients with traumatic optic neuropathy (34,50,51,77), but unlike the flash VEP, steady fixation is required and testing unresponsive patients is not typically feasible. The PhNR of the full-field ERG is also reduced in patients with optic atrophy due to trauma (65).

Optic Nerve Head Drusen

Prognosis of refractile nodules or drusen of the optic nerve head is generally favorable, and the diagnosis is usually made by ultrasound. As a reflection of impaired ganglion cell function, reduced N95 component of the pattern ERG may be found up to nearly 80% of eyes with optic nerve drusen while the P50 component is less likely to be affected (78). Reduced and prolonged VEP responses may also be found (78–80).

Hereditary Optic Neuropathies

Inheritance patterns of hereditary optic neuropathies include autosomal dominant, autosomal recessive, and maternal through mitochondrial DNA. All hereditary optic neuropathies result in bilateral visual loss and optic atrophy, and except in Leber hereditary optic neuropathy, the visual loss is often slow and progressive. The optic neuropathy may occur in isolation or as part of an inherited systemic syndrome. The more common hereditary optic neuropathies include Leber hereditary optic neuropathy and dominant optic atrophy.

Leber hereditary optic neuropathy is caused by mitochondrial DNA mutations with changes at positions 11778, 3460, or 14484, being found in at least 90% of affected persons. Although mitochondrial DNA is inherited maternally, 80–90% of symptomatic persons are male. Some carriers of the mutant mitochondrial DNA, especially females, may never become symptomatic. Symptoms start with acute or subacute painless loss of central vision in one eye followed by the involvement of the second eye usually within weeks to months. Spontaneous visual improvement may occur gradually or suddenly up to 10 years after onset of visual loss. During the acute stage, circumpapillary telangiectatic microangiopathy, swelling of the peripapillary nerve fiber layer, and absence of leakage from the disc or papillary region on fluorescein angiography may occur, but up to 40% of patients may not have any visible abnormalities. Subsequently, optic atrophy develops over weeks. The diagnosis is confirmed by mitochondrial DNA analysis, and electrophysiologic tests are of limited value except when desired for documenting optic nerve dysfunction. In Leber optic neuropathy, full-field ERG is normal and pattern ERG demonstrates reduced N95 with a normal or attenuated P50 indicating retinal ganglion cell dysfunction (52,81). Flash and pattern VEP shows reduced amplitude and increased latency (81–83). Carriers or presymptomatic persons with Leber optic neuropathy may or may not have impaired VEP responses (83–85).

Patients with dominant optic atrophy have progressive central vision loss with developing optic atrophy that typically begins insidiously in the first decade of life. Multiple genotypes may produce dominant optic atrophy. In OPA1, mutations of the OPA1 gene are found on chromosome 3. Diagnosis of dominant optic atrophy is based on clinical features, family history, and genetic testing. Electrophysiologic findings document optic nerve dysfunction but are non-specific (86). Pattern ERG reports from a series of 87 patients from 21 pedigrees with dominant optic atrophy showed preferential N95 reduction early in the disease with P50 reduction as the disease progressed (87,88). However, the pattern ERG remained detectable even in advance cases. The VEP responses may be non-detectable in more advanced cases, and when detectable, most VEP responses are mildly to moderately delayed (87,89,90).

CENTRAL NERVOUS SYSTEM DISORDERS

Cortical Blindness

Cortical blindness refers to bilateral dysfunction of the visual pathways anywhere along the lateral geniculate body to the occipital cortex. Because the lesions are not always isolated to the cortex and the degree of visual impairment in cortical blindness is highly variable and rarely complete, the term "cortical visual impaired" has been suggested (91). Cortical visual impairment may be caused by a spectrum of conditions including stroke, infections, neurodegenerative diseases, metabolic and toxic insults, tumors, and trauma.

The diagnosis of cortical visual impairment is made on the basis of ophthalmic examination and abnormal findings on diagnostic tests such as MRI and VEP. If the patient is able to perform visual fields, the homonymous nature of the visual loss may be detected. In some cases, full-field ERG is necessary to rule out occult ocular disorders such as paraneoplastic retinopathy, previous retinal vascular occlusions, achromatopsia, and Leber congenital amaurosis. The VEP is helpful to establish visual pathway dysfunction in cortical visual impairment, and a high correlation between visual acuity and VEP is found in some studies (92,93). Flash VEP improvement may precede clinical recovery in cortical visual impairment and may serve as a prognostic indicator in disorders such as encephalopathy, hydrocephalus, basilar artery occlusion, and trauma (94–96). In children with cortical visual impairment, sweep VEP is a valid method for measuring grating acuity (97). However, caution should be exercised in making a diagnosis of cortical visual impairment in infants with a reduced flash VEP because of the possibility of delayed visual pathway maturation. In addition, children with central nervous system diseases but normal vision may demonstrate abnormal flash VEP responses (98). On the other hand, in some cases of complete cortical blindness, a residual flash VEP response may still be present (99,100).

Spinocerebellar Ataxia, Olivopontocerebellar Atrophy, and Friedreich Ataxia

Spinocerebellar ataxia may occur sporadically or as an autosomal dominant disorder. Autosomal dominant spinocerebellar ataxia is genetically heterogenous and is associated with genetic expansion of repeat trinucleotide CAG. For example, SCA1 is due to increased CAG repeats of the ataxin-1 gene on chromosome 6p23; SCA2 is associated with CAG repeats of the ataxin-2 on chromosome 12p24; SCA6 is related to CAG repeats of the alpha-1A calcium channel subunit gene on chromosome 19p13; and SCA12 is caused by CAG repeats of the gene encoding a subunit of the protein phosphatase PP2A on chromosome 5. SCA1 is also known as olivopontocerebellar atrophy 1. Aside from signs of progressive cerebellar dysfunction such as gait ataxia and dysarthria, patients may also have optic atrophy, progressive retinal degeneration, and decreased corneal endothelial density (101–104). Symptoms and signs of the disease are highly variable with the number of CAG repeats being inversely correlated with age of disease onset. Abe et al. (101) found reduced full-field ERG b-wave and oscillatory potentials in patients with SCA1 (101). The same investigation group also demonstrated macular degeneration with reduced central multifocal ERG responses and rare impaired full-field cone ERG responses in patients with SCA7 (105). In addition, generalized impairment of the full-field ERG including the a-wave and b-wave is found in many patients with olivopontocerebellar atrophy type II (106). Other forms of olivopontocerebellar atrophies distinct from spinocerebellar ataxia have also been described. Taken together, progressive macular or generalized retinal dysfunction may occur in this group of patients as demonstrated by ERG responses. Further, impaired VEP responses have been reported in SCA1 and SCA2 patients with normal retinal appearance, but whether these abnormal responses are due to early retinal dysfunction or central visual pathway dysfunction has not been clarified (107).

Friedreich ataxia is an autosomal recessive disorder characterized by degeneration of the spinocerebellar tracts, dorsal columns, pyramidal traits, cerebellum, and medulla. Clinical manifestations include progressive cerebellar dysfunction, hypoactive deep tendon reflexes, dysarthria, and nystagmus. Impaired VEP responses implying central visual pathway dysfunction are found in many affected patients (108,109).

Alzheimer Disease

Described in 1907 by Alzheimer (110), Alzheimer disease is the most common form of dementia. The disorder may be sporadic or inherited as an autosomal dominant trait. Progressive dementia and histologic finding of neurofibrillary tangles of the central nervous system are some of the features of Alzheimer disease. Ocular findings may include impaired visual acuity, visual field, color perception, contrast sensitivity, and eye movement (111).

Despite numerous studies, the clinical utility of visual electrophysiologic testing in Alzheimer disease is uncertain. Focal and full-field ERG responses are normal (112,113). Loss of retinal ganglion cells with axonal degeneration of the optic nerve is found on postmortem studies of patients with Alzheimer disease (114). Although some of these changes may be attributable to normal aging (115), retinal nerve fiber layer thickness as measured by optical coherence tomography has been found to be reduced in patients with Alzheimer disease when compared to age-matched control subjects (116). However, studies of pattern ERG, a measure of ganglion cell function, have revealed mixed results. Some studies showed normal pattern ERG responses in Alzheimer patients (112,117); while other studies demonstrated abnormal pattern ERG responses (116,118). These conflicting results are likely due to differences in patient population and methodology as well as the possible effect of defocusing in Alzheimer patients as compared to normal subjects (119,120).

Likewise, VEP studies in Alzheimer disease are equally conflicting. While some studies reported delayed pattern VEP in Alzheimer patients and demonstrated a correlation between delayed flash VEP and dementia (121–123), no correlation between pattern or flash VEP and the degree of dementia was shown in one study (124) and another study noted normal VEP responses (113). Of interest, in one study, impairment of the visual association cortices was found (125).

Parkinson Disease

After Alzheimer disease, Parkinson disease is the second most common neurodegenerative disorder. The condition is due to loss of dopaminergic neurons particularly in the basal ganglia and substantia nigra. Clinical features include tremor, rigidity, bradykinesia, and dementia. Full-field ERG responses are generally mildly to moderately impaired in Parkinson patients with improved responses after oral or intravenous levodopa administration (126,127). The EOG abnormalities such as delay in reaching the light-peak as well as reduced light-peak have also been reported (128). Pattern ERG and VEP responses are also delayed even in the early tage of Parkinson disease with pattern ERG being more delayed and more reversible with levodopa treatment than VEP (129). Visual processing deficits in Parkinson disease are also evident on onset/offset pattern VEP and chromatic VEP (130,131). Utility of intraoperative VEP monitoring during pallidotomy on Parkinson patients has been demonstrated (132,133). The procedure is performed on patients who are not responding adequately to medical treatment and involves making a lesion in the globus pallidus internus near the optic tract. Intracranial recording of VEP with electrode stimu lation determines the location of the optic tract and allows accurate targeting of the globus pallidus internus.

Leukodystrophies

Leukodystrophies is a group of genetically heterogeneous disorders characterized by degeneration of the white matter of the central nervous system. Examples of leukodystrophy include adrenoleukodystrophy (X-linked), metachromatic leukodystrophy (recessive), and various lyposomal disorders (recessive). The VEP responses may be impaired due to demyelination and white matter degeneration (134–138). For instance, in adrenoleukodystrophy, Kaplan et al. (139) using pattern VEP, magnetic resonance imaging, and clinical examination, found 63% of patients had visual pathway abnormalities involving the optic nerve head, optic nerves, lateral geniculate bodies, optic radiations, and parietal-occipital cortex (139). The same authors noted that 17% of the affected males had abnormal pattern VEP which did not improve with medical treatment that reduced very-long-chain fatty acid levels (140).

REFERENCES

1. Kass MA, Heuer DK, Higginbotham EJ, Johnson CA, Keltner JL, Miller JP, Parrish RK, II, Wilson MR, Gordon MO. The ocular hypertension treatment study. A randomized trial determines that topical ocular hypertensive medication delays or prevents the onset of primary open-angle glaucoma. Arch Ophthalmol 2002; 120:701–713.

2. Papst N, Bopp M, Schnaudigel OE. Pattern electroretinogram and visual evoked cortical potentials in glaucoma. Graefes Arch Clin Exp Ophthalmol 1984; 222:29–33.

3. Ringens PJ, Vijfvinkel-Bruinenga S, van Lith GH. The pattern-elicited electroretinogram, I. A tool in the early detection of glaucoma? Ophthalmologica 1986; 182:171–175.

4. van den Berg TJ, Riemslag FC, de Vos GW, Verduyn Lunel HF. Pattern ERG and glaucomatous visual field defects. Doc Ophthalmol 1986; 62:335–341.

5. Howe JW, Mitchell KW. Simultaneous recording of the pattern electroretinogram and visual evoked cortical potentials in a group of patients with chronic glaucoma. Doc Ophthalmol Proc Ser 1984; 40:101–107.

6. Ohta H, Tamura T, Kawasaki K. [Negative wave in human pattern ERG and its suppression in glaucoma]. Nippon Ganka Gakkai Zasshi 1986; 90:882–887.

7. Weinstein GW, Arden GB, Hitchings RA, Ryan S, Calthorpe CM, Odom JV. The pattern electroretinogram (PERG) in ocular hypertension and glaucoma. Arch Ophthalmol 1988; 106:923–928.

8. Bömer TG, Meyer JH, Bach M, Funk J. Pattern electroretinogram and computerized optic nerve-head analysis in ocular hypertension—interim results after 2.5 years. Ger J Ophthalmol 1996; 5:26–30.

9. Graham SL, Drance SM, Chauhan BC, Swindale NV, Hnik P, Mikelberg FS, Douglas GR. Comparison of psychophysical and electrophysiological testing in early glaucoma. Invest Ophthalmol Vis Sci 1996; 37:2651–2662.

10. Martus P, Korth M, Horn F, Junemann A, Wisse M, Jonas JB. A multivariate sensory model in glaucoma diagnosis. Invest Ophthalmol Vis Sci 1998; 39:1567–1574.

11. Ruben ST, Hitchings RA, Fitzke F, Arden GB. Electrophysiology and psychophysics in ocular hypertension and glaucoma: evidence for different pathomechanisms in early glaucoma. Eye 1994; 8:516–520.

12. Ruben ST, Arden GB, O'Sullivan F, Hitchings RA. Pattern electroretinogram and peripheral colour contrast thresholds in ocular hypertension and glaucoma: comparison and correlation of results. Br J Ophthalmol 1995; 79:326–331.

13. Parisi V, Manni G, Centofanti M, Gandolfi SA, Olzi D, Bucci MG. Correlation between optical coherence tomography, pattern electroretinogram, and visual evoked potentials in open-angle glaucoma patients. Ophthalmology 2001; 108:905–912.

14. Martus P, Junemann A, Wisse M, Budde WM, Horn F, Korth M, Jonas JB. Multivariate approach for quantification of morphologic and functional damage in glaucoma. Invest Ophthalmol Vis Sci 2000; 41:1099–1110.

15. Bayer AU, Maag KP, Erb C. Detection of optic neuropathy in glaucomatous eyes with normal standard visual fields using a test battery of short-wavelength automated perimetry and pattern electroretinography. Ophthalmology 2002; 109: 1350–1361.

16. Bayer AU, Erb C. Short wavelength automated perimetry, frequency doubling technology perimetry, and pattern electroretinography for prediction of progressive glaucomatous standard visual field defects. Ophthalmology 2002; 109:1009–1017.

17. Bach M, Speidel-Faux A. Pattern electroretinogram in glaucoma and ocular hypertension. Doc Ophthalmol 1989; 73: 173–181.

18. Pfeiffer N, Bach M. The pattern-electroretinogram in glaucoma and ocular hypertension: a cross-sectional and longitudinal study. Ger J Ophthalmol 1992; 1:35–40.

19. Pfeiffer N, Tillmon B, Bach M. Predictive value of the pattern electroretinogram in high-risk ocular hypertension. Invest Ophthalmol Vis Sci 1993; 34:1710–1715.

20. Porciatti V, Falsini B, Brunori S, Colotto A, Moretti G. Pattern electroretinogram as a function of spatial frequency in ocular hypertension and early glaucoma. Doc Ophthalmol 1987; 65:349–355.

21. Graham SL, Wong VA, Drance SM, Mikelberg FS. Pattern electroretinograms from hemifields in normal subjects and patients with glaucoma. Invest Ophthalmol Vis Sci 1994; 35:3347–3356.

22. Bach M, Sulimma F, Gerling J. Little correlation of the pattern electroretinogram (PERG) and visual field measures in early glaucoma. Doc Ophthalmol 1997; 94:253–263.

23. Neoh C, Kaye SB, Brown MS, Ansons AM, Wishart P. Pattern electroretinogram and automated perimetry in patients with

glaucoma and ocular hypertension. Br J Ophthalmol 1994; 78:359–362.

24. O'Donaghue E, Arden GB, O'Sullivan F, Falcao-Reis F, Moriarty B, Hitchings RA, Spilleers W, Hogg CR, Weinstein G. The pattern electroretinogram in glaucoma and ocular hypertension. Br J Ophthalmol 1992; 76:387–394.

25. Trick GL, Bickler–Bluth M, Cooper DG, Kolker AE, Nesher R. Pattern reversal electroretinogram (PRERG) abnormalities in ocular hypertension: correlation with glaucoma risk factors. Curr Eye Res 1988; 7:201–206.

26. Salgarello T, Colotto A, Falsini B, Buzzonetti L, Cesari L, Iarossi G, Scullica L. Correlation of pattern electroretinogram with optic disc cup shape in ocular hypertension. Invest Ophthalmol Vis Sci 1999; 40:1989–1997.

27. Hood DC, Zhang X. Multifocal ERG and VEP responses and visual fields: comparing disease-related changes. Doc Ophthalmol 2000; 100:115–137.

28. Hood DC, Zhang X, Greenstein VC, Kangovi S, Odel JG, Liebmann JM, Ritch R. An interocular comparison of the multifocal VEP; a possible technique for detecting local damage to the optic nerve. Invest Ophthalmol Vis Sci 2000; 41:1580–1587.

29. Hood DC, Greenstein VC, Holopigian K, Bauer R, Firoz B, Liebmann JM, Odel JG, Ritch R. An attempt to detect glaucomatous damage to the inner retina with the multifocal ERG. Invest Ophthalmol Vis Sci 2000; 41:1570–1579.

30. Klistorner AI, Graham SL, Martins A. Multifocal pattern electroretinogram does not demonstrate localised field defects in glaucoma. Doc Ophthalmol 2000; 100:155–165.

31. Holopigian K, Greenstein VC, Seiple W, Hood DC, Ritch R. Electrophysiologic assessment of photoreceptor function in patients with primary open-angle glaucoma. J Glaucoma 2000; 9:163–168.

32. Viswanathan S, Frishman LJ, Robson JG, Walters JW. The photopic negative response of the flash electroretinogram in primary open angle glaucoma. Invest Ophthalmol Vis Sci 2001; 42:514–522.

33. Hasegawa S, Takagi M, Usui T, Takada R, Abe H. Waveform changes of the first-order multifocal electroretinogram in patients with glaucoma. Invest Ophthalmol Vis Sci 2000; 41:1597–1603.

34. Galloway NR, Barber C. The pattern evoked response in disorders of the optic nerve. Doc Ophthalmol 1986; 63:31–36.

35. Halliday AM, McDonald WI, Mushin J. Delayed visual evoked response in optic neuritis. Lancet 1972; 1:982–985.

36. Plant GT, Hess RF, Thomas SJ. The pattern evoked electroretinogram in optic neuritis: a combined psychophysical and electrophysiological study. Brain 1986; 109:469–490.

37. Porciatti V, Sartucci F. Retinal and cortical evoked responses to chromatic contrast stimuli: specific losses in both eyes of patients with multiple sclerosis and unilateral optic neuritis. Brain 1996; 119:723–740.

38. Frederiksen JL, Petrera J. Serial visual evoked potentials in 90 untreated patients with acute optic neuritis. Surv Ophthalmol 1999; 44(suppl 1):S54–S62.

39. Trauzettel-Klosinski S, Diener H-C, Dietz K, Zrenner E. The effect of oral prednisolone on visual-evoked potential latencies in acute optic neuritis monitored in a prospective, randomized, controlled study. Doc Ophthalmol 1996; 91:165–179.

40. Leys MJ, Candaele CM, de Rouck AF, Odom JV. Detection of hidden visual loss in multiple sclerosis: a comparison of pattern-reversal visual evoked potentials and contrast sensitivity. Doc Ophthalmol 1991; 77:255–264.

41. Halliday AM, McDonald WI, Mushin J. Delayed pattern-evoked responses in optic neuritis in relation to visual acuity. Trans Ophthalmol Soc UK 1973; 93:315–324.

42. Celesia GG, Kaufman DI, Brigell M, Toleikis S, Kokinakis D, Lorance T, Lizano B. Optic neuritis: a prospective study. Neurology 1990; 40:919–923.

43. Asselman P, Chadwick DW, Marsden DC. Visual evoked responses in the diagnosis and management of patients suspected of multiple sclerosis. Brain 1975; 98:261–282.

44. Fillipini G, Comi G, Cosi V, Bevilacqua L, Ferrarini M, Martinelli V, Bergamaschi R, Filippi M, Citterio A, D'Incerti L. Sensitivities and predictive values of paraclinical tests for diagnosing multiple sclerosis. J Neurol 1994; 241:132–137.

45. Hume AL, Waxman SG. Evoked potentials in suspected multiple sclerosis: diagnostic value and prediction of clinical course. J Neurol Sci 1988; 83:191–210.

46. Lee KH, Hashimoto SA, Hooge JP, Kastrukoff LF, Oger JJ, Li DK, Paty DW. Magnetic resonance imaging of the head in the diagnosis of multiple sclerosis: a prospective 2-year follow-up with comparison of clinical evaluation, evoked potentials, oligoclonal banding, and CT. Neurology 1991; 41:657–660.

47. Matthews WB, R W-BJ, Pountney E. Evoked potentials in the diagnosis of multiple sclerosis: a follow up study. J Neurol Neurosurg Psychiatry 1982; 45:303–307.

48. Gronseth GS, Ashman EJ. Practice parameter: the usefulness of evoked potentials in identifying clinically silent lesions in patients with suspected multiple sclerosis (an evidence-based review). Report of the Quality Standards Subcommittee of the American Academy of Neurology. Neurology 2000; 54:1720–1725.

49. McDonald WI, Compston A, Edan G, Goodkin D, Hartung HP, Lublin FD, McFarland HF, Paty DW, Polman CH, Reingold SC, Sandberg-Wollheim M, Sibley W, Thompson A, van den Noort S, Weinshenker BY, Wolinsky JS. Recommended diagnostic criteria for multiple sclerosis: guidelines from the International Panel on the diagnosis of multiple sclerosis. Ann Neurol 2001; 50:121–127.

50. Kaufman DI, Lorance RW, Woods M, Wray SH. The pattern electroretinogram: a long-term study in acute optic neuropathy. Neurology 1988; 38:1767–1774.

51. Seiple W, Price MJ, Kupersmith M, Siegel IM, Carr RE. The pattern electroretinogram in optic nerve disease. Ophthalmology 1983; 90:1127–1132.

52. Holder GE. The pattern electroretinogram in anterior visual pathway dysfunction and its relationship to the pattern visual evoked potentials: a personal clinical review of 743 eyes. Eye 1997; 11:924–934.

53. Berninger TA, Heider W. Pattern electroretinograms in optic neuritis during the acute stage and after remission. Graefes Arch Clin Exp Ophthalmol 1990; 228:410–414.

54. Holder GE. The incidence of abnormal pattern electroretinography in optic nerve demyelination. Electroencephalogr Clin Neurophysiol 1991; 78:18–26.

55. Falsini B, Bardocci A, Porciatti V, Bolzani R, Piccardi M. Macular dysfunction in multiple sclerosis revealed by steady-state flicker and pattern ERGs. Electroencephalogr Clin Neurophysiol 1992; 82:53–59.

56. Bobak P, Bodis-Wollner I, Harnois C, Maffei L, Mylin L, Podos S, Thornton J. Pattern electroretinograms and visual-evoked potentials in glaucoma and multiple sclerosis. Am J Ophthalmol 1983; 96:72–83.

57. Thompson PD, Mastaglia FL, Carroll WM. Anterior ischaemic optic neuropathy. A correlative clinical and visual evoked potential study of 18 patients. J Neurol Neurosurg Psychiatry 1986; 49:128–135.

58. Froehlich J, Kaufman DI. Use of pattern electroretinography to differentiate acute optic neuritis from acute anterior ischemic optic neuropathy. Electroencephalogr Clin Neurophysiol 1994; 92:480–486.

59. Sorensen PS, Trojaborg W, Gjerris F, Krogsan B. Visual evoked potentials in pseudotumor cerebri. Arch Neurol 1985; 42:150–153.

60. Falsini B, Tamburrelli C, Porciatti V, Anile C, Porrello G, Mangiola N. Pattern electroretinograms and visual evoked potentials in idiopathic intracranial hypertension. Ophthalmologica 1992; 205:194–203.

61. Halliday AM, Halliday E, Kriss A, McDonald WI, Mushin J. The pattern-evoked potential in compression of the anterior visual pathway. Brain 1976; 99:357–374.

62. Genovesi–Ebert F, Di Bartolo E, Lepri A, Poggi V, Romani A, Nardi M. Standardized echography, pattern electroretinography and visual-evoked potential and automated perimetry in the early diagnosis of Graves' neuropathy. Ophthalmologica 1998; 212(suppl 1):101–103.

63. Spadea L, Bianco G, Dragani T, Balestrazzi E. Early detection of P-VEP and PERG changes in ophthalmic Graves' disease. Graefes Arch Clin Exp Ophthalmol 1997; 235:501–505.

64. Bobak P, Friedman R, Brigell M, Goodwin J, Anderson R. Visual evoked potentials to multiple temporal frequencies. Use in the differential diagnosis of optic neuropathy. Arch Ophthalmol 1988; 106:936–940.

65. Gotoh Y, Machida S, Tazawa Y. Selective loss of the photopic negative response in patients with optic nerve atrophy. Arch Ophthalmol 2004; 122:341–346.

66. Salvi M, Spaggiari, E, Neri F, Maculuso C, Gardini B, Ferrozzi F, Minelli R, Wall JR, Roti E. The study of visual evoked potentials in patients with thyroid-associated ophthalmopathy identifies asymptomatic optic nerve involvement. J Clin Endocrinol Metab 1997; 82:1027–1030.

67. Setala K, Raitta C, Valimake M, Katevuo V, Lamberg B-A. The value of visual evoked potentials in optic neuropathy of Graves' disease. J Endocrinol Invest 1992; 15:821–826.

68. Tsaloumas MD, Good PA, Burdon MA, Misson GP. Flash and pattern visual evoked potentials in the diagnosis and monitoring of dysthyroid optic neuropathy. Eye 1994; 8:638–645.

69. Ambrosio G, Ferrara G, Vitale R, De Marco R. Visual evoked potentials in patients with Graves' ophthalmopathy complicated by ocular hypertension and suspect glaucoma or dysthyroid optic neuropathy. Doc Ophthalmol 2003; 106:99–104.

70. Parmar DN, Sofat A, Bowman R, Bartlett JR, Holder GE. Visual prognostic value of the pattern electroretinogram in chiasmal compression. Br J Ophthalmol 2000; 84:1024–1026.

71. Levin LA, Beck RW, Joseph MP, Seiff S, Kraker R. The International Optic Nerve Trauma Study Group. The treatment of traumatic optic neuropathy. Ophthalmology 1999; 106: 1268–1277.

72. Abraham FA, Spierer A, Blumenthal M. Optic nerve trauma with prolonged blindness followed by visual-evoked potential. Ophthalmologica 1987; 194:40–43.

73. Fuller DG, Hutton WL. Prediction of postoperative vision in eyes with severe trauma. Retina 1990; 10:520–534.

74. Mahapatra AK. Visual evoked potentials in optic nerve injury—does it merit to be mentioned. Ind J Ophthalmol 1991; 39:20–21.

75. Tandon DA, Thakar A, Mahapatra AK, Ghosh P. Transethmoidal optic nerve decompression. Clin Otolaryngol 1994; 19:98–104.

76. Cornelius CP, Altenmuller E, Ehrenfeld M. The use of flash visual evoked potentials in the early diagnosis of suspected optic nerve lesions due to craniofacial trauma. J Craniomaxillofac Surg 1996; 24:1–11.

77. Mashima Y, Oguchi Y. Clinical study of the pattern electroretinogram in patients with optic nerve damage. Doc Ophthalmol 1985; 61:91–96.

78. Scholl GB, Song HS, Winkler DE, Wray SH. The pattern visual evoked potential and pattern electroretinogram in drusen-associated optic neuropathy. Arch Ophthalmol 1992; 110:75–81.

79. Mustonon E, Sulg I, Kallanranta T. Electroretinogram (ERG) and visual evoked response (VER) studies in patients with optci disc drusen. Acta Ophthalmol (Copenh) 1980; 58: 539–549.

80. Vieregge P, Rosengart A, Mehdorn E, Wessel K, Kompf D. [Drusen papilla with vision disorder and pathologic visual evoked potentials]. Nervenarzt 1990; 61:364–368.

81. Shibata K, Shibagaki Y, Nagal C, Iwata M. Visual evoked potentials and electro retinograms in an early stage of Leber's hereditary optic neuropathy. J Neurol 1999; 246:847–849.

82. Nikoskelainen E, Sogg RL, Rosenthal AR, Friberg TR, Dorfman LJ. The early phase in Leber hereditary optic atrophy. Arch Ophthalmol 1977; 95:969–978.

83. Livingstone IR, Mastaglia FL, Howe JW, Aherne GE. Leber's optic neuropathy: clinical and visual evoked response studies in asymptomatic and symptomatic members of a 4-generation family. Br J Ophthalmol 1980; 64:751–757.

84. Carroll WM, Mastaglia FL. Leber's optic neuropathy: a clinical and visual evoked potential study of affected and asymp-

tomatic members of a six generation family. Brain 1979; 102:559–580.

85. Mondelli M, Rossi A, Scarpini C, Dotti MT, Federico A. Leber's optic atrophy: VEP and BAEP changes in 16 asymptomatic subjects. Acta Neurol Scand 1991; 84:366.

86. Berninger TA, Jaeger W, Krastel H. Electrophysiology and colour perimetry in dominant infantile optic atrophy. Br J Ophthalmol 1991; 75:49–52.

87. Holder GE, Votruba M, Carter AC, Bhattacharya SS, Fitzke FW, Moore AT. Electrophysiological findings in dominant optic atrophy (DOA) linking to the OPA1 locus on chromosome 3q 28–qter. Doc Ophthalmol 1998–1999; 95:217–228.

88. Votruba M, Fitzke FW, Holder GE, Carter AC, Bhattacharya SS, Moore AT. Clinical features in affected individuals from 21 pedigrees with dominant optic atrophy. Arch Ophthalmol 1998; 116:351–358.

89. Harding GF, Crews SJ, Pitts SM. Psychophysical and visual evoked potential findings in hereditary optic atrophy. Trans Ophthalmol Soc UK 1979; 99:96–102.

90. Kline LB, Glaser JS. Dominant optic atrophy: the clinical profile. Arch Ophthalmol 1979; 97:1680–1686.

91. Good WV, Jan JE, DeSa L, Barkovich J, Groenveld M, Hoyt CS. Cortical visual impairment in children. Surv Ophthalmol 1994; 38:351–364.

92. Crighel E, Botex MI. Photopic evoked potentials in man in lesions of the occipital lobe. Brain 1966; 69:311–316.

93. Kooi KA, Sharbtough FW. Electrophysiological findings in cortical blindness. Electroencephalogr Clin Neurophysiol 1966; 2:260–263.

94. Abraham FA, Melamed E, Levy S. Prognostic value of visual evoked potentials in occipital blindness following basilar artery occlusion. Appl Neurophysiol 1975; 38:126–135.

95. Duchoway MS, Weiss IP, Majlessi H, Barnet AB. Visual evoked response in childhood cortical blindness after head trauma and meningitis. A longitudinal study of six cases. Neurology 1974; 24:933–940.

96. Kupersmith MJ, Nelson JI. Preserved visual evoked potential in infancy cortical blindness relationship to blindsight. Neuro-Ophthalmol 1986; 6:685–694.

97. Good WV. Development of a quantitative method to measure vision in children with chronic cortical visual impairment. Trans Am Ophthalmol Soc 2001; 99:253–269.

98. Frank Y, Torres F. Visual evoked potentials in the evaluation of "cortical blindness" in children. Ann Neurol 1979; 6: 126–129.

99. Barnet AB, Manson JI, Wilner E. Acute cerebral blindness in childhood. Neurology 1970; 20:1147–1156.

100. Bodis-Wollner I, Atkin A, Raab E, Wolkstein M. Visual association cortex and vision in man: pattern-evoked occipital potentials in a blind boy. Science 1977; 198:629–631.

101. Abe T, Abe K, Aoki M, Itojama Y, Tamai M. Ocular changes in patients with spinocerebellar degeneration and repeated trinucleotide expansion of spinocerebellar ataxia type 1 gene. Arch Ophthalmol 1997; 115:231–236.

102. Drack AV, Traboulsi EI, Maumenee IH. Progression of retinopathy in olivopontocerebellar atrophy with retinal degeneration. Arch Ophthalmol 1992; 110:712–713.

103. Traboulsi EI, Maumenee IH, Green WR, Freimer ML, Moser H. Olivopontocerebellar atrophy with retinal degeneration. A clinical and ocular histopathologic study. Arch Ophthalmol 1988; 106:801–806.

104. Gouw LG, Kaplan CD, Haines JH, Digre KB, Rutledge SL, Matilla A, Leppert M, Zoghbi HY, PtÃcek LJ. Retinal degeneration characterizes a spinocerebellar ataxia mapping to chromosome 3p. Nat Genet 1995; 10:89–93.

105. Abe T, Tsuda T, Yoshida M, Wada Y, Kano T, itoyama Y, Tamai M. Macular degeneration associated with aberrant expansion of trinucleotide repeat of the SCA7 gene in 2 Japanese families. Arch Ophthalmol 2000; 118:1415–1421.

106. To KW, Adamian M, Jakobiec FA, Berson EL. Olivopontocerebellar atrophy with retinal degeneration. An electroretinographic and histophatologic investigation. Ophthalmology 1993; 100:15–23.

107. Perretti A, Santoro L, Lanzillo B, Filla A, De Michele G, Barbieri F, Martino G, Ragno M, Cocozza S, Caruso G. Autosomal dominant cerebellar ataxia type 1: multimodal electrophysiological study and comparison between SCA1 and SCA2 patients. J Neurol Sci 1996; 142:45–53.

108. Carroll WM, Kriss A, Baraitser M, Barrett G, Halliday AM. The incidence and nature of visual pathway involvement in Friedreich's ataxia. A clinical and visual evoked potential study of 22 patients. Brain 1980; 103:413–434.

109. Pelosi L, Fels A, Petrillo A, Senatore R, Russo G, Lonegren K, Calace P, Caruso G. Friedreich's ataxia: clinical involvement and evoked potentials. Acta Neurol Scand 1984; 70:360–368.

110. Alzheimer A. Ueber eiene eigenartige Erkrankung der Himrinede. Allg Z Psychiat Med 1907; 64:146–148.

111. Sadun AA, Borchert M, DeVita E, Hinton DR, Bassi CJ. Assessment of visual impairment in patients with Alzheimer's disease. Am J Ophthalmol 1987; 104:113–120.

112. Kergoat H, Kergoat MJ, Justino L, Chertkow H, Robillard A, Bergman H. Visual retinocortical function in dementia of the Alzheimer type. Gerontology 2002; 28:197–203.

113. Rizzo J, III, Cronin-Golomb A, Growdon JH, Corkin S, Rosen T, Sandberg MA, Chiappa KH, Lessell S. Retinocalcarine function in Alzheimer's disease. A clinical and electrophysiological study. Arch Neurol 1992; 49:92–101.

114. Hinton DR, Sadun AA, Blanks JC, Miller CA. Optic-nerve degeneration in Alzheimer's disease. N Engl J Med 1986; 315:485–487.

115. Curcio CA, Drucker DN. Retinal ganglion cells in Alzheimer's disease and aging. Ann Neurol 1993; 33:248–257.

116. Parisi V, Restuccia R, Fattapposta F, Mina C, Bucci MG, Pierelli F. Morphological and functional retinal impairment in Alzheimer's diseae patients. Clin Neurophysiol 2001; 112:1860–1867.

117. Strenn K, Dal-Bianco P, Weghaupt H, Koch G, Vass C, Gottlob I. Pattern electroretinogram and luminanace electroretinogram in Alzheimer's disease. J Neural Transm Suppl 1991; 33:73–80.

118. Trick GL, Barris MC, Bickler-Bluth M. Abnormal pattern electroretinograms in patients with senile dementia of the Alzheimer type. Ann Neurol 1989; 26:226–331.

119. Prager TC, Schweitzer FC, Peacock LW, Garcia CA. The effect of optical defocus on the pattern electroretinogram in normal subjects and patients with Alzheimer's disease. Am J Ophthalmol 1993; 116:363–369.

120. Nesher R, Trick GL. The pattern electroretinogram in retinal and optic nerve disease. A quantitative comparison of the pattern of visual dysfunction. Doc Ophthalmol 1991; 77:225–235.

121. Philpot MP, Amin D, Levy R. Visual evoked potentials in Alzheimer's disease: correlations with age and severity. Electroencephalogr Clin Neurophysiol 1990; 77:323–329.

122. Wright CE, Harding GF, Orwin A. The flash and pattern VEP as a diagnostic indicator dementia. Doc Ophthalmol 1986; 62:89–96.

123. Visser SL, Van Tilburg W, Hooijer C, Jonker C, De Rijke W. Visual evoked potentials (VEPs) in senile dementia (Alzheimer type) and in non-organic behavioural disorders in the elderly: comparison with EEG parameters. Electroencephalogr Clin Neurophysiol 1985; 60:115–121.

124. Haupt WF, Dietz E, Mielke R, Kessler J. Visual evoked potentials in Alzheimer's disease: investigations in a PET-defined collective. Int J Neurosci 1994; 79:59–66.

125. Celesia GG, Villa AE, Brigell M, Rubboli G, Bolcioni G, Fiori MG. An electrophysiologic study of visual processing in Alzheimer's disease. Electroencephalogr Clin Neurophysiol 1993; 87:97–104.

126. Ellis CJK, Allen TG, Marsden CD, Ikeda H. Electroretinographic abnormalities in idiopathic Parkinson's disease and the effect of levodopa administration. Clin Vision Sci 1987; 1:347–355.

127. Jaffe MJ, Bruno G, Campbell G, Lavine RA, Karson CN, Weinberger DR. Ganzfeld electroretinographic findings in parkinsonism: untreated patients and the effect of levodopa intravenous infusion. J Neurol Neurosurg Psychiatry 1987; 50:847–852.

128.   Ikeda H, Head GM, Ellis CJ. Electrophysiological signs of retinal dopamine deficiency in recently diagnosed Parkinson's disease and a follow up study. Vision Res 1994; 34: 2629–2638.

129.   Peppe A, Stanzione P, Pierelli F, De Angelis D, Pierantozzi M, Bernardi G. Visual alterations in de novo Parkinson's disease: pattern electroretinogram latencies are more delayed and more reversible by levodopa than are visual evoked potentials. Neurology 1995; 45:1144–1148.

130.   Bandini R, Pierantozzi M, Bodis-Wollner I. Parkinson's disease changes the balance of onset and offset visual responses: an evoked potential study. Clin Neurophysiol 2001; 112: 976–983.

131.   Buttner T, Kuhn W, Muller T, Heinze T, Puhl C, Przuntek H. Chromatic and achromatic visual evoked potentials in Parkinson's disease. Electroencephalogr Clin Neurophysiol 1996; 110:443–447.

132.   Yokoyama T, Suglyama K, Nishizawa S, Yokota N, Ohta S, Uemura K. Visual evoked potentials during posteroventral pallidotomy for Parkinson's disease. Neurosurgery 1999; 44:815–822.

133.   Tobimatsu S, Shima F, Ishido K, Kato M. Visual evoked potentials in the vicinity of the optic tract during stereotactic pallidotomy. Electroencephalogr Clin Neurophysiol 1997; 104:274–279.

134.   De Meirleir LJ, Taylor MJ, Logan WJ. Multimodal evoked potentials studies in leukodystrophies of children. Can J Neurol Sci 1988; 15:26–31.

135.   Markland ON, Garg BP, DeMyer WE, Warren C, Worth RM. Brain stem auditory, visual and somatosensory evoked potentials in leukodystrophies. Electroencephalogr Clin Neurophysiol 1982; 54:39–48.

136.   Wulff CH, Trojaborg W. Adult metachromatic leukodystrophy: neurophysiologic findings. Neurology 1985; 35: 1776–1778.

137.   Mamoli B, Graf M, Toifl K. EEG, pattern-evoked potentials and nerve conduction velocity in a family with adrenoleuco-

dystrophy. Electroencephalogr Clin Neurophysiol 1979; 47:411–419.

138. Tobimatsu S, Fukui R, Kato M, Kobayashi T, Kuroiwa Y. Multimodality evoked potentials in patients and carriers with adrenoleukodystrophy and adrenomyeloneuropathy. Electroencephalogr Clin Neurophysiol 1985; 62:18–24.

139. Kaplan PW, Kruse B, Tusa RJ, Shankroff J, Rignani J, Moser HW. Visual system abnormalities in adrenomyeloneuropathy. Ann Neurol 1995; 37:550–552.

140. Kaplan PW, Tusa RJ, Shankroff J, Heller J, Moser HW. Visual evoked potentials in adrenoleukodystrophy: a trial with glycerol trioleate and Lorenzo oil. Ann Neurol 1993; 34:169–174.

141. Hood DC, Greenstein VC, Odel JG, Zhang X, Ritch R, Liebmann JM, Chen CS, Thienprasiddhi P. Visual field defects and multifocal visual evoked potentials: evidence of a linear relationship. Arch Ophthalmol 2002; 120:1672–1681.

142. Fortune B, Bearse MA, Cioffi GA, Johnson CA. Selective loss of an oscillatory component from temporal retinal multifocal ERG responses in glaucoma. Invest Ophthalmol Vis Sci 2002; 43:2638–2647.

Index